CURRICULUM BUILDING
IN NURSING

a process

CURRICULUM BUILDING IN NURSING

a process

EM OLIVIA BEVIS, R.N., B.S., M.A., F.A.A.N.

Professor and Coordinator, Graduate Nursing Program,
Medical College of Georgia, Savannah Satellite,
Savannah, Georgia

SECOND EDITION

with 87 illustrations

THE C. V. MOSBY COMPANY

Saint Louis   1978

RT
73
.B4
1978

SECOND EDITION

The C. V. Mosby Company
11830 Westline Industrial Drive, St. Louis, Missouri 63141

Library of Congress Cataloging in Publication Data

Bevis, Em Olivia.
    Curriculum building in nursing.

    Bibliography: p.
    Includes index.
    1. Nursing—Study and teaching. 2. Curriculum
planning. I. Title. [DNLM: 1. Education, Nursing.
2. Curriculum. WY18 B572c]
RT73.B4   1978   610.73'07'11   77-13045
ISBN 0-8016-0668-3

GW/M/M   9 8 7 6 5 4 3

To

Honor Beecroft Dufour

supportive

facilitative

creative

communicative

motivating

loving

FRIEND

When I dwell in my pit called despair
My sensitized soul is all aware
Of man's depraved, bestial, brutalization of men.

And then

Quite by accident my leadened self will find
Some quiet, sudden sample of how man's mind
Has worked some logical design that bares
the humanism of men

Again.

Em Olivia Bevis

PREFACE

The purpose of this book is to provide a source for those engaged in the process of nursing curriculum formation, revision, or study. The text is based on the assumption that most of the difficulties of curriculum building stem from two basic causes: (1) the problems arising from lack of procedural knowledge about curriculum building process in nursing and (2) the problems inherent in changing.

This book is designed to facilitate the work of the curriculum builder by providing a guide through the maze of curriculum theory and by making direct, explicit applications to nursing curriculum problems. The book is predicated on the assumption that the key to successful curriculum building or change is the involvement of all those who must live and work with the changes; thus examples of devices for involving people are placed at the end of each chapter. These example heuristics are merely tools or devices; like any heuristic they can be used if appropriate or can be stimulants to the imaginations of curriculum builders for devising their own heuristics for curriculum change.

I have tried to pare curriculum theory to the essentials, to define terminology, and to provide examples, illustrative figures, and models for clarity and practicality, since as a graduate student and as a curriculum builder, I found the literature abundant but difficult to apply to nursing.

I have attempted to deal with the difficult subject of nursing theory because its direct relationship to nursing curricula seems very important to me, and it was obscure when I first began to struggle with curriculum building. The decade of the 1970s has seen an explosion of nursing theories. The 1980s will see many more generated, and their sum will make curriculum content in nursing easier to form into holistic nursing patterns.

This book is not intended as a thorough source on curriculum theory; specialists in the field of education are available for that. This is a "how to" book designed to help those who need concrete ideas about how to use curriculum theory in nursing education and how to involve the total faculty in developing their own ideas and facilitate the translation of those ideas into a workable curriculum.

In 1968 the United States Department of Health, Education, and Welfare, Public Health Service, awarded a training project grant, "Identifying the Core Content of an Advanced Nursing Curriculum," to California State University, San Jose. The experiences gained with this curriculum endeavor gave me the motivation to write this book. I am grateful both to the university and to the Public Health Service for the opportunity they gave me to participate in curriculum change.

Since that date my colleagues across the United States and Canada have generously shared with me the problems and joys of their curriculum change attempts. Participation with them has added to my knowledge of the curriculum development process. I offer my sincere and deepest appreciation to the following friends and colleagues who have helped me.

Dr. Shepard Insel contributed greatly to my personal growth and helped me learn to facilitate curriculum change. Dr. June Bailey and Dr. Frederick McDonald have been mentors and friends and have provided direction and substance to thoughts and ideas.

Dr. Margaret Jacobson has been a constant in my life since I began to work in curriculum change. She is warm, reinforcing, knowledgeable, and generous with her expertise and with herself. Her contributions to this book are immeasurable.

Mrs. Fay Bower, my close friend and colleague, provides me with support and motivation when I lag. She has an unerring eye, provides dependable, believable feedback, and keeps me honest.

Mrs. Judy Deal Spencer, who from love and friendship read and critiqued the first edition manuscript in the midst of moving and coping with a family, has my warm gratitude. She made her contribution during an author's most harried time—the last minutes before sending the manuscript for final typing. Judy corrected 2,347 spelling errors. Her help was sorely missed during the preparation of this second edition.

My friends and fellow teachers at the Department of Nursing, San Jose State University, San Jose, California, have my expressed affection and gratitude for the work we did together for the five years of the Curriculum Project, 1968 to 1973. I loved their ability to dream of better ways to teach nursing, their readiness to take the risks necessary to make the dreams reality, and their ability to change changes as new forms and shapes emerged; in this way they made real the process of curriculum change. It was impossible for me to be a member of this group and not grow. I am grateful to these friends for the rich gift of themselves they make to the students, to each other, and to the process of curriculum change. I learned a great deal from them.

I am grateful to Dr. Dorothy T. White who, with very few constraints, gave me carte blanche to try all my wild, weird, and wonderful (depending on one's perspective) ideas at the Medical College of Georgia, Savannah Satellite. She provided support, reinforcement, and administrative clearance that freed me to do what I love to do: teach, develop curriculum, and structure courses and learning activities. The continued testing of ideas and personal growth made possible by this freedom is reflected in this edition.

Mrs. Martha Anderson Coleman and Mrs. Joyce Popham Murray, my two colleagues and friends at the Savannah Satellite, give me love, support, and stimulation on a daily basis. They are a bonus in my life. I truly never go to work without a feeling of gladness that I am fortunate enough to work with them. This edition inevitably has their mark on it.

Miss Marsha Brandon, at Medical College of Georgia, gave her Thanksgiving vacation to take the vague directions and messy manuscript I gave her and with intelligent enthusiasm reorganized the first five chapters into the new format of this second edition. Thank you, Marsha.

Mrs. Verle Hamilton Waters, knowledgeable, wise, mature, and good, has taught me so much about curriculum that I cannot begin to communicate it all. She has an endless supply of love that nourishes growth. I am fortunate that some fell on me and thereby into this book.

Since the advent of the first edition, my grandmother, Mrs. Annie Bullock, who was my constant supporter, died at age 93. "Miss" Annie originally encouraged me to write this book. Margaret Mead says that grandmothers are the inseminators of culture. For me this was certainly true, and I consider this book partly Grandmother's.

Dr. Shirley Chater, whose ideas I so much admire, has influenced my thinking about curriculum. It was she who pointed out to me that conceptual frameworks could logically be categorized into setting, student, and subject. She made her early thoughts and writings on the subject available to me and provided me with stimulation, support, and friendship. Her conceptual framework model on the cover of this book is a tribute to her impact on my thinking.

Last, I thank my husband, Julian, who is a blessing in my life. His love, support, protection, and egalitarianism help me continue to feel good about writing. His love of words, like mine, is a source of joy to us both, and our stimulating discussions add a dimension of precision to this book.

Em Olivia Bevis

CONTENTS

CURRICULUM BUILDING IN NURSING
a process

INTRODUCTION

Once there was a knight riding across England's roads and byways. He was gloriously armored and gauntleted and looking for good deeds to do, fair maidens to rescue, Holy Grails to quest for, and dragons to slay. So far he had found none. As he rode along he noticed a small brown sparrow lying on its back in the dust of the road with its spindly little legs sticking up, stiff and straight into the air. The knight reined in his mighty mount and hailed the sparrow.

"What ho? what ho? little sparrow. Why do you lie in the road dust with your spindly little legs sticking up stiff and straight into the air?"

"Oh dear knight sir," replied the sparrow, "haven't you heard? The sky is going to fall."

"And you think you can hold it up all by yourself with those spindly little legs?" bellowed the knight sir.

A deep sigh escaped the sparrow as he replied, "One does what one can, kind sir, one does what one can."

What nurse educator cannot identify with the frantic little sparrow? Sometimes it looks as if the sky *is* going to fall in on nursing. Nursing care demands are exploding in kind, quality, and quantity; for many, health care is unavailable or maldistributed; health care costs are escalating beyond inflation into the ridiculous; massive health problems endanger the world; all health workers' jobs, requirements, and constraints are being legislated to the point of confusion; and health care delivery systems and health worker educational systems are grossly obsolete

and inadequate. Health care consumers are demanding better quality care and more humanistic care. Nursing is responding to the threat of a falling sky in all the many ways that people and organizations respond to stress: some are stunned into immobility, some are confused and going in circles, some are engaged in change activities, but all are "doing what one can, kind sir, doing what one can."

The rapidity of change in nursing has resulted in what Toffler has named "future shock."[1] Nursing has passed through the phase of immobility and into the phase of fermenting activity. Nursing educators all over the nation are "doing what one can." The fermenting activity manifests itself in a universal restlessness among nursing educators, nursing practitioners, and nursing students.

Restlessness is the behavior of anxiety— that ill-defined feeling that something is wrong somewhere, that something threatens, that a need is unmet, a problem unsolved, or things simply are not as they could be.

Nursing schools are restless; faculties find themselves a little dissatisfied; teachers have an uneasy feeling that they could be doing a little better job or that there are health problems to which students are unprepared to respond.

This restlessness manifests itself in a desire to change what is now being done to something else in the belief that after the change things will be better somehow.

The need to change—the restlessness— has its basis not in the dreamer's fantasy of a better world but in the reality of

1

life. In a situation where there are many constants and few variables, little change is necessary to produce the conditions that provide for satisfaction, stability, and low human anxiety. In a situation where there are many variables and few constants, change becomes a way of life and necessary to the productive, satisfied state of being. There are few constants and many variables in all facets of life today. The multiplicity of the variables affecting human institutions made itself felt explosively in the 1960s in violent attempts to change social institutions that were contrived for maintaining stability, in other words, organized so that they would change little. By the middle 1970s social institutions were learning how to respond to social need and accommodate the many variables efficiently. The restlessness of nursing faculties and the pursuit of curriculum change are attempts to accommodate, constructively and efficiently, to the variables in society that affect health. It is hoped that the outcome will be more effective than the solution which the sparrow devised, but the motivation is the same—nursing faculties and organizations are "doing what they can."

According to Chapter 2, conceptual frameworks are derived from factors in three areas: knowledge or subject, setting, and students. Alterations in any of these elements alter the conceptual framework and, in the viable curriculum, alter the curriculum. Changes in all three of these areas are occurring so rapidly that curriculum innovation in nursing is epidemic. This epidemic has a multitude of etiologies, only a few of which will be discussed here.

KNOWLEDGE EXPLOSION

The twentieth century scientific and technological "knowledge explosion" has forced educators everywhere to reexamine their curricula. Nursing applies theories from numerous scientific fields and is rapidly building a body of knowledge uniquely its own. Updating the curriculum through the simple technique of adding that which is new is no longer feasible.

There exists no conclusive evidence about what information or skills are necessary to conduct the business of nursing. Nursing leaders, through the professional organizations and through the official publications of those organizations, have expressed some common agreement about the characteristics of nurses that they believe are necessary to perform nursing functions and fulfill nursing roles. The described characteristics are congruent with the educated mind.[2] It is therefore paradoxical that after so many years of describing the processes necessary to nurse, nursing curricula still focus on the information necessary to nurse rather than on the processes necessary to develop the desired characteristics. This can be accounted for, at least in part, by the success of most schools of nursing in producing a high percentage of students who pass state board examinations for licensure after completing a curriculum based on the ability to "recall" data.

The "knowledge explosion" has placed educators in the untenable position of teaching to a built-in obsolescence. Much of the theoretical or informational material communicated to students is obsolete before it has been in use for five years. Much more material is outdated within one half of the graduate's professional life, and only a small part of the information presented to students is useful throughout the professional life span. The great dilemma of nursing educators is that no one knows what information will survive in the rapid validation and generation process now occurring in the physical, biological, social, and nursing sciences. Another difficult problem for the information-oriented curriculum is that for many years learning psychologists have demonstrated definitively that less than 25% of content material "learned" is available for recall in two years,[3] unless it is used and reinforced regularly or organized around meaningful life processes.[4] Thus the knowledge explosion, taken alone, mandates the use of modern technology for enabling students to have the greatest possible informational input with the least possible expenditure of time and effort and the minimum amount of direct teacher contact.

HOLISM AND THE NURSING MODEL

Another powerful impact on nursing is an increased awareness of the shortcomings of the medical model for either teaching nursing or providing care. Nurses are seeking to build a nursing model that addresses itself to nursing's domain of practice, to the care of human beings as wholes, and to organismic responsiveness in the delivery of nursing services. Dualism, the division of man and the sciences that explains him in terms of mind and body, seems better suited to the disease-oriented systems of medicine than it does to nursing. Nursing's domain of practice is what happens to people before, during, and after health problems. Medicine's domain of practice is the diagnosis and treatment of diseases in people. Nurses work with humans as wholes, since in nursing's domain of practice the whole person responds to health needs and this holistic response demands organismic nursing care. Nursing science is currently seeking ways to elaborate this within its practice domain; therefore it is generating theories about its practice domain that have holistic perceptions of clients and organismic nursing care responses. These new theories entice educators to take a new look at curriculum.

SETTING CONSUMERS' DEMANDS

Population growth, human longevity, health insurance, governmental commitment (subsidies, grants, Medicare, and so forth), and consumer expectations and demands have combined to place a strain unequalled in history on the nation's health facilities. Hospitals and health agencies have expanded services and facilities rapidly to meet the needs of the growing population. Nursing service requirements have been expanded both qualitatively and quantitatively, and there is no apparent end in sight for the expanding role of the nurse.

Accompanying the vastly increased demand for nursing services is a change in the philosophy about where the responsibility for educating nurses lies. Currently, educational philosophy places the responsibility for nursing education in institutions, the functions of which are primarily educational. Consequently, hospitals are closing their schools of nursing, and more and more colleges are opening programs. In its early years the transition of educational and training responsibility from hospitals to colleges created an identity crisis in nursing that set off a thirty-year period of self-examination and search for identity. The establishment of a nursing identity separate and apart from medical education and hospital apprenticeship enabled nursing to acclaim its independence without knowing how to achieve a content discipline uniquely its own. The firm entrenchment of nursing in institutions of higher learning has enabled nurses to use the academic tools of research and educational methodology to identify, select, and organize nursing's body of knowledge interdependently with other relevant disciplines.

INFLATION IN NURSE PREPARATION COST

Nationally accepted average teacher-student ratios of 1:8 in nursing have proved to be unacceptably expensive to colleges and universities. The expense of educating associate and baccalaureate degree nursing students threatens the existence of many collegiate nursing programs. Expensive programs are receiving close examination by college authorities beset by alumni and taxpayers who, in response to the educational revolution, inflation, and the "tight money" market, are urging financial cutbacks. Nursing programs have received financial backing from federal and state sources in the form of grants to students and faculty. This financial backing has, to date, allowed many programs to exist; however, current federal funding trends threaten to curtail most forms of student training grants.

College administrative personnel are justly pressuring nursing administration and faculty to find more efficient ways to teach so that nursing school budgets may be brought more in line with other college program budgets in expenditures per full-time student. An increasing proportion of students are selecting nursing as a major, and nursing faculties are being expected to increase their student load while still maintaining safe student supervision in nursing settings.

Services and facilities, expanded and altered to serve the needs of a rapidly growing population with altered care demands, have placed a strain on existing educational facilities. There is emerging a vastly different kind of graduate to fill nursing position vacancies. Nurses are more assertive, independent, and willing to speak out in behalf of themselves and their clients, and, consequently, nursing salaries have increased substantially. This series of events has made the nursing major a more desirable choice for students, and most nursing schools have many more applicants than spaces. Thus nursing educators are increasingly exploring curriculum innovations that will improve nursing education efficiency while making it more responsive to current health care needs.

NURSE REGISTRATION AND LICENSURE

The wide variety in the length of time and type of educational program required for a nursing student to qualify for the same licensure examination is nursing's most startling paradox. Two years in an associate of arts degree program, three years in a hospital program, or four or five years in a baccalaureate college or university qualifies a candidate for the same licensing examination and thereby the same legal practice privileges. This custom defies logic and produces such confusion in the consumer public that legislators are now seeking to pass laws more closely regulating nurse education and licensure. Some states are resolved to alter the whole licensure structure, creating two levels of nursing—associate of arts degree nursing and baccalaureate degree nursing. Resolutions about this choice are stimulating debates and examination of the licensure structure. These issues affect curriculum planning.

Florence Nightingale predicted in the late 1800s that if nursing adopted a system of state licensure, the result would be to "stereotype mediocrity." Although more benefits than liabilities have been derived from the state licensure system, Nightingale's fear has been realized. Nursing, however, not the law, is responsible for the lack of delineation of practice characteristics and licensure requirements. The demands of the public, through political pressure groups, for equal education and employment opportunities combined with the social legislation that is increasing medical care to larger numbers of the population make legislators ready to enact laws that will gravely affect nursing curricula and practice. Nursing resists change in the licensure structure because that very structure provides social, employment, and monetary rewards to the "registered nurse" regardless of any preparation or practice criteria. Changes in the licensure structure to reflect the quality and quantity of job preparation threaten the status and pocketbook of the largest segment of nursing practitioners.

Nursing curriculum architects must not only work at developing the best possible nursing curriculum for their particular setting but also must concomitantly work toward a system of state licensure that is designed to evaluate varying types of nursing job preparation. To do this, nursing must decrease the status and monetary threat to the majority of nursing practitioners by devising ways whereby continued preparation will enable the nurse to qualify for successive licensure examinations.

Nursing curricula cannot be developed in a legal vacuum. One of the basic commitments of any nursing education program is that the graduate be eligible to stand the licensure examination with the reasonable expectation of passing it. A change in the licensure structure would not change the process of curriculum building; it would change one of the outcomes of that process.

STUDENTS

Curriculum patterns are altering drastically to respond to the needs of students. Many nursing school faculties are sincerely reaching for ways to facilitate student progress through the maze of possible programs. Open curriculum efforts embrace the idea that nursing need not be an obstacle course, one type of program discounting another and forcing students to repeat content learned in other schools leading to lesser degrees. Open curriculum proponents believe that nursing education can facilitate the progress of nurses from lower diplomas and degrees to higher ones without undue redundance and that the nursing academic obstacle course can be changed into a racecourse without jeopardizing the quality of education or the skills required of graduates. Other programs are innovative in expediting students' achievement through continuous progress programs such as that pioneered by Arizona State College in Tempe, Arizona, and external degrees by examination, pioneered by the State University of New York. Two plus two programs, second step programs, continuous progress programs, external degree programs, degree by examination, and the generic masters' programs are among the options open to faculties who are attempting to respond to students' needs as exhibited by the kinds of preparation students can have, their individual learning styles and pace, and their career goals.

Students' characteristics alter with trends. Those who teach in post–high school programs find students more aware of their rights, less doubtful and willing to submit to the tyranny of the system without redress, more assertive, and less hostile than a few years ago. Television provides exposure to a wider range of stimuli than ever before, and students come to nursing more sophisticated and more aware of social and political currents affecting nursing. The movement of society toward sexual equality in rights, privileges, and responsibilities is probably the social factor most influential in nursing today. Nursing is departing from its sex-role stereotype to be equal partners-colleagues with others in health care. Autonomy, accountability, and authority are the hallmark of the new nurse. Nursing curricula are including elements that reinforce this trend and utilize its momentum for nursing.

The process of curriculum building is the same regardless of the problems encountered and regardless of the difference in program objectives. The content one introduces into process varies, depending on factors unique to each nursing program; therefore the curriculum outcome also varies.

This book deals with the process of curriculum building for nursing in the hope that the process itself can be adapted by faculties and students to the development of nursing curricula which will improve the quality of patient care regardless of the type or setting of the nursing program.

NOTES

1. Toffler, Alvin: Future shock, New York, 1970, Bantam Books, Inc., pp. 10-12.
2. Western Interstate Commission for Higher Education: The graduate of baccalaureate degree nursing programs: a description of the expected competencies, roles, and behaviors, Boulder, Colo., 1968, The Commission.
3. Pressey, Sidney L., and Robinson, Francis P.: Psychology in education, ed. 3, New York, 1959, Harper & Row, Publishers, pp. 262-263.
4. McDonald, Frederick J.: Educational psychology, Belmont, Calif., 1966, Wadsworth Publishing Co., Inc., pp. 227-240.

1

COMMON FRAME OF REFERENCE:
THE NATURE OF NURSING

OVERVIEW

This book describes the curriculum-building process and its specific application to nursing curricula. It supplements, but does not replace, educational reference books on curriculum building. Nurse educators, whether in generic, postgraduate, in-service, continuing education, or client-teaching aspects of nursing education, have had to struggle to apply the abstractions of curriculum theory to the practice-oriented discipline of nursing. Most curriculum theory books are geared to the needs of primary and secondary education and to the needs of the general subjects curricula such as social studies, history, and literature. Therefore, to meet the special needs of nursing educators, this book approaches the curriculum-building process from the point of view of the practice discipline of nursing and provides a practical approach to curriculum development.

The initial question that faculties ask when they seek to change their curriculum is, "How do we begin?" In actual fact, two questions are being asked: "On what task do we begin?" and "How do we organize for going about curriculum change and development?" This book discusses both questions. It starts with what tasks to do, gives examples of how to accomplish the tasks, and suggests some organizational strategies for involving appropriate others in the effort.

This chapter does not examine curriculum building but begins to develop a common vocabulary and a common curriculum-building model. To accomplish this goal the chapter defines curriculum, outlines a system for curriculum development, and discusses some of the basic premises on which the book rests. This chapter also discusses the nature of process, since the book suggests that curriculum building is a process and overtly supports process-oriented curriculum designs and teaching operations. The reader is introduced to one conceptualization of nursing and is provided with a brief operational definition that is elaborated in later chapters. Another important area that is discussed is theory building, which is approached from two directions: (1) nursing as theory and (2) theory building and learning. These two aspects of theory building provide a premise for continued use throughout subsequent chapters. An introduction to the conceptual framework of a curriculum as the keystone on which all subsequent curriculum-building work rests concludes the chapter.

COMMON FRAME OF REFERENCE

A key problem in beginning curriculum building is to establish among faculty a common vocabulary and similar frames of reference. Common meanings for essential concepts and common frames of reference enable intrafaculty communication, the basic component of every step in the curriculum-building process. This step provides some cohesion, unity of purpose, and direction, and the ability to identify, negotiate, and resolve differences. Semantic entanglements can be a major stumbling block to progress. Semantic problems can never be avoided entirely, although they can be minimized by anticipating and exploring concepts and the vocabulary necessary to discuss curriculum building. Absence of a common vocabulary and a common frame of reference isolates individuals so that each faculty member develops a curriculum in a personal and private way, not through selfishness but through the inability to "touch base" with colleagues.

Each faculty group will devise its own list of concepts and items to be defined according to its own needs. A simple vocabulary list with definitions will not serve, since it is the discussion and negotiation of definitions that lays the foundation for mutual understanding, clarification, and tacit agreement. This book takes the same format, in that this chapter elaborates some concepts basic to curriculum building to establish a common reference point with the reader. These concepts are (1) the nature of process, (2) process and systems, (3) systems theory and holism, (4) the nature of nursing, and (5) theory development.

CURRICULUM DEFINED

The curriculum is the learning activities that are designed to achieve specific educational goals. The basic problems of the curriculum-building process are to (1) determine the behaviors desired of the product, (2) devise a system of experiences that will produce the specified desired behaviors, and (3) discover whether the product exhibits the desired behaviors. These problems require solutions based in a conceptual construct usually called *a conceptual framework,* which is the decision-making guide for the curriculum-building process. The curriculum is the holistic manifestation of many composite parts and factors, which together enable the achievement of nursing educational goals that have been carefully identified, selected, and articulated.

Nature of process

Since curriculum building is a process, since nursing is a process, and since all components of nursing practice are subprocesses, it is essential to begin curriculum construction with a clear understanding of the nature of process so that curriculum building can be operationalized.

Processes have three characteristics: (1) inherent purpose, (2) internal organization, and (3) infinite creativity. Thus, by definition, process is the core phenomenon of all human knowledge and activities. Process is a series of acts or progressive changes toward a desired end or goal[1]; it is any phenomenon that shows a continuous change in time toward some objective.

Processes are not mutually exclusive; they overlap, feed into each other, articulate, support, cooperate, and interact, as well as conflict, oppose, or inhibit each other. Processes are mutually inclusive and are in all ways part of larger functioning wholes. For example, the process of assessment is integral to the process of problem solving. A problem cannot be identified until the process of assessment has been employed successfully. Yet the process of assessment is a process in and of itself, with an objective, a system, and a creative element that is "a continuous change in time." The same can be said for evaluation or for the formulation of alternative actions. Just as a throttle is a functioning unit yet is part of the "whole" automobile and can be used in a wide variety of sizes, makes, and models of cars, so processes such as assessment and evaluation are individual, yet parts of functioning wholes.

The first characteristic of process is the *purpose* of the phenomenon, sometimes called the subjective aim. Each process has a reason for existing. This reason is the end or goal toward which the series of actions or operations lead. The aim or purpose is what the process accomplishes. Growth is an example of a process. One subjective aim of the process of human growth is Maslow's "self-actualization."[2]

Similarly, the subjective aim of the process of problem solving is the best possible decision and subsequent action; the subjective aim of the process of nursing is the optimal level of wellness or health for every individual.

The second characteristic of process is its *organization,* which is the "series of actions or operations" that accomplishes the given aim. In other words, a process has a goal and an organizational structure that enables the goal to be accomplished. In the process of "growth," the internal organization could be Erikson's "central task of development."[3] These tasks prescribe the order and sequence of human development. Erikson also describes the conditions necessary to the accomplishment of the order and sequence of the central tasks of development. Another example is seen in problem solving. The internal organization of problem solving is evident in the sequential order of the scientific method or the explicit system of problem-solving operations expounded by educational psychologists. These psychologists have carefully described the steps necessary for identifying the problem, gathering data relevant to the problem, formulating meaningful predictive principles from the data, listing alternatives, assessing probabilities and risks, making decisions, and evaluating results.

The order or organization of each process is inherent in the process; it is discovered, not invented, and through reality testing and validation, new discoveries are constantly being made about each process. This constant collection of empirical data gradually changes man's ideas about the internal structure of each process so that each revision of ideas about the order of operation more nearly approximates the true nature of the process.

The third characteristic of process is *infinite creativity.* Creativity is the "progressing," or "advancing," or "continuous change in time." It is ongoing innovation, the infinite production of something that, although it may be essentially the same, is in some way unique or different from its predecessors. Whitehead[4] states that "it lies in the nature of things that many enter into complex unity." He proposes that *many* uniting together to form *one* distinct new entity is the normal universal phenomenon. The result of this unification is truly novel, different from all its predecessors, and distinctively unique from the many parts from which it was comprised. The creative aspect of process is illustrated by a kaleidoscope: a tube with many tiny parts of colored glass and mirrors that, when held to the eye and twisted, form an infinite variety of forms and patterns, each unique from the other but all formed of the exact same "many parts."

In the example of the process of growth, the creative characteristic is evidenced in the birth of a new and unique human being who is essentially the same yet separate and evolutionary from his many antecedents. In the process of problem solving, creativity is expressed in the experientially based evolving skill of innovating solutions to problems from many components. In nursing, the element of creativity is seen in the dynamics of evolving uniquely more effective and efficient nursing activities for the achievement of optimal health from many contributing parts.

Processes exist that have not yet been discovered, and no discovered process has been so completely operationalized that it is fully and finally understood. The builders of nursing curricula can utilize the discoveries of the specialists in other fields about processes and apply these discoveries to nursing. Eclecticism is ideally suited to synthesize seemingly conflicting theories into useful processes. This is a creative aspect of "process."

Everyone uses process; each person uses many processes, some of them quite well. The object of conscientiously studying a given process, identifying its subjective purpose, and trying to discover the order and sequence of its inherent organization and the manifestation of its creativity is to make it more fully applicable to its appropriate task and more easily and successfully taught to another person. This cognitive availability of information about a given process, added to practice in the use of the process, increases the extent and frequency of successful achievement of the objectives of that process. For example, the ability to articulate the subjective aim of problem solving, the ability to recall and use the inherent organization in a logical sequential order, enables the individual to adapt the process of problem solving to a wide variety of different problems with a high degree of success.

Skill in the ability to operationalize process can be equated to driving a car. Few people who drive a car can build one. Even many experts or professional drivers cannot build a car as well engineered and constructed as the one they can buy. However, people who know the principles involved in automobile mechanisms can use automobiles more effectively. These people can modify engines, redesign the body, adapt other parts, install racing clutches, alter the fuel, and make all manner of innovations to better fit the basic machine to their particular needs. It is also possible for these people to repair the car when it breaks down. Very knowledgeable people can also build automobiles for specific purposes. Like the mechanic-driver, the person who understands processes, their nature and use, can adapt them to specific needs, modify the currently accepted sequence and order of their inherent organization, diagnose and repair them when they fail to function, and build better process tools (heuristic devices).

Many ancient philosophers were "process" oriented. Almost all Eastern philosophy reflects elements of the "unity of parts," the "creative purpose," the "'one' being greater than and different from the sum of the parts." The Bible is filled with references to the elements of process philosophy. Paul, in his Epistles, repeatedly refers to "the many members" that are of "one Body." His most explicit description of "holistic" or "process" philosophy, as he applies it to the early Christian Church, can be found in 1 Corinthians 12.

The twentieth century concept of "wholes" was first expounded in the 1920s in South Africa by Smuts.[5] His book, *Holism and Evolution*, although about biological evolution, sparked a concern in the philosophical world and rekindled human interest in the essential nature of phenomenon. Smuts coined the word "holism," which was taken from the Greek word ὅλος, meaning "whole."

Smuts defines holism as a "unity of parts" so mutually supportive and intense that the whole is greater than and entirely different from the sum of the parts. He states that all the activities and products of the many parts are directed toward central ends; thus there is unified action of the organism. The individual parts are not suppressed, swallowed up, or lost; instead, there is more perfect individuation and specialized development, which are directed specifically toward the central ends and accomplish these ends through unified action or creative synthesis. In summary, there are many parts, unified in activity, organized for a specific purpose, that through synthesis become one "whole," creative and self-renewing, which in turn brings about new structural groupings. The process continues dynamically into infinity.[6]

Other philosophers have evolved Smuts' "holism" into a galaxy of hypotheses. The value of his thesis can be seen in the works of Bruner, Burton, Parker and Rubin, Rogers, Taba, Whitehead, and, indeed, all educators whose actions reflect a commitment to process education, the philosophical commitment to holism, process, and creativity.

The beauty of process education is the practical, systematic reality focus. This reality orientation offers, with pride, a curriculum that is devised to teach "how to" formulas that can be examined, tested, evaluated, and reformulated.

Nursing research is in the most exciting phases of its evolution. The generation of nursing theories is gathering momentum and increasing in volume and will eventually provide a substantial theoretical base for nursing. These theories will give rise to nursing processes that are clearly identified and definitive and will be separate, individual, functioning parts of the purposeful, systematically organized, creative, holistic nursing process. Process curricula will be able to accommodate these new theories with learning activities appropriate to the theory and to the curriculum, without a major curriculum revision, because by its very nature the process curriculum is dynamic. Since processes and theories are discovered, not invented, new discoveries only add to the effectiveness of the process; they do not change the purpose. The teaching strategies may alter, because of new discoveries, but the whole of a process curriculum need not change.

It is not possible to review all who have made outstanding contributions to education through their commitment to process. Each nursing faculty engaged in the pursuit of a process curriculum will, through necessity, study at length and in detail the works of process educators. The essential task of nursing curriculum builders is to search out and select processes that are applicable to nursing and to design instructional strategies that will enable students to learn those processes in the most efficient and effective way possible.

Process and systems

Banathy[7] defines system as "deliberately designed synthetic organisms, comprised of interrelated and interacting components which are employed to function in an integrated fashion to attain predetermined purposes." In common usage the word "process" and the word "system" are used interchangeably.

Systems structure is the functional implementation of process philosophy. It is man's recent discovery of a way to design a process so that it is efficiently and reliably achievable. While reading about systems and systems analysis, one often thinks, "There is nothing new here; I am familiar with this as a process; it's the language that's different and perhaps the organization." As mentioned previously, processes exist, they are discovered and gradually uncovered, and man increases his ability to organize himself and his activities so that his use of each evolving system more closely approximates existing dynamic processes. Therefore it is not strange that once one gets beyond the barrier of new vocabulary, the actuality of systems themselves is comfortable and familiar.

Systems analysis techniques have permitted processes to be broken into definitive tasks so that they can become consistently, specifically operational, with a high probability of success. Table 1 aligns the components of systems language under the three categories of process to clarify their mutual identity.

"Systems" has its origins in industry. Its initial purpose was to enable industry to break a job down into manageable bits and pieces so that several departments of

Table 1. Systems arranged under the components of process

Purpose	Organization	Innovation
Input	Throughput	Output
Objectives	Content-concepts	Goods
End-product criterion needs	Components tasks	Behaviors
Systemic linkages	Accomplishment strategies	Services
Information	Choice alternatives and potential consequences, probability risks, and value estimates	Products
	Implementation of test for workability	Evaluation
		Alter to improve retest
		Realter to improve to infinity
		Systemic linkages

different firms could work together toward a common goal with some degree of certainty that the goal would be met. Systems analysis came into popular use in World War II, and weapons systems were the prime movers and the major outcome. In the postwar and current computer age, systems analysis techniques enable human beings to do the thinking and machines to do the work. Systems analysis techniques have been applied to problem solving in an attempt to diagram human thought processes so that machines might synthesize these thought processes. Cybernetics, then, is the outcome, the interlinking of human being and machine, resulting in highly reliable problem solving.

Systems theory and holism

This is the age of holism. Ecologists deal with the interrelatedness of nature and all living things, proving to scientists that no part of the world is so isolated or independent as not to be intimately tied to all other living things in mutual maintenance, growth, life, and destiny. The only exceptions are closed systems, and they are rare and almost all are artificially created.

One of the scientific mechanisms that has made possible the age of holism is general systems theory, which seeks to define how wholes function in relationship to each other. It takes "objects" that are wholes—divergent, different, complex, and variable—and discovers how these wholes are interdependent and what the relationships are between and among objects of differing properties and attributes. This theory is particularly relevant for nursing curricula, since nurse educators are attempting to define humans as holistic. Holistic concepts of humans means that they must be conceived and related to as a total system whose parts function interdependently and whose whole is inclusive of their environment. Furthermore, holism implies that humans cannot be treated as sums of parts. Holism is a step beyond "comprehensive nursing care."

Comprehensive nursing care is treating all the parts—parts referred to in the neo-integrated jargon as biopsychosocial. Systems theory enables educators to move beyond the dualistically bound theories and concepts and to categorize parts of humans in more meaningful ways. This short introduction to systems theory will only attempt to define some of the language so that language can be used in this book to aid in curriculum-building activities.

A system is anything that functions as a unit of "wholes" because its parts are interdependent.[8] There are two kinds of systems—open and closed. Closed systems are isolated from their environments and are therefore limited in their energy, their functions, and their life expectancy. The usual example of a closed system is a chemical reaction in a sealed container. The law of entropy applies to open and closed systems but is highly characteristic of closed ones. In practice this means that there is a leveling of all differences. The materials and/or factors in the closed system tend to move toward and eventually attain a state of homogeneity. If one places two fluids of differing densities into a closed container separated by a semipermeable membrane, the fluids will move from the side of lesser density to the side of greater density until the two fluids are of equal density. This is the attainment of homogeneity. In living systems there are no true closed systems. However, in some nursing programs, isolated from reality and social stimulation, there tends to be a sameness or leveling of all differences among the students, faculty, and type of nursing care. Entropy, then, is a limited amount of energy causing an equilibrium (stabilization) toward homogeneity.

The opposite of entropy is negative entropy, called negentropy. Negentropy means that energy and matter are imported from other systems, and the free exchange causes the system to achieve more complexity and heterogeneity. True homogeneity is never reached in open systems, but a "steady state" can be reached. The steady state is a condition of the organism where the composition, components, and functions of the organism remain constant but there is always a flow of materials, energy, and components from and to other systems, and thereby some changes are constantly taking place within the system.

In the preceding paragraphs, exchanges with other systems and other organisms have been discussed. This presumes some interconnection with other systems and leads to another property of open systems. All open systems have subsystems (except the smallest ones), and all but the largest systems have suprasystems. All systems, then, except those unimaginable, infinitesimal, and gargantuan ones, are in hierarchies of suprasystems and subsystems. Systemic linkages interlock systems into complex systems.

Other properties of systems are that every system has factors which are called variables. These variables affect the structure and function of the system. When the factor or variable is in the environment of the system, it is called a parameter.

Every system has a boundary that separates it in some way from its environment. Sometimes boundaries are hard to distinguish. Every system has an environment, which has two aspects: proximal (close) and distal (remote). Actually, proximal environments are those environments of which the system is aware and distal environments are those of which the system is unaware; both environments affect the behavior of the system.

Systems have inputs (energy and information going into the system) and outputs (energy and information going out of the systems). In nursing, as in many systems, the output is goods and services, behaviors, and acts of nursing care.

There are other characteristics of systems—self-regulation and equifinality.

Self-regulation is the ability of the organism to reestablish another steady state after being stimulated or affected by external conditions. The characteristic of self-regulation implies that open systems have order and are predictable. This is in some opposition to the philosophical viewpoint of the existentialist, who believes that life is ultimately unpredictable.

Equifinality means that there is a characteristic state for all things and that, starting from different conditions and using different factors, similar organisms will achieve or assume for each successive stage of development a similar state which is typical or characteristic for the organism. Note that the state is typical or equal, not identical. Only rarely does nature make an "identical."

Since life is whole and not fractured as presented by scientists, life processes are interrelated, mutually interdependent, and mutually inclusive. Studying life processes in their separate states is much like the committee of blind men examining the elephant. Is an elephant like a rope, like a tree trunk, or like a snake? Of course, the elephant is like the elephant, but a detailed study of his tail, leg, or trunk will never reveal that. Human beings are growing in their ability to study wholes. The study of individual parts, such as learning capacity, socialization behavior, and physiology, has finally led to the conclusion that the knowledge gained by studying the parts is incomplete, contradictory, and inadequate to explain the phenomenon of man; a new way of bringing the parts together is now in use. Systems theory provides the framework for viewing processes as open systems interlinked to provide a whole that acts as one ecological unit. Processes are concerned with wholes; systems are concerned with the organization of the whole or with how the parts interact to make the whole. This has caused the words "process" and "system" to be used interchangeably. Commonly, systems comprise an operationalization of a process. Fig. 1-1 is a diagram of a process, revealing the three basic components of all true processes.

Note that Fig. 1-1 emphasizes the dynamic nature of process by arranging the components around a feedback matrix,

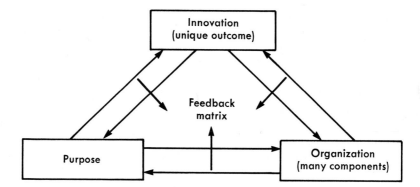

Fig. 1-1. Three basic components of all true processes.

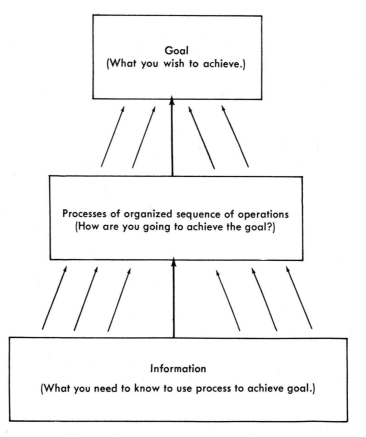

Fig. 1-2. Content in a process curriculum.

which is a device that permits feedback from any stage of the process to be shuttled to the appropriate components so that ongoing changes can occur. This makes innovation a constant characteristic of the outcome. Changes feed back and alter the whole process, if only in miniscule ways, so that the process is continually changing. For educational purposes a system is an operational design of a process for achieving a specific purpose. Processes or systems are fluid, dynamic, and always

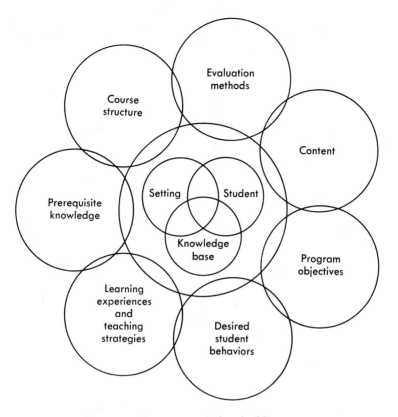

Fig. 1-3. Nursing care curriculum-building system.

new, just a little different from any prior moment. A process is much like a river—to examine it, it must be frozen. Thus one begins to discover its "system," its "interrelated and interacting components," and begins to employ this system to attain the predetermined or "subjective purposes," that is, goods, behavior, products, and services.

Content-process problem of teachers. Processes and systems do not exist in an information vacuum. For instance, problem solving is a process that can be systematized. It has purpose, organization, and innovation. To utilize the process, a goal or purpose must exist. For problems to be solved and goals achieved, the system must be utilized around the "content" information to be processed through the problem-solving system sequence. The content of any system is determined by the subject of the "problem," or "goal." In an educational system, content is *information and processes* necessary to achieve an educational goal. The goal of the content system, then, determines the selection of information (input) and the educational processes to be used. Fig. 1-2 is a diagram of this concept.

In other words, process is the *use* of the information. One can separate information from its *behavioral use,* but when combined with the process, the two become the content of a subject. If educational goals are expressed behaviorally, information must be geared to "how it is useful in achieving those behaviors." Once translated into its behavioral potential, information loses its esoteric character and becomes functional. Once it becomes functional, it becomes content, that is, process and information which is goal oriented.

Curriculum building as process. Curriculum building is a process, and because it is a process it has purpose, system (or organization), and innovation. The system, or organization, of the curriculum-building process exists solely to accomplish the purpose, and because it is a system, the internal organization for the process of curriculum building can be analyzed and arranged and ordered in a way that will facilitate the accomplishment of the purpose. *The purpose of curriculum building in nursing is to provide learning experiences that will enable students to develop nursing behaviors that promote the greatest possible health for every individual in society.*

The system or organization of the curriculum-building process can be arranged in a series of groups of operations. Each group of operations is called a subsystem; taken together, these subsystems comprise

the system (or internal organization) of the curriculum-building process for nursing. This system, together with curriculum-building processes of other health workers, comprises the greater overall system called the suprasystem of the education of all those disciplines concerned with the health of people. Fig. 1-3 is a diagram of the nursing care curriculum-building system.

Nursing is just beginning to develop an ability to use cybernetic systems for nursing processes. The first step is the deliberate use of process or systems flow for solving nursing problems; the second step is the careful identification and analysis of the kinds of subsystems or subprocesses inherent in nursing processes. Fig. 1-4 is a model of one concept of nursing process presented in a systems flow chart.

The following is a definition and brief explanation of Fig. 1-4.

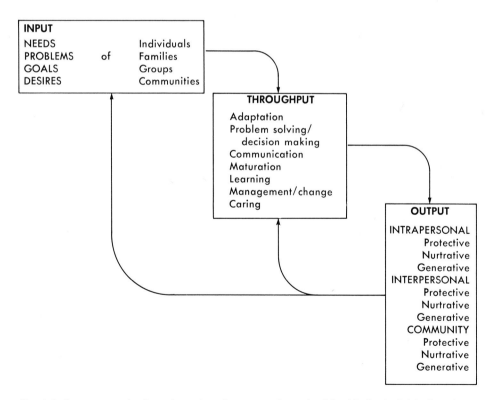

Fig. 1-4. System organization of nursing. System goal: optimal health for individuals, groups, and committees.

Nature of nursing

For the purpose of this book, and as an example for curriculum builders of the kind of definition that must be devised by a faculty, nursing is defined as follows:

Nursing is a process: Its purpose is to promote optimal health through protective, nurtrative,[9] and generative activities. These activities are carried out with three client systems— the intrapersonal system, the interpersonal system, and the community system. Nursing's role is to facilitate maturation and adaptation in these client systems. The tools with which nurses function are the subprocesses of communicating, caring, problem solving/decision making, managing/changing, and teaching. Nurses are autonomous health care givers within the limits of employment contracts, collaborating with other members of the health care team for the benefit of clients. They are accountable for their activities, they monitor and regulate the quality of the nursing care given and provide each other with mutual protection, nurturing, and facilitation of growth.

Nursing is a process and has the three characteristics inherent in any process, that is, purpose, organization, and innovation. As a process, its system can be analyzed and its structure designed.

The purpose of the process of nursing is the highest possible level of health or self-actualization for each individual. Regardless of where nurses practice, what role they are enacting, what their educational preparation or experience, or how independent or dependent their functions, the paramount raison d'être is to promote optimal health.

Health or high-level wellness, however defined by educational programs, is the purpose of the nursing process and central to the whole system. The goals of nursing are specifically aimed at individuals, families, other groups, and communities.

Input. Input for the nursing system comprises the needs, goals, problems, and desires of clients and nurses. The clients (target systems) are intrapersonal (individuals), interpersonal (groups, families, agencies), and/or communities. The input includes assessment data and information necessary to work with the problems, needs, goals, and desires.

Throughput. Throughput consists of the theories, processes, concepts, and conceptual constructs selected from nursing and from appropriate fields of the sciences and arts and synthesized into content useful to the practice discipline of nursing.

Rogers states that "Science seeks to make intelligible the world of man's experiences. Nursing science seeks to make intelligible knowledge about man and his world that has special significance for nursing. The phenomenon central to nursing's conceptual system is the life process in man."[10] She further states that "Nursing's conceptual system is (neither) static nor inflexible. Quite the contrary. In its evolution it is properly subject to reformulation and change as empirical knowledge grows, as conceptual data achieve greater clarity, and as the interconnectedness between ideas takes on new dimensions."[11] The creative element of nursing process is not only, as Rogers states, within the theories themselves but inevitably within the intrapersonal, interpersonal, and/or community system wherein nursing is practiced.

Whitehead's[4] description of creativity presented earlier in this chapter has special significance for the nursing process. That which is uniquely nursing is the output or nursing act or intervention which is novel or different and the result of the synthesis of the many throughput components. The "many" that come together to make nursing activities are the five subprocesses, or subsystems, which are the tools nurses use and the two areas of humans with which nurses are concerned. These are as follows:

Tools
   Problem solving/decision making
   Caring
   Learning
   Communication
   Management/change
Areas
   Adaptation
   Maturation

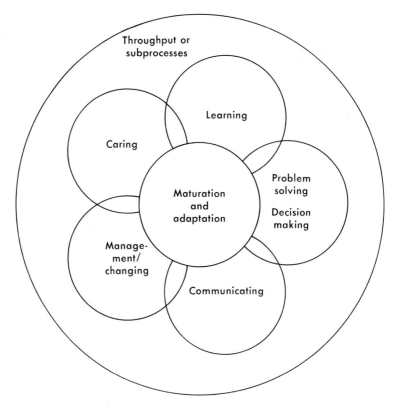

Fig. 1-5. Throughput or subprocesses of nursing's system.

These seven subprocesses are the result of the synthesis of life processes that, when utilized in the practice of nursing, makes change toward optimal health inevitable. Each utilization of these subprocesses in nursing practice calls for a unique synthesis of the theories that funnel into the feedback matrix, renovating the specific purposes and organization. Fig. 1-5 is a schematic presentation of the throughput component of nursing process.

Output. Output comprises the behaviors and services, roles, functions, and skills of nursing. These behaviors attain the goals the system. Nursing behaviors are classified into the following three categories, which are adapted alterations of Leavell and Clark[12] and are not sequential:

1. **Protective behaviors**—nursing measures that prevent disease or diminishing health, or, expressed positively, maintain and promote health

2. **Nurtrative behaviors**—nursing measures that nurture or are therapeutic, curative, and comforting
3. **Generative behaviors**—nursing measures that are innovative, productive, reproductive, and/or rehabilitative

These three categories of behaviors are enacted in the three target systems or client systems of nursing. In other words, both input and output are geared to the target (client) system, whereas throughput, although relevant to the client system, is in fact more intimately concerned with the content of the data than the targets of the data. The client systems are as follows:

1. **Intrapersonal system**—the target of protective, nurtrative, and/or generative nursing behaviors that promote the optimal functioning of all internal life processes. This includes all growth processes, individual personality formation, and anything that is the expression of one person.

2. **Interpersonal system**—the target of protective, nurtrative, and/or generative nursing behaviors that promote the optimal functioning of two or more people. This includes the nurse and client, the nurse and other health persons, the nurse and other professionals, the nurse and agencies, the nurse and the client family, and the nurse and surrogate families (such as communes and some religious orders).

3. **Community system**—the target of protective, nurtrative, and/or generative nursing behaviors that promote the optimal functioning of communities. Community is here defined as "a group of people having common organization and mutual interest." The common organization facilitates the creation of institutions and agencies for the common good and mutual interest and enables the enactment and enforcement of rules that further those interests. Nurses engage in activities in communities, whether the community be local, as in a town or city, or worldwide, which involves working with health care systems, governmental agencies, citizen groups, and proprietary agencies. Any nursing activity that reduces threat to the health of the community or promotes the health of communities is a community activity. Any activity that the nurse engages in that promotes community coping or maturation qualifies as a community activity.

This book does not presume to cover completely the seven life processes inherent in nursing. Chapter 5 will present a brief discussion of the kinds of theories categorized into these processes. From the seven processes, only learning and change will be discussed at any length because these two processes are specifically necessary to the process of building nursing curricula.

Theory development in nursing

Nursing is a practice discipline, and, as in all disciplines that function in reality, theories selected to be included in curricula are chosen with their practice implication as the most essential criterion. Historically, nursing moved slowly into the theoretical arena, since most nursing content was appropriated from medicine. The

nursing curriculum was watered-down medical information with a few hints about "nursing implications" thrown in to sweeten the dose of "medicine." A major step occurred after many nurses, with no doctoral study in nursing available, earned doctorates in other disciplines. These people contributed the theories and the research methodologies of their disciplines to nursing—the applied field. Nursing was seen during this era as having no claim to theory on its own but being "applied" and therefore using theories from all other disciplines. Nurse scientist programs sprang up wherein nurses could obtain advanced degrees in sciences and concentrate on the nursing applications while they were about it. These programs made and continue to make valuable contributions to nursing's body of knowledge.

Today theories for nursing are rapidly being generated and validated. More and more nurses believe that there remains a largely undiscovered body of nursing theory. Nurses from all aspects of nursing are seeking, developing, and formulating theories of nursing.

McKay states, "It is evident that nursing is not all science: the ethical and aesthetic elements cannot be disregarded. As a profession grows all three areas change—value assumptions are redefined, knowledge is extended, and skill is perfected—but it is the acquisition of knowledge and the organizing of it into meaningful patterns which enriches professional practice."[13] When speaking of "the acquisition of knowledge and the organizing of it into meaningful patterns," McKay was describing theories. Nursing researchers and educators are speaking about the need for theory development in nursing and working toward that end. Some nurses speak of "a" theory of nursing. Leininger[14] states that that kind of thinking is "magical" and unrealistic and that a single theory would box nursing in and be unnecessarily restricting. She makes a case that multiple theories, conceptual frameworks, and models are a healthy diversity that stimulate new areas of research and the generation of new theory. Individual schools generally select one or more theory constructs or conceptual constructs to formulate an umbrella type of framework for curriculum. These conceptual frameworks tend to have some common denominators. From this scant evidence one could conjecture that there could be developed, using the general systems theory model, a systemization of theories and concepts of nursing that would allow for Leininger's diversity while enabling some unanimity. That is not present reality, however, and nursing is currently in the stage of rapidly generating new and diverse theories, each valuable in nursing's steady progress toward its own clearly defined body of knowledge.

Curriculum construction involves selecting and arranging content in an order that will promote the most efficient learning of a given subject. Curriculum is constantly changed because faculties desire to select different content, arrange content differently, or find a new content-organizing strategy in the hope that a new selection and/or arrangement will result in more effective learning. One of the most helpful things in revising or developing a curriculum is a clear picture of how thinking develops and how theories develop in a practice discipline such as nursing. Content that is analyzed to determine the presence of the successive stages of theory development can be arranged for learning so that each stage of theory development can be taught for every selected concept. In this way the practice or reality implementation of each theory can be an optimally learned and fully developed behavior. There is an analogy for theory evolution in Erikson's theory of human development. Human development theory maintains that success in life, or human maturity, is attained when each central task of development is accomplished, at least in part, in its proper order. Furthermore, full maturity is not attained until these tasks of development are accomplished. In the same manner the attainment of the highest level of theories or practice depends on the successful learning of each prior level of that theory.

Definitions of theory and its components.[15] A theory is a human invention that is evolved to explain what something is, what its characteristics and attributes are, how it relates to other things, what will make it behave in certain ways, what will keep it from behaving in certain ways, and how it can be used in a life situation. In other words, theory is a collection of concepts, facts, postulates, propositions, laws, principles, and hypotheses related into a meaningful whole so that it is useful for explaining phenomena and guiding behavior. There are hierarchies of theory complexity or maturity, and names for the stages of their development. The names used to label various hierarchical levels of theory depend on whose jargon or what framework is used to label them. There are presented here some general definitions used by theorists followed by a simplified summary of theory development as perceived by Dickoff, James, and Wiedenbach.

Facts are basic, irreducible objects, conditions, or occurrences. They are held to be immutable—things that are true, that exist, that have occurred. Facts are building blocks of all other words used to describe theory. They are observations, descriptions, and depictions of the world of events as perceived and validated by one or more humans; for example, bacteria cause infections in wounds.

Concepts are groups of ideas, objects, or facts that are abstract generalizations based on some common denominator. They are mental filing systems for ideas that are held together by meaningful aspects or likenesses; for example, wound damage to the body by trauma, an injury that damages, destroys, or disrupts tissue. A hole made by a bullet or scalpel as well as a bruise or scrape caused by a fall are both classified in the general conceptual category of wound. As another example, *bacteria* (microorganism, yeast, *Parame-*

cium, spirochetes, coccidia, molds, fungi) are all classified in the conceptual category of microorganisms.

Conceptual constructs are a means of grouping data by using concepts. Conceptual constructs comprise some rational, sequential, or useful ordering of concepts. Most nursing conceptual frameworks are constructs. For example, infection can become a whole conceptual construct, its subconcepts are contamination, sterilization, antisepsis, asepsis, cleanliness, susceptibility, resistance, inflammation, etc.

Postulates are only a step removed from concepts; they too are abstract ideas. However, they are premises which underlie assumptions; they are statements of logic which are assumed truths; and they are different from facts in that the truth is not known, just assumed. They generally have universal significance, can be documented from the literature, and have the strength of logic or reasoning; for example, wound infections occur more readily when the surrounding tissue is damaged or bruised.

Propositions are different from postulates in that whereas postulates are assumed to be true, propositions are offered so that they can be tested. Propositions are declarations (always a declarative sentence), statements about something that is offered for consideration, argument, acceptance, or refutation. It is an idea to be proved; for example, infections occur more frequently in operating rooms than in delivery rooms.

A *hypothesis* is a statement of relationships among or between facts, concepts, and/or propositions. Hypotheses are expected relationships and are predictive; they predict behavior, consequences, and occurrences. They are causal or correlative by nature and are constructed by chaining concepts and constructs in logical sequence for predictive and explanatory purposes. They are offered to be proved or refuted and used as a basis of problem solving and research. For example, susceptibility to infection is controlled by three variables:

(1) the virulence of the infective organism, (2) the resistance of the host, and (3) the dosage of the infection. Wound infection incidence is significantly changed by altering one or more of the three variables.

Principles are a general or fundamental truth, law, or assumption and are like postulates. The word is from the Latin *principium* and means first-fundamental. A more complex type of principle is a *predictive principle,* which is like a simple hypothesis. It is a proposition or postulate that is connected to some logical consequence. It is an "if"/"then" connection. A predictive principle is "a set of circumstances, conditions, or behaviors that produces a given, definable outcome . . . it expresses relationships of facts, concepts, or circumstances to consequences."[16] For example, thoroughly washing the hands by the attending nurse decreases the amount of bacteria on the hands and thereby decreases the number of wound infections carried by the nurse.

Laws originate as postulates, become hypotheses, and are proved or validated to be accepted as laws. They are generalizations of the behavior of factors from observations of repeatable facts and occurrences. They are not drawn from one occurrence or by chance but by rigid standards of observation, experimentation, and proof. In the grand scheme of science there are relatively few laws. Whereas facts are single statements of truths, laws are generally cause-and-effect statements of truths. The social sciences have few if any laws; the biological sciences have more than the social sciences but still relatively few; the physical sciences, being the most measurable science area, have the most laws; for example, fluids and gases in a confined space exert pressure equally and undiminished in all directions.

Theory is a cogent, generally lengthy group of facts, concepts, conceptual constructs, laws, propositions, postulates, and hypotheses in any combination that are logically intertwined into a whole and are statements about expected relationships among phenomena or are tentative explanations of phenomena or occurrences. A theory does not have to be proved; it need only be logical, testable, usable. Examples are the theory of relativity and the theory of the conservation of energy.

An *operational definition* is a definition of a concept or phenomenon that is arranged in sequential order so that the definition itself describes the progressional sequence in which the phenomenon occurs. The definition can then be followed as a recipe either to analyze or to re-create the phenomenon. Operational definitions of concepts that are processes are the ones most easily devised and most useful to nursing. For example, each of the processes used in this chapter as components of nursing is an operational definition that is developed in progressive stages.

Operational definitions, like theory development, are extremely useful for nursing curriculum because they enable concepts or processes to be systematized and content to be derived from that system. They also indicate in what order the process can best be learned and used and thereby can provide guidelines for focus or emphasis for courses of increasing complexity. (The five subprocesses or tools nurses use have been operationalized in Chapter 4.)

Four levels or phases of theories in practice disciplines. Dickoff, James, and Weidenbach[17] sort theory development into four levels, which provide excellent guidelines for sorting content into levels of complexity. Therefore the four levels provide help for writing course and learning activity objectives and are helpful in deriving evaluation criteria. In combination with definitions of facts, concepts, constructs, laws, propositions, postulates, hypotheses, and theory given in the preceding paragraphs, theory levels of development can be the curriculum builder's most useful tool.

Four stages of development are necessary for a theory to reach its full maturity and thus be optimally useful to nurses. Each stage indicates that the theory has evolved successfully through the preceding phases. Every level of theory is still correctly labeled theory whether or not the theory has attained maturity—the fourth phase.

Level 1: Factor-isolating theories. Level 1 has two activities: (1) naming, or labeling, and (2) classifying, or categorizing.

The basic stage is the activity of naming, or labeling. The function of naming allows an idea or object to be perceived and talked about or referred to. One must isolate identifying aspects or factors to recognize that a thing is what it is and not something else, thus the title of this level—factor-isolating theories. Names may be chosen for a variety of reasons, such as the order of discovery or occurrence (for example, the Caribbean hurricanes are labeled alphabetically "Angela," "Betty," "Carol," "Doris," and so on), the person who discovered or invented it (Cushing's disease or Bowman's capsule), its function (heart-lung machine or walkie-talkie), its similarity to other things that have already been identified and named (kidney basin or kidney bean), or by description (the black-backed, three-toed woodpecker).

The second activity in Level 1 is classifying, that is, the sorting, categorizing, or grouping of things according to some commonality. Classifying by commonality requires that the factors or attributes of an object, idea, or thing be isolated. This second activity is not possible unless the first activity, that of naming or labeling, has occurred. Categorizing requires one to identify what something is and what it is not. Categories can be grouped just as single items can be grouped, and this grouping of categories is possible because of some common denominator or unifying factor. Thus a hierarchy of categories is formed. (Acute inflammatory response is a large category that contains subcategories, one of which is fever; another is local edema.)

Level 2: Factor-relating theories. There are two activities in this level of theory building: (1) depicting or describing and (2) relating factors. This level describes or depicts how one single-named and classified thing (factor) relates to another single-named and classified thing (factor); thus the title—factor-relating theories. For example, a description of the face requires communication of how the eyes sit in relation to the nose, mouth, ears, and forehead. This level of theory describes relationships to other factors; in other words, it is a "natural history" of any given subject. Any descriptive science, such as anatomy, is an example of factor-relating theory.

Level 3: Situation-relating theories. This level of theory is concerned with causal relationships. It relates one situation to another in a way that allows for prediction. One of its essential ingredients is causal-connecting statements that give a basis for the prediction. Prediction is a statement of causal or consequential connections between two states of affairs or two concepts. This level of theory reveals what conditions, circumstances, or behavior (what the cost in time, energy, effort, pain, and/or what factors) will promote or inhibit the occurrence of another situation. Dickoff, James, and Wiedenbach[17] call this level of theory building of "incredible importance" to practice. Douglass and Bevis[16] state that principles (predictive and inhibiting theories) are guides for developing realistic alternatives of action. They further describe predictive theories as being essential to problem solving and decision making (the fourth level of theory building).

Simply stated, Level 3 theory tells one that if "a" occurs, "b" will occur. It tells one what promotes, accelerates, has a catalytic effect, retards, inhibits, or stops an occurrence. Promoting or inhibiting theories indicate under what circumstances things will occur and with what speed and effort.

Level 4: Situation-producing theories. Situation-producing theory, also called goal-incorporating theory and prescriptive theory, is the level of theory that specifies precisely how situations described, de-picted, and predicted in lower levels of theory can be produced or made to occur. Situation-producing theory is a design of how the content and goals of the theory can be realized. It has several important ingredients: (1) conceptualization and stating of a goal or goals and (2) conceptualization and articulation of prescriptions.

Prescriptions are directives or commands that are directed toward the goal and specifically devised for a particular agent or agents. According to Dickoff, James, and Wiedenbach, the content of the prescription follows a survey list as a matter of "judgment." The agent's judgment, a combination of experience, wisdom, or practical insight, is used in selecting the content of the directives that follow a survey list. Most of nursing now uses problem solving/decision making as the tool that enables the agent to have "good" judgment. The survey list of Dickoff, James, and Wiedenbach[17] has six aspects:

1. Who (or what) does the activity?
2. Who (or what) receives the activity?
3. What is the environment or context of the activity?
4. What is the activity's end point?
5. What is the technique, procedure, or protocol that guides the activity?
6. What or where is the energy source for the activity?

Theory building and learning. Gagne[15b] lists eight types of learning, which have a remarkable similarity to Dickoff, James, and Wiedenbach's[19] four levels of theories. This is understandable when one considers that the logical evolution of a theory must naturally follow the serially organized development of learning. Gagné states that seven of the eight types of learning are sequential and the development of each type increases in complexity and requires that the antecedent types of learning be mastered as prerequisites. The listed types of learning have such a similarity to Dickoff, James, and Wiedenbach's four levels of theories that one is tempted to draw the conclusion that the conditions necessary for learning are nearly the same as the

Table 2. Comparison of levels of theories in a practice discipline and sequential varieties of learning

Levels of theories (Dickoff, James, and Wiedenbach)	Sequential varieties of learning (Gagné)
1. Factor-isolating a. Naming b. Simple categories	1. Stimulus-response connections (type 2) 2. Verbal associations (type 4) or other chains (type 3)
2. Factor-relating a. Describing b. Depicting c. Relating	3. Multiple discrimination (type 5) 4. Concepts (type 6)
3. Situation-relating a. Predictive b. Promoting and inhibiting	5. Principles (type 7)
4. Situation-producing (prescriptive)	6. Problem solving (type 8)

conditions necessary for a fully developed or mature practice-oriented theory.

Table 2 gives a comparison of Gagné's sequential varieties of learning and Dickoff, James, and Wiedenbach's four levels of theories in a practice discipline. The levels are listed from most simple to most complex.

Theory building is a process, the ultimate purpose of which is to provide a guide for action or practice. It has inherent organization as illustrated by the systematic progression of the four levels of theories, and it has the characteristic of innovation in its many components and variety of factors that combine into one unique situation-producing theory that varies for each situation in a self-renewing and self-fulfilling manner. Curricula that trace nursing theory components through the four stages and ensure that students are taught essential factors from each successive stage of theory building produce graduates who can utilize theories in nursing practice. Nursing courses need not be solely responsible for each stage of theories, but nursing faculty engaged in building curricula are responsible for inventorying all courses for essential theory components to ensure that the hierarchy of selected theories is in-

cluded in the curriculum, either in non-nursing or nursing courses.

SYSTEM AND SUBSYSTEMS OF CURRICULUM BUILDING IN NURSING

The process of curriculum building in nursing has been pragmatically organized into a system, which has been invented to provide goal orientation and a natural logical sequence of tasks to achieve this goal.

The sequential arrangement of tasks presented in the following outline is suggested as appropriate to nursing.

PROCESS AND SUBPROCESSES

Objective of the system: To select and devise learning experiences that will foster nursing behaviors that enable persons completing the experiences to promote optimal health.

Contributing subsystems

I. Conceptual framework
  A. Philosophy
    1. Devise a narrative statement of belief based on the philosophy of the sponsoring agency and the philosophical agreements of the faculty.
  B. Setting
    1. Prognosticate the working environment of the graduate for the 15 to 20 years of expected active nursing, e.g., the community, area, state, and nation (all characteristics and statistics that influence nursing).
    2. Describe the current community, the environment in which health care is provided.
    3. Describe the educational environment of the school of nursing.
    4. Describe the current and projected major health problems of the area.
  C. Students
    1. Survey the demographic characteristics of the students who are currently enrolled in the school of nursing.
    2. Assess the personality and personal preferences of the students.
    3. Assess the educational and nursing attainments and needs of the students.
    4. Determine what, if any, differences are desired in the following:
      a. The type of students accepted into the program.
      b. The characteristics desired on exit from the program.

5. Formulate a list of concepts, postulates, propositions, principles, and theories of learning that are congruent with student and faculty characteristics.
6. Assess and describe the faculty of the school of nursing.

D. Knowledge or subject matter
   1. List the concepts deemed important to the faculty, students, and university that are applicable to the practice of nursing.
   2. Survey the literature for constructs and theories useful to nursing.
   3. Select or devise a conceptual construct or theories of nursing that can be used in nursing practice and/or education.

II. Course vivification

A. Conceptual framework
   1. List the definitive curriculum commitments explicit or implicit in the theoretical and philosophical statements as an implementation or functional checklist.

B. Aims
   1. Describe essential nursing behaviors (graduate).
   2. Establish program objectives.

C. Content
   1. Pattern course configuration.
   2. Select content* based on the following:
      a. The processes inherent in nursing.
      b. The information of nursing.
   3. Arrange the content in a pattern considering the following:
      a. Natural groupings.
      b. Level of complexity.
   4. Devise courses as follows:
      a. Establish course objectives (these are desired behaviors that are building blocks in achieving the curriculum objectives).
      b. Select learning activities that will provide the content necessary to accomplish the objectives.

D. Evaluation
   1. Establish minimal competencies or mastery criteria directly from the objectives.
   2. Make grading decisions and establish grading policies consistent with institutional guidelines, faculty philosophy, and selected learning theories.

Curriculum building is a process, and therefore it can be organized as a dynamic system. No one task is completed in its entirety prior to beginning the next task. Many tasks are in progress simultaneously in various stages of development. Curriculum builders utilize many feedback systems and go back and forth among tasks, adding, deleting, and changing components and ideas in a continuous growth toward a better system for learning.

INTRODUCTION TO CONCEPTUAL FRAMEWORK AS THE CURRICULUM KEYSTONE
Orientation

A conceptual framework is an interrelated system of premises that provide guidelines or ground rules for making all curricular decisions—objectives, content, implementation, and evaluation. The conceptual framework is variously referred to as the curriculum framework or the framework for curriculum development,[20] the conceptual system,[21] the curriculum theory,[22] a theory of education,[23] and the theoretical framework.[24] Regardless of the name, it is the *conceptualization and articulation of concepts, facts, propositions, postulates, theories, phenomena, and variables relevant to a specific nursing educational system.* It comprises concepts, facts, hypotheses, theories, and/or other crucial elements or ideas on which a nursing curriculum is based and the relationship these concepts have to each other and to the nursing curriculum in a specific educational situation. The frame of reference, or a conceptual framework, is the structure that provides the map for all curriculum matters. It is like the framing of a house in that it furnishes the specifications and decision-making guidelines for the walls, rooms, form, and function of the house. The conceptual framework provides the perimeters (limits and constraints) and parameters (values) for curriculum development, giving consistency and integrity to the learning plan. The frame of reference, or conceptual framework, of each school of nursing differs, at least slightly, from that of every other school of nursing, even though large areas of similarity will exist because of the nature of nursing.

Just as each person has a frame of reference that is influenced by his life ex-

---

*For use in this book, content is defined as the processes and information of a given subject.

periences, his ethnicity, his philosophy, and his personality, so each school of nursing's conceptual framework is influenced by its "culture," that is, its philosophical set, educational setting, the community it serves, the students who attend, and the characteristics of its faculty—their beliefs about nursing, learning, and people. These elements comprise an implied and expressed value system and provide explicit decision-making rules for curriculum.

Much nursing literature, when referring to a conceptual framework for nursing curriculum, seems to refer only to the knowledge base of nursing, and most authors communicate concepts and theories relevant to this area to the exclusion of other factors that are equally influential in curriculum decision making. According to Chater[25] there are three areas that provide concepts, theories, and decision-making guidelines for curriculum building. The context or setting of the school of nursing, including both the educational setting and the broader civic setting, comprises one area of conceptual framework materials, and the students, their characteristics, personal preferences, and the learning theories most likely to be successful with them comprise a second area. These two areas, with the knowledge base of concepts and theories, provide the three areas of data necessary to a complete and therefore useful conceptual framework.

Some of the factors that comprise the conceptual framework from which the curriculum design is derived simply exist and must be either described or discovered. These include the following:

1. The present and projected health problems and their probable solution for the geographical area served, viewed within the context of life conditions that will exist during the working life of the graduate
2. The educational setting and the objectives or purposes of the sponsoring institution (hospital, associate of arts college, university, and so forth)

3. The characteristics of the students either in attendance or anticipated
4. The characteristics of the faculty

Other factors that comprise the conceptual framework of the curriculum must be defined by each member of the faculty and negotiated for a compromise that serves the whole. These factors include the following:

1. The nature of nursing, including a description of roles and/or functions
2. Valued nursing behaviors
3. Theories that contribute to the attainment of the valued nursing behaviors
4. Theories of learning most useful to the faculty

The conceptual framework of the curriculum must be recorded in a statement of basic curricular assumptions in a clear and concise manner. Formulating a conceptual framework is merely an intellectual exercise if it is not used as a source for deriving criteria for content, teaching methods, evaluation methods, and human relationships. Thus the conceptual framework becomes a dynamic document, not carved in marble but always tentative and provisional. For instance, when a curricular decision is to be made, one looks back at the statement of conceptual framework for guidelines. If needed explicit statements are absent, items should be added; if use or growth demonstrates that parts of the conceptual system are nonfunctional or incongruent with what is being done, the document should be altered. Thus the conceptual framework becomes the "constitution" for curriculum development and is altered and changed as the conditions, information practices, and people who generated it change.

CURRICULUM DEVELOPMENT HEURISTICS

Two basic problems confront the group members at the beginning of curriculum change:

1. The problem of isolation, or people feeling they are alone in their fantasies, fears, hopes, dreams, and anxieties about impending change

2. The problem of semantics, or words meaning different things to different people

This discussion will present a brief picture of each problem and some suggested heuristics for handling the problems. Only one or two heuristics will be given as examples. Curriculum innovators and faculty rapidly generate their own devices once they begin to feel free to create. Some heuristics work in specific instances and not in others. One of the advantages of tools and devices is that they can be tried and discarded and others substituted without disrupting the process.

Problem of isolation

Curriculum change is a frightening thing for several reasons: (1) there is an anticipated rapid shifting of known landmarks and a consequential form of cultural shock in that the familiar educational structure that provides the necessary orienting cues may disappear or become obscure; (2) there is an expected loss of something in which one has invested energy, time, and thought, and a resulting separation anxiety and grief; (3) because the future structure is unknown, there is a stimulation of fantasies about what that future structure may or may not offer in the realization of hopes or nightmares; and (4) in any faculty there are traditional faculty battle lines or power groups and cliques formed around course structure, clinical specialty area, personality conflict, or philosophical views. The forces of curriculum change threaten the existence of such power cliques through destroying the issues or courses around which they have organized. This threat can create an anticipated loss of identity and power base and a consequent aloneness.

The truth is that there will be some shifting of the curriculum structure and a resulting cultural or "curriculum" shock, and there will be a sense of loss as the old course structure disappears. However, fantasies, and aloneness in those fantasies, can be avoided.

Heuristic: *Hopes, dreams, and nightmares.*
Activity. Make a form with directions as given in the example on p. 28. Faculty will record their desires about curriculum changes as they see them at this time and under the present conditions. They will also record those things that they wish to avoid. In each set of requested responses, group those that have commonalities. Have a typist transcribe the comments verbatim. The grouped "commonality" com-

ments should be transcribed first, followed by those that are "unique." Distribute the composite transcribed work back to the faculty. Discuss the many things in all categories that people seem to have in common. Some discussion of the differences in responses can also be included. However, the responses usually show more common desires and fears than unique ones. The commonalities should remain the focus of the discussion. If differences become the focus of debate, suggest that the settling of differences may be premature. Be explicit that the purpose of this exercise is to identify the similarities rather than the differences among faculty hopes, dreams, and fears. One can take the completed agreed-on statements and use the list of those things perceived as "wrong" and least desired as those things to avoid in working on the new curriculum. The list of those things perceived as "right" and desired (hopes and dreams) become the goals toward which to work in curriculum change.

Materials. Questionnaire for each faculty member.

Procedure
1. Formulate a questionnaire on the format suggested by the example.
2. Distribute copies to faculty with a due date, or ask them to sit in a group and respond.
3. Collect questionnaires.
4. Using scissors, cut the questionnaires, sorting each question into a pile.
5. Taking each question, cut responses into single concept or thought format.
6. Group all those that say essentially the same thing; group those that say substantially the direct opposite; group those that are unique.
7. Have the typist copy verbatim all the responses in the above order.
8. Distribute copies of transcribed, categorized responses to all faculty.
9. Have a group meeting at which you discuss the likenesses and differences of responses.

Puissance
1. Seeing the tangible evidence that the fantasies, hopes, and desires of others are similar to one's own lessens the feeling of aloneness.
2. Verbalization of fantasies makes them less frightening.
3. Touching base with those of like beliefs begins the reformation of power bases so necessary to reduce the sense of impending powerlessness.
4. Getting concrete ideas on paper begins to make the future less mysterious.
5. Thinking about curriculum change in terms of reality is initiated.
6. Commonalities of the faculty are focused on.
7. Providing a reference point enables the faculty to see changes in perspective.

Contingencies
1. May crystallize curriculum change plans prior

Example

To: Faculty
From: _____
Re: Curriculum wishes

The following is a form designed to help communicate where we are in our thinking about curriculum change. The responses will be compiled into a single document so we can get a composite picture of the faculty's wishes as a total group. However, individual comments will not be lost. There is no need for you to sign your name. Please return this form by Friday so it can be compiled and distributed to you by _____ (date).

What do you think is wrong in our curriculum, wish to see changed, hope will be dropped, hope we can get away from?

What do you see right about our curriculum, hope we can retain, wish to see kept, would hate to see dropped or changed?

What would you like to see in a new curriculum, fondly hope and dream about, have always wanted, wish we could do here, would do if there were no constraints?

What are the things you would least like to see happen, hope do not happen, dread happening, fear will happen, have nightmares about?

to the proper groundwork being laid (not probable but possible).
2. May harden win-lose power lines.
3. Can be misused as a head count about who wants what.

Problem of word definition

Almost every teacher has had some exposure to the language of curriculum and therefore has some "sets" about what specific words in curriculum and nursing jargon mean. The sets differ from person to person. There are some definite problems involved when language differs: (1) people using the same word may not know that they mean two different things, and (2) people using different words may not know that they are talking about the same idea.

The problem of semantics is seldom the "difficult" problem it is viewed as being. Seman-

tic differences is a catchall category for hidden agenda and other interaction problems. If semantic problems begin to absorb the group's time unduly, the group leader needs to help the group determine if there are other issues that are inherent in the discussion.

Heuristic: *Words and concepts central to curriculum development*

Activity. Make an initial list of words and concepts necessary to the problem of curriculum development. This list can be added to as development of curriculum moves from phase to phase. Ask each faculty member to define, without use of resources (even dictionaries), the words on the list. Provide space on the list for individual definitions. Circulate respected resources definitions or discussions of each word or concept to the group. Discuss which definitions or parts of definitions have meaning and relevancy for the group. Build a definition for each word or concept the group feels it can live with for a while. Label

Example

To: Faculty

Below are some words we will be using in revising our curriculum. Look over the list. If you think of additional words, add them in the space provided. Define these words without the use of any resources—try to communicate what each word or concept means to you right now. On the page indicated, put any references you have or know about that will provide us with resource material for any of the listed concepts. All answers will be compiled and distributed to the faculty. Discussions from authoritative sources will also be distributed to the faculty. After discussion we will formulate some provisional definitions of these words and concepts. These definitions will express tentatively the way we agree to use the words for purposes of our curriculum discussions. Do not put your name on your papers.*

concept	independent learning	practicum
theory	individualized learning	simulation
content	self-paced learning	environment
core	educational game	curriculum
process	criterion-referenced evaluation	course
module	normative-referenced evaluation	evaluation
learning activity	proposition	grading
learning episode	postulate	mastery
team teaching	principle	contract
nursing	conceptual construct	negotiation
health		patient
behavior		client
objective		learning
specialty area		learner
nursing arena		teacher
clinical		role blurring

Add other words you think we need to consider.
Please share your resources with the rest of the faculty.

In the space provided below, please give the bibliographical reference and page number (if you have it) for sources you think would be useful for the faculty to have in discussing the words listed above. The semantics task force will excerpt or extract the appropriate content for distribution to the faculty.

*Cross through those words you do not think we need to discuss.

the definitions: *Provisional definitions.* Agree to change or alter definitions as the group changes its concepts or use of the words.

Materials
1. A beginning list of words or concepts
2. A well-documented discussion (on paper) of various authorities' use or definition of a word or concept

Procedure
1. Compile a list of words and concepts (leave writing space between them).
2. Distribute with clear directions (see example).
3. To diminish the constraints on participants, ask for no names.
4. Collect completed forms.
5. Compile the responses for each word.
6. Research resources and provide short concise

documented explanations of concepts and/or words from these resources. Conduct a discussion of each word or phrase.
7. Formulate (together) an acceptable definition for each word.
8. Place a 10- to 15-minute discussion time limit on each word. Those which cannot be finished in that length of time may need to be delayed or tabled until another meeting, or assigned to a task group for basic defining (to be brought back to the main group for alteration and acceptance). Tabling, delaying, or assigning to task groups can be effective for unlocking and removing the win-lose aspect of discussions, and/or providing time lapses so necessary for self-appropriation of meanings by members of the group.

Puissance
1. Semantics is a neutral ground for faculties to begin discussions of curriculum and constitutes a "warm-up" period.
2. Discussion of concepts central to curriculum development constitutes a safe and easy way to review and internalize materials that often have not been thought about since graduate school curriculum courses.
3. Words and concepts provide faculty with an easy way to "touch base" with each other, identify differences and commonalities in viewpoint and philosophy, and enable the beginning of important patterns of group discussion behaviors: legitimizing differences, negotiating, compromising, making tentative agreements, building "trial" or "working" definitions and agreements to unlock, delay, holding over or shelving discussions that become win-lose.

Contingencies
1. Members of the group may use semantics to block, delay, filibuster, or lock the group into this safe activity at the expense of moving on to other areas.
2. Some will want to get dictionary definitions of words and move on to "doing something" more important.
3. The group can "bog down" and wheelspin.

NOTES

1. Gove, Philip B., editor: Webster's third new international dictionary of the English language unabridged, Springfield, Mass., 1971, G. & C. Merriam Co., Publishers.
2. Maslow defines self-actualization as acceptance and expression of the essential self, the ability to fully develop personal potential, and the ability to act on readily available and fully developed human and personal essence. He states that the self-actualization concept implies minimal ill health or behavior that would in any way restrict or diminish the basic human and personal capacities and capabilities. Maslow, Abraham H.: Toward a psychology of being, ed. 2, New York, 1968, Van Nostrand-Reinhold Co., pp. 97-98, 103-109, 145.
3. Erikson, Erik H.: Childhood and society, ed. 2, New York, 1963, W. W. Norton & Co., Inc., Publishers.
4. Whitehead, Alfred N.: Process and reality, New York, 1969, The Free Press, pp. 31-32.
5. Smuts, Jan C.: Holism and evolution, New York, 1926, The Macmillan Co.
6. Ibid., pp. 82-83, 86-87, 118-119, 314, 337-345.
7. Banathy, Bela H.: Instructional systems, Palo Alto, Calif., 1968, Fearon Publishers, pp. 2-3.
8. This section on general systems theory is taken from the following sources:
   a. Bertalanffy, Ludwig von.: General systems theory, New York, 1968, George Braziller, Inc.
   b. Gray, William, Duhl, Frederick, and Rizzo, Nicholas, editors: General systems theory and psychiatry, Boston, 1969, Little, Brown & Co., Inc.
   c. Hall, A. D., and Fagan, R. C.: General systems. In Bertalanffy, Ludwig von and Raporport, Aratol: Yearbook of the Society for the Advancement of General Systems Theory, Ann Arbor, Mich., 1950, Braun Brumfield.
   d. Hazzard, Mary E.: An overview of systems theory, Nursing Clinics of North America **6:** 385-394, 1971.
   e. Killeen, Maureen: General systems theory and nursing. In Bower, Fay L., and Bevis, Em O., editors: Fundamentals of nursing practice, St. Louis, 1978, The C. V. Mosby Co.
   f. McKay, Rose: Theories models and systems for nursing, Conference on the Nature of Science in Nursing, Nursing Research **18:**393-394, Sept.-Oct., 1969.
   g. Marmor, Judd: The relationship between systems theory and community psychiatry, Hospital and Community Psychiatry **26:**807-811, 1975.
   h. Messick, Janice, Singh, Amar J., and May, P. R.: A systems analysis approach to planned change in a clinical psychiatric program, Journal of Psychiatric Nursing and Mental Health Services **13:**7-11, July-Aug., 1975.
   i. Sedgwick, Rae: The family as a system: a network of relationships. Journal of Psychiatric Nursing and Mental Health Services, **12:**17-20, March-April, 1974.
9. Nurtrative is a coined word, meaning of or (related to nurturing,) caring for, sustaining, supporting, and promoting growth.
10. Rogers, Martha: An introduction to the theoretical basis of nursing, Philadelphia, 1970, F. A. Davis Co., p. 83.
11. Ibid., p. 84.
12. Leavell, H., and Clark, E. G.: Preventive medicine for the doctor in his community, ed. 3, New York, 1965, McGraw-Hill Book Co.
13. McKay, p. 393.
14. Leininger, Madeline: Introduction: nature of science in nursing, Conference on the Nature of Science in Nursing, Nursing Research **18:**388-389, Sept.-Oct., 1969.
15. The materials on theory used for this section were derived from the following sources:
    a. Abdellah, Fay G.: The nature of nursing science, Conference on the Nature of Science in Nursing, Nursing Research **18:**390-393, Sept.-Oct., 1969.
    b. Gagné, Robert M.: The conditions of learning, New York, 1965, Holt, Rinehart & Winston, Inc., pp. 31-61.
    c. Jacox, Ada: Theory construction in nursing:

an overview, Nursing Research **23:**4-13, Jan.-Feb., 1974.
  d. Johnson, Dorothy E.: Development of theory: a requisite for nursing as a primary health profession, Nursing Research **23:**372-377, Sept.-Oct., 1974.
  e. Kimball, William H., Roland B., and Wing, Richard L.: Education for effective thinking, New York, 1960, Appleton-Century-Crofts, pp. 100-104.
  f. McKay, pp. 393-399.
  g. Vaillot, Sister Madeleine C.: Nursing theory, levels of nursing, and curriculum development, Nursing Forum, **9:**235-249, 1970.
16. Douglass, Laura M., and Bevis, Em O.: Nursing leadership in action: principles and application to staff situations, ed. 2, St. Louis, 1974, The C. V. Mosby Co., p. 11.
17. Dickoff, James, James, Patricia, and Wiedenbach, Ernestine: Theory in a practice discipline, Nursing Research **17:**415-435, 1968.
18. Douglass and Bevis, pp. 9-11.
19. Dickoff, James, and Wiedenbach, pp. 419-423.
20. Alberty, Elsie: Toward a framework for curriculum development, Theory and Practice **6:**204-208, 1967.
21. Goodlad, J. L.: Toward a conceptual system for curriculum problems, School Review **66:**392-396, 1958.
22. Herrick, V. E., and Tyler, R. W.: Toward improved curriculum theory, Supplementary Educational Monograph no. 71, Chicago, 1950, University of Chicago Press, p. 1.
23. Leeper, Robert, editor: Curriculum change: direction and process, Washington, D.C., 1966, Association for Supervision and Curriculum Development, National Education Association, p. 18.
24. Taba, Hilda: Curriculum development: theory and practice, New York, 1962, Harcourt, Brace & World, Inc., pp. 420-421.
25. Chater, Shirley S.: A conceptual framework for curriculum development, Nursing Outlook **23:**428-433, July, 1975.

BIBLIOGRAPHY

Alberty, Elsie: Toward a framework for curriculum development, Theory and Practice **6:**204-208, 1967.
Arpin, Kathleen E., and Parker, Nora I.: Developing a conceptual framework, Nursing Papers **7:**28-34, Winter, 1976.
Banathy, Bela H.: Instructional systems, Palo Alto, Calif., 1968, Fearon Publishers.
Burton, William H., Kimball, Roland B., and Wing, Richard L.: Education for effective thinking, New York, 1960, Appleton-Century-Crofts.
Chater, Shirley S.: A conceptual framework for curriculum development, Nursing Outlook **23:**428-433, July, 1975.
Department of Baccalaureate and Higher Degree Programs: Curriculum in graduate education in nursing. Part I. Factors influencing curriculum in graduate education in nursing, New York, 1975, National League for Nursing.
Dickoff, James, James, Patricia, and Wiedenbach, Ernestine: Theory in a practice discipline, Nursing Research **17:**415-435, 1968.
Douglass, Laura M., and Bevis, Em O.: Team leadership in action: principles and applications to staff nursing situations, ed. 2, St. Louis, 1974, The C. V. Mosby Co.
Erikson, Erik H.: Childhood and society, ed. 2, New York, 1963, W. W. Norton & Co., Inc., Publishers.
Fawdry, M. Kaye: Curricular theories for nursing as process, Nursing Papers **7:**35-38, Winter, 1976.
Gagné, Robert M.: The conditions of learning, New York, 1965, Holt, Rinehart & Winston, Inc.
Goodlad, J. L.: Toward a conceptual system for curriculum problems, School Review **66:**392-396, 1958.
Herrick, V. E., and Tyler, R. W.: Toward improved curriculum theory, Supplementary Educational Monograph no. 71, Chicago, 1950, University of Chicago Press.
Jacox, Ada: Theory construction in nursing: an overview, Nurs. Res. **23:**4-12, Jan.-Feb., 1974.
Kramer, Marlene: Identification of needs affecting curriculum in graduate education in nursing. In Department of Baccalaureate and Higher Degree Programs: Curriculum in graduate education in nursing. Part I. Factors influencing curriculum in graduate education in nursing, New York, 1975, National League for Nursing, pp. 10-20.
Leavell, H., and Clark, E. G.: Preventive medicine for the doctor in his community, ed. 3, New York, 1965, McGraw-Hill Book Co.
Leeper, Robert, editor: Curriculum change: direction and process, Washington, D.C., 1966, Association for Supervision and Curriculum Development, National Education Association.
Maslow, Abraham H.: Toward a psychology of being, ed. 2, New York, 1968, Van Nostrand-Reinhold Co.
Rogers, Martha: An introduction to the theoretical basis of nursing, Philadelphia, 1970, F. A. Davis Co.
Smuts, Jan C.: Holism and evolution, New York, 1926, The Macmillan Co.
Taba, Hilda: Curriculum development: theory and practice, New York, 1962, Harcourt, Brace & World, Inc.
Torres, Gertrude, and Yura, Helen: Today's conceptual framework: its relationship to the curriculum development process, National League for Nursing Department of Baccalaureate and Higher Degree Programs, Publication no. 15-1529, New York, 1974, National League for Nursing.
Tyler, R. W.: Basic principles of curriculum and instruction, Chicago, 1950, University of Chicago Press.
Whitehead, Alfred N.: Process and reality, New York, 1969, The Free Press.

2

CONCEPTUAL FRAMEWORK: PHILOSOPHICAL BASE

PHILOSOPHY OF NURSING

Traditional curriculum theory would have the process of curriculum development proceeding from philosophy, through objectives, content, and evaluation. This progression suggests that philosophy is the keystone, or foundation, of the curriculum and that all other components flow from this fountainhead. In reality the conceptual framework provides the foundation and the materials from which the total curriculum structure is devised, and the philosophy provides the picture window through which the world is viewed. *Philosophy, in other words, provides a point of view; it is a belief construct, a speculation about the nature and value of things.* Values are based in philosophy, since philosophy inquires into the ideal possibilities and the significance of things. Whereas philosophy explores values, science seeks to describe facts. Science breaks things into their component parts to study, describe, and explain how things operate. Science answers *how, when,* and *where.*

Philosophy looks at wholes and their relationship to other wholes. It answers the question *why* and queries the *worth* of an experience. Durant says that "Science tells us how to heal and how to kill; it reduces the death rate in retail and then kills us wholesale in war; but only wisdom—desire coordinated in the light of all experience—can tell us when to heal and when to kill."[1]

When philosophical concepts move into the realm of theory, philosophical thought is translated into hypotheses that can be tested. Thus the conceptual construct is no longer philosophy; it is theory.

Much curriculum building is still devised around philosophy. But rapid generation of knowledge and increasing sophistication of human ability to test hypotheses leave fewer curriculum keystones in the realm of "belief" and more in the realm of "theory." For example, most nursing school philosophies, objectives, and courses contain reference to and activities centered around problem solving. The *belief* that problem solving is somehow valuable to nurses has been replaced with theories about effective problem-solving strategies, effective ways of teaching problem solving, and the impact of problem-solving ability on nursing practice. Ways of testing these theories are being devised, and therefore problem solving as a component is moving from a *value-belief* to a conceptual, or theoretical, component of the curriculum.

Philosophy alone is a weak keystone for curriculum development, but in conjunction with other components of the curriculum framework it strengthens the curriculum conceptual construct. Values, beliefs, and points of view do exist, and the articulation of these facilitates direct coping with them and reduces the possibility of irrelevant and unrelated battles over them.

Philosophical base of nursing practice

Clear statements of conceptual constructs drawn from the three categories of setting, clients, and knowledge provide the conceptual and theoretical basis for nursing practice. But only philosophy, a clear conception of values, can provide the rationale or wisdom for making the choices about what is important in those concepts, which concepts shall have priority, and how they will be used. All choices are made from one's value system.

Historically, nursing's value system contains many elements. Four basic ones will be discussed: asceticism, romanticism, pragmatism, and humanistic existentialism. Each of these four rose into prominence at differing periods in nursing's development and gave rise to different choices. None of them ever entirely disappeared from nursing's decision-making system, and traces of them are found in modern nursing. These values are, in subtle ways, enculturated into novices so that their continuation is assured in generation after generation of practicing nurses. Each one of the four philosophical perspectives will be explored and its impact on nursing discussed.

Selecting a descriptive word to label a trend in nursing philosophy is difficult. Perhaps asceticism and romanticism as philosophies do not exist. However, they are labels for periods of art, architecture, and religion. They adequately describe the attitudes, values, and behaviors of a period of nursing history; therefore asceticism and romanticism are the titles given to periods of nursing just as if they were legitimate philosophical structures like pragmatism and existentialism.

These four philosophical periods of nursing history, although reflecting society's values and attitudes, did not parallel the periods when the philosophies were popular in society. Asceticism existed from nursing's inception. It was very strong in pre-Nightingalian times and continued as a strong system of motivation for nursing through 1910 or into 1920. It did not disappear then but was joined by romanticism. In the 1920s, 1930s, and early 1940s romanticism was dominant. Post–World War II saw the ascendancy of pragmatism, and it held the focus until the early 1960s when humanistic existentialism began to be felt as an important force in nursing. As each of the four schools of thought entered nursing's consciousness, the former value system did not die but only became less important than the current one. Former value systems still operated, still influenced judgments and decisions, and still provided some material for nursing practice and

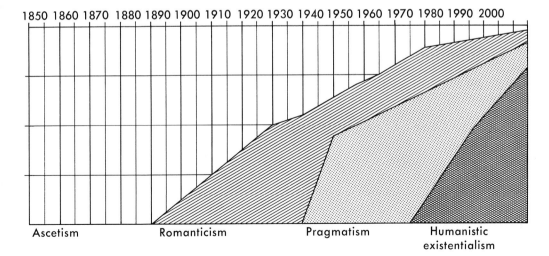

1850 1860 1870 1880 1890 1900 1910 1920 1930 1940 1950 1960 1970 1980 1990 2000

Ascetism   Romanticism   Pragmatism   Humanistic
                                          existentialism

Fig. 2-1. Chronology of four philosophical systems which affect nursing.

educational behaviors. Fig. 2-1 demonstrates the dates of rise of influence of each of the four philosophical systems.

Asceticism. Asceticism is a way of life that centers on self-denial. It is closely identified with Christianity, beginning with the martyrs and early Christians who were willing to sacrifice their lives, safety, and comfort for the ideal of religion. It became an avenue for salvation and/or achievement of higher spiritual states throughout Christianity's history. Many other religions use self-denial and deprivation to achieve higher spirituality, and many of the early Christian saints were ascetics. This way of life proposes that rigorous self-discipline and self-denial are valued ways to achieve internal harmony on earth and rewards in the hereafter. Ascetics try, through self-denial, to rise above physical needs, passion, caring, interdependence on others, and love of humans. Love of God and pursuit of the ideal, dedication to a task that is felt to be a God-given mission, and martyrdom to that task, role, or ideal are all attributes of the ascetic.

Early nurses gave up home, family, and fortune and often devoted themselves to nursing through holy orders. From Nightingale on there was less insistence on complete self-denial, but there was still a strong emphasis on devotion to duty to the exclusion of self. Nursing was viewed as a "calling." Nurses worked seven days a week with only one afternoon off and were enculturated to believe that duty to one's patients and to one's calling required self-denial and dedication without thought for one's own comfort, self-development, security, or personal needs. This philosophical structure was exploited by employers (clients, physicians, health agencies). Nurses would not assert themselves for adequate salaries, fringe benefits, and improved working conditions because all of those goals were outside the value system of the ascetic philosophy that was dominant in nursing.

Asceticism was the basis for a nursing framework that was concerned about neither the approach to care nor the emphasis on a perception of the client's health. The client was seen as a spiritual being, and his salvation was most important. In reality the true emphasis of the nurse was on self—on the enrichment of her own spiritual growth and attainment. Duty was important, more important than client advocacy, treating the client as a whole, or the development of nursing science. Since nurses concentrated primarily on service, self-denial, and spiritual growth, little importance was given to the development of a curriculum. There were few formal classes, training was done on the units while care was given to patients, and explanations about care were offered as an unplanned bonus from physicians. Nightingale instituted planned courses of study, which departed from the hit-and-miss (mostly miss) curriculum that emphasized the duty and hard labor aspect of nursing. But except for the Nightingale tradition and other scattered centers of nursing learning, and because of the ascetic philosophy, ordered systems of thought and decision making about nursing care remained undeveloped. As late as the mid-1950s, the American Nurses' Association House of Delegates walked out on Shirley Titus of the California delegation while she pleaded for the organization to support nurses seeking decent wages and benefits. This was one of the last great rumbles of asceticism.

Romanticism. Romanticism was a natural, logical transition for nursing philosophy. Nurses must have tired of the drudgery of self-denial, of asceticism and the narrow confines of its religious and spiritual goals. Romanticism provided an easy escape. It rose in the eighteenth century and continued to be in vogue in art, literature, music, writing, poetry, and architecture through the nineteenth century.

Romanticism supports behavior without factual basis in logical precision. Romantics take very few facts and elaborate them beyond reality into fancy. The word "fanciful" describes the whole Gothic phenomenon of romanticism. Romanticism means to operate from a visionary or quixotic viewpoint. It is full of feelings, attitudes of romance, adventure, and escape from reality and practicality. The romantic notion of Florence Nightingale as The Lady With The Lamp is a reflection of this attitude. Cherry Ames and Sue Barton were the characterization of nursing's romantic period in literature.

If it was offensive to nurses to continue to practice self-denial for their spiritual growth, they now could continue to conform to social expectations for nurses by doing it for the romance of loyalty to a physician, to an alma mater (school of nursing), and to patients. Personal glory, pride in devotion, and "knowing I have done my best for my client, been a credit to my school, and the doctor is proud of me" were the romantic notions that motivated action and influenced decisions. This value system influenced the adoption of a conceptual framework of curriculum and practice that conformed to medical models and hospital patient housing patterns. The motivation for this was not based on any pragmatic outcome or rational basis; it simply conformed to the romantic ideal of what the authority people (physicians and hospital administrators) perceived as best for nursing.

Romanticism supported and sustained a dependence on physicians and a lack of autonomy, assertiveness, or independence. It supported the most subservient and idealized traits of women. It remains a primary reason why nursing is so intricately tied to women's problems, since with the idealistic romanticized view of women came the idealistic romanticized view of nursing. These factors still influence nursing's value system and thereby nurses' decisions and choices in their behavior as a professional group and as individuals. The romanticist nurse is the physician's helper. With him she will save the world. Behind every good man is a good woman. Behind every great physician is a great nurse. Nursing, to the romanticist, is a

dependent occupation that finds glory and adventure in service to others. World War I was the epic adventure for nursing's romantic era.

More recently, curriculum manifestations of romanticism have taken the form of nurses aspiring to be junior doctors. Nurses assume more and more of the functions of physicians without rational examination of the appropriateness of those functions for nursing. One need only examine how many nursing programs now have courses or units called "physical assessment," "physical diagnosis," or the "physical exam." Even the name ties nursing to the medical model and confirms that the romantic era continues still in this, the latter half of the twentieth century. Programs, not philosophically grounded in romanticism, label similar courses and content, such as nursing assessment, nursing history and physical, etc.

World War II came, and reality impacted nurses. War was no longer a romantic adventure, and postwar nurse shortages thrust nursing into the age of pragmatism.

Pragmatism. Pragmatism comes from the Greek word *pragmata,* which means acts, affairs, or business. It is a method of logic for determining the meanings of intellectual concepts. Its two leading proponents were Charles Sanders (1839-1914) and William James (1842-1910). It requires its adherents to look at specific practical consequences of acts, ideas, or concepts. The question is always asked in any debate or decision, "What practical behavioral difference does it make?" If an idea makes no practical difference, it is not significant. Pragmatism is a method for looking directly at a question to determine its use, its function, and whether or not it serves a purpose, thus its practicality. Pragmatism holds that no idea has meaning unless there is some direct or indirect application of it to something real. Value, then, is based in practical use and consequences.

This philosophy was a natural for a practice discipline such as nursing, which was faced with the emergency of World War II. The severe shortage of nurses during and after the war forced them to become very pragmatic in dealing with the problems of nursing care. It was war-created nursing shortages that stimulated the rise of ancillary nursing groups. Since there were not enough registered nurses, non-nurse personnel were given short courses or informal, on-the-job training and placed under the supervision of a nurse. Operating room technicians, nursing assistants, nursing aides, vocational or practical nurses, emergency technicians, cast or orthopedic technicians, psychiatric technicians, respiratory therapists, and many other specialized technical groups made their appearance because they solved the immediate problem facing nursing—how to get enough people to do the work. Nursing became largely a group of teachers and supervisors, and much of the actual caring for patients was done by ancillary personnel under the supervision of nurses. Nursing still suffers from removal from direct client care in many agencies.

Another pragmatic decision was for nursing personnel to remain a group of health care workers that responded to physician needs rather than client needs. It was easy and more expedient, it worked, and it did not seem to make a great deal of practical difference to nurses. Hospitals were organized around physicians-specialty areas. There were no intensive care areas, few ambulatory care units, and few convalescent units. A client was admitted to the unit of his physician's specialization. Nurses who cared for him on that unit specialized in medical specialty areas. Clients were often referred to by their diagnosis or the part of the body affected, that is, "the paraplegic in room 842 and the arm in room 843." The focus was on the problem, the disability, the disease, and the diagnosis, not on the person, his family, his needs, his wholeness, or his humanity.

Hospitals began to add patient care areas based on the client's stages of illness in the mid-1950s. Intensive care units arose to provide special *nursing* care for those who were acutely ill and in need of constant expert care. Convalescent and rehabilitation units, which focused on the return of the client to optimal health, came into being. Ambulatory care units for the treatment of clients who did not need hospitalization assumed significant size and use. Hospitals were finally responding to the nursing needs of clients. As health care moved to be more responsive to the nursing needs of people, nursing moved to reexamine its basic position. The pragmatism of nursing motivated nursing personnel to investigate the consequences of the decision to follow medicine into dualism, to divide clients into medical specialty parts, and to be attentive only to his illness. In other words, pragmatic values moved nursing toward humanism, and holism. The rise of humanism in nursing caused nurses to begin viewing clients in new ways that would eventually make a significant difference in the quality, distribution, and effectiveness of nursing care. The essential difference was that the client, not the physician or the agency, became the most important "other" to nursing.

Transition to humanism. At the same time nonhospital settings for nursing care of clients began to increase in prominence and the community in all its complexity rose as a primary place where clients received nursing care. Families and neighborhoods became important to nursing, and nursing moved into service to groups in a new way. This progressive alteration of practice shifted because of a basic shift in nursing's value system.

Nurses became increasingly concerned with wholes—the whole person, the whole family, the whole community. Humans became the most important factor to nurses, not spiritual salvation, not service to God, country, and physician, and not disease and diagnosis but what happens to people in all their possible groupings and environments. Nursing curricula altered through creating a model for clients that was holistic rather than divided physical, psychological, and social systems.

Medical specialities were doubted as *the* appropriate organizing strategy for nursing curriculum.

Abdellah's twenty-one nursing problems and Maslow's hierarchy of needs, rather than medical or hospital specialties, were early nursing models for assessing clients' needs. These innovations gave rise to content integration as a curriculum format for teaching nursing.

The early movement in nursing to develop a nursing model commenced with Abdellah's introduction of twenty-one nursing problems as a way to view *nursing care*. This first attempt to focus nursing on nursing rather than on medicine revolutionized curriculum in the late 1950s and dominated curriculum revision during the 1960s. The associate of arts programs were beginning to grow and spread, and this nursing framework provided the perfect vehicle for them to reorganize nursing content into a new and different time allotment. The late Ruth Matheney, working with many others, elaborated Abdellah's work and was instrumental in its wide use among college-based programs.

The movement seeking a holistic model for nursing resulted in the development of two types of curriculum organization: the early integrated model and the late integrated model, which reflect nursing's gradual shift from dualism to holism and from pragmatism to humanistic existentialism. These two models rose from the pragmatic period and reflect pragmatisms virtues. They herald the humanistic existentialism that had begun to be felt as a small but significant force in nursing. The early integrated model was essentially the medical model with "threads" of things that needed to be taught in every course woven throughout the medical specialty areas (Fig. 2-2). The late integrated model hyphenated the specialties as though through the hyphen the fractured whole of dualism could be put together again. "Concepts" came into popularity, and concepts and "threads" were woven throughout "patient-centered" problems. The patient problems tended to follow physiological and psychological systems, tying the old dualism to nursing's new need to provide care to the whole person. The term "comprehensive" nursing care became popular, and it meant to give care that considered all of the patient's aspects—physical, mental, spiritual, and social. Biopsycho-social care (the ultimate in hyphenated words) is the new way to say comprehensive. It was not holistic; it was summative dualism (adding all the parts trying to make them equal the

	Medical nursing	Surgical nursing	Obstetrical nursing	Pediatric nursing	Gynecological nursing	Eye, ear, nose, and throat	Neurological nursing	Orthopedic nursing
Pharmacology								
Nutrition								
Diet therapy								
First aid								
Public health								
Epidemiology								

Fig. 2-2. Early integrated model.

	Growth and development	Perception	Grief and loss	Oxygenation and metabolism	Fluid and electrolyte balance	Ingestion, digestion, and elimination	Pain	Motion-locomotion	Orientation and cognition
Psych-mental health									
Medical-surgical nursing									
Maternal-child health									
Community health									

Fig. 2-3. Late integrated model.

whole). Fig. 2-3 represents the late integrated model.

When nurses began to be accountable to clients (the central focus of their care) rather than to physicians, they could no longer pass the buck for the responsibility for their own decisions and actions to paternalistic physicians—physicians all too willing to trade being responsible for nursing care for the complete loyalty and subservience of the nurse. When clients are central to nursing, the responsibility trade-off with physicians stops. The stage was set, through pragmatic logic, for the rise of humanistic existentialism.

Humanistic existentialism. Existentialism is a modern philosophical term. It arose after World War I in Germany and became popular in the United States after World War II. Most existentialists trace their origins to Soren Kierkegaard, a Danish philosopher who lived and wrote from 1813 to 1855. His work, largely neglected in his lifetime, was influential after being translated into German between 1904 and 1914, and it remains the touchstone for existentialism.

Existentialism holds that each person is unique and inexplicable by scientific or metaphysical systems. It is a natural part of holistic philosophy and proposes that the whole of a human being is different from his parts. Science studies human parts but cannot explain or understand the human being. Furthermore, existentialism proposes that humans are thinking beings who make choices. A basic tenet is that a human is free—freedom to choose being the most basic of all freedoms. From this freedom springs two other attributes. Freedom of choice makes a human being a suffering individual—and unpredictable. The whole area of a human being as an individual who has freedom to choose and who is a thinking being implies accountability. If one makes one's own choices, then each person is accountable to self and fellow humans for the consequences.

Humanism is a system of thought that arose during the Middle Ages and helped give impetus to the Renaissance. Springing from the study of classical Greek and Latin culture, it emphasized the importance of humans and the centrality of human beings above that of science or religion. Humanism emphasized the value, beauty, and importance of being human and a concerned action geared to human ideals, human existence, and quality of life. It is characterized by a value system that places great importance and high priority on caring about people.

Humanistic existentialism seems to be the natural maturational philosophy for nursing. It implies orientation to people as the central and basic priority of all nursing activity. It proposes that a human being is an organismic whole, complete and unified, that cannot be treated as component parts. The parts do not explain the whole and the mystery of the whole, how it works, and its ultimate unpredictability. It does not absolve nursing from trying to predict responses and from basing nursing care on scientific principles that provide a way of predicting consequences. What it does is to make acceptable individual deviations from the expected or "scientific" norms. It makes it acceptable for each individual client to make personal choices about nursing care, alternative healing methods, ways to achieve goals, and the use of medical and nursing health advice. It puts nursing squarely in the middle of accountability, placing essential value on making one's own choices as best one can in the interest of the client and standing accountable for those choices. Once the precept of accountability is accepted, the step to autonomy is a short one. If one is to be accountable for one's actions and not an automaton responding to physicians' orders, then one must have the freedom to make choices and decisions about one's area of expertise, freedom which does not require that persons outside the profession be blindly followed. Colleague consultation is sought, but ultimate decisions are made about nursing care by nurses, and nurses stand accountable for these decisions. The current philosophy that is swaying nursing thought and action is humanistic existentialism, a long slow walk from asceticism.

PHILOSOPHY AS A SOURCE OF PROFESSIONAL POWER

There exists in the world today all the evidence or clues one needs to know about everything, and yet so little actually is known and half of what is known is wrong; the sad part of it is that no one knows which half. But for philosophy, human beings would indeed be in difficult straits. Philosophy is the art of reason; reason is an attempt to put what is perceived about life's phenomena together, both the right and the wrong halves, and make sense of it. When an individual makes sense of "it all" in a manner that is satisfactory to himself, he has a feeling of knowing who he is, what he is about, and where he is going. This sense of assurance is one of the major sources of human power. Individual or group power is remarkable in that it cannot be taken away by another person or group. Power is never taken; it is surrendered. Nurses often surrender to others their power, their self-identity, and the direction of their own affairs. Powerlessness, or a sense of powerlessness, has many roots: ignorance, lack of confidence, lack of technology, lack of resources, lack of unity or organization. Nursing shows increasing signs of an awakening sense of power. As nursing finds unity in the articulation of a common philosophy, self-appropriated, self-experienced, and dynamically applied to practice, there will be active collaboration with other groups in the solution of common problems and much greater control over its own future and affairs. A unification of some common philosophical elements for all of nursing may be a source of power that will help nursing make sense of the world and nursing's place in that world. It will be a foundation for a sense of identity, security, and confidence and ultimately will enable a clear or a better identification of *purpose,* evolution of a *system* to achieve that purpose, and *creation* of new approaches to nursing problems. Each school of nursing must produce from its own setting, faculty, and students its philosophical commitments.

The philosophy is a component of the conceptual framework. It should be detailed enough so that it can act as a checklist for curriculum implementation. It should be written so that any knowledgeable person reading it can understand it. Attempts to shorten it will make it nebulous and less meaningful to the reader who has not participated in its creation. Traditionally, faculties desire a philosophy that they can put in a few paragraphs, insert in a bulletin, and expose for public view. There is a need to display to the public reader some clues about the philosophical commitments of each nursing program so that the individual nature of each program can be clearly expressed. However, a philosophical abstract can be distilled from the conceptual framework when needed. For usefulness in curriculum building there needs to be a clear and detailed statement of philosophy so that it is useful as a chart for curriculum decisions. The purposes achieved by extracting a philosophical statement for public use are: (1) emphasis of certain aspects; (2) summarization in a concise statement; and (3) facilitation of distribution to the public through catalog or bulletin.

Some issues addressed by a philosophy

Each school of nursing has a different list of essential philosophical issues, depending on the priority of values for that school of nursing. There are several central issues that almost all schools of nursing address in their statement of philosophy: (1) What is the nature of the client? (2) What is the nature of nursing? (3) What is health? (4) What are the basic commitments of this nursing educational enterprise?

This book addresses each of these issues in succeeding chapters. This chapter merely introduces the issues and suggests that faculties wrestle with the ideas so that a statement of the values of the school and the faculty appears which is (1) congruent with the philosophy of the sponsoring agency, (2) apparent in the rest of the conceptual framework, (3) representative of the consensus of the faculty, and (4) conclusive enough to provide the value system for the structure of the concepts and theories and the system of teaching and learning of the curriculum.

Faculties often have difficulty arriving at consensus in a statement of philosophy. The following discussion is designed to provide stimulation to the faculty group about some points that faculties usually find easy to agree on and some points that they often have difficulty agreeing on. Other philosophical points, especially those about nursing, health, the client, and the educational enterprise are elaborated elsewhere.

Philosophical points of agreement. As nursing defines its divisions and sorts and delegates its roles and functions to the various divisions, it will be easier to see the unity of belief because the competition and sensitivity over the finer points of application will decrease. Even though the following philosophical propositions are suggested as generally agreed on, there is little agreement among nurses in their implications or in their implementation.

However, even a cursory review of nursing literature over the past ten years suggests that there is actually much more common agreement than one would have initially expected. The following points of general agreement are suggested:

1. *The individual has intrinsic value, and there is worth inherent in human life.* This general belief seems to be self-evident in the very nature of a group whose social role is one of nurturing individuals and concerning themselves with the welfare of people, their health, comfort, optimal productivity, adequate life adjustment, and longest possible life.

Nursing works with people, intrapersonally, interpersonally, and in communities. Regardless of how mechanical nursing services become for some nurses, nursing service is a "people" service, and as such it is concerned with human welfare.

To be concerned with human welfare is to act out a belief in the worth of the individual and the worth of life. The "worth of human life" commitment implies client equality. Therefore sex, color, and religion concern nursing functions only as ethnic considerations for tailoring nursing more nearly to fit the needs of the individual. This commitment further implies that health is a human right and that finances, living arrangements, transportation, and other impediments to adequate health care cannot be allowed to hinder the uniform availability of optimum nursing care. Therefore nurses not only work to ensure this but they render nursing services in any environment where there are people.

2. *Nursing is a rational activity.* Throughout the literature the appearance of problem solving and decision making as central and systematic nursing activities implies that nursing process is cognitive and nursing functions are natural outcomes of cognitive processes. Nursing functions require the exercise of critical thinking processes, logic, judgment, or any of the pseudonyms given for the problem-solving, decision-making process. All kinds of nursing activities in all settings require both strategic and tactical decisions. The time is past when the nurse, as a dependent practitioner, could, with impunity, pass the responsibility "buck" to a physician. The nurse is a legally and morally accountable individual. The definition of nursing functions as distinct from physician functions has left some shades of gray between the two professions because both are clearly working to achieve health, although in different ways. The educational implications of the rationality of nursing actions are that the third and fourth levels of theory building form the basis of nursing content, and nursing skills become a means of carrying out decisions.

3. *Nursing's uniqueness is in the way the basic social and biological sciences are synthesized in functions that promote health.* Nursing programs commonly require some exposure to sociology, psychol-ogy, bacteriology, anatomy, physiology, and chemistry, regardless of the breadth or depth of the exposure. The simple fact that, generally, nursing programs in hospital schools, associate of arts colleges, and baccalaureate programs require varying degrees of content in these areas attests to the philosophical belief that nursing functions relate the physical and social sciences in some unique way to produce a science of nursing. Whitehead's many-to-one principle (Chapter 1) of process is extremely applicable here. Nursing has often been called an applied discipline, and so it is. But "applied" often refers to one science, that is, applied psychology, applied physics, and so forth, as opposed to pure science. With nursing, as with most service-oriented disciplines, the application is not of one science but of components of almost all sciences—social, physical, and biological. Almost every nursing practice act is the *unique* amalgamation of many science fields. The simple nurtrative behavior of placing a client who is in congestive heart failure in a more comfortable position for breathing applies physics, anatomy, physiology, and chemistry.

4. *The individual nurse-citizen has some control over and responsibility for the political and social milieu in which she lives.* The participation of the nurse-citizen in community affairs attests to the almost universal commitment of nurses to this idea. Nurses seem to believe that they can influence the direction of social change through the established channels of government. The participation of nurses on city, county, state, and federal committees, commissions, and legislative action groups speaks to this philosophical commitment. Nurses have had successes in all levels of government, which reinforces their belief in the ultimate worth and workability of the democratic process. As nurses have become more sophisticated in working for social and political changes, they have learned how to use the change process more effectively. Civic activities with clubs, established organizations, and sponta-

neous concerned groups of citizens are forums for nurses seeking an organized basis for changes that will influence health care.

The whole idea of nurse advocacy is built on the belief that nursing responsibility entails speaking for people who cannot speak for themselves, who desire or request nurses to speak for them, or who depend on nurses as experts in health affairs to speak in behalf of needs.

5. *Nursing is a process with a central subjective purpose, an inherent organization or system, and dynamic creativity.* Although the wording varies throughout nursing literature, there seems to be a consensus about the existence of nursing process. There is divergence about the nature of that process. The operationalized analysis of the process of nursing offered in Chapter 1 is *one* attempt to discover the nature of nursing process and to write a description of it that is useful. All the components of nursing process listed on pp. 17 through 19 are generally agreed on in a wide variety of sources, although few of them identify the components as part of nursing process. The divergence comes in the order, use, and importance of the components.

Philosophical points of divergence. Points of difference receive more attention than points of commonality, since no one seems to feel the need to discuss at length something about which there is general agreement. But with disagreement comes the need to proselyte, to sell a point of view to others, and to defend the correctness of "rightness" of a point of view. The issues of divergence are not really more in number than the points of agreement; they only receive more time and attention, thus giving the impression of being more numerous. Some of the points about which there seems to be disagreement among nurses are listed here. Whether or not nursing as a whole need resolve these issues is a moot point; however, faculty groups devising a unified curriculum need openly to discuss and negotiate some work-

ing agreement so that the curriculum has some consistency and curriculum conflicts due to individual philosophical differences are minimized.

1. *Nursing functions are independent and interdependent or collaborative.* The degree of independence or dependence of nursing functions is widely debated in nursing circles. For some nurses, complete independence is necessary to professionalism, and to others the nurse is the physician's assistant or helper. The 1965 American Nurses' Association's position paper, *Educational Preparation for Nurse Practitioners and Assistants to Nurses*, states and reaffirms the position that the direction of nursing by nurses was a central and enduring belief of Florence Nightingale.[2] The position paper further develops this theme by stating that "Professional nursing practice coordinates and synchronizes medical and other professional and technical services that affect patients."[3] This statement implies a collaborative position in lieu of nursing dependence or independence. The official position of the American Nurses' Association has not put an end to the debate and there seems to be little imminent resolution of the problem. Faculties must resolve this issue so that the curriculum reflects the independence, dependence, or collaborative position of the nurse and role confusion is lessened for the student. The continuation of a dichotomized view of this issue increases the difficulty the student has in identifying herself as a nurse. The usual pattern of teaching students that the role of the nurse in the acute setting is a dependent functioning role and the nurse in the home and community is an independent functioning role is inconsistent with the belief that nursing is nursing regardless of the environment in which it occurs.

2. *Nursing is a holistic unit with central and common philosophy, purposes, knowledges, and functions.* This view is the antithesis of the concept of nursing as an articulated group of specialty areas and is one of the disputes that has the

widest ramifications in nursing practice and education. Both the Western Interstate Commission for Higher Education for Nursing[4] and the Southern Regional Education Board[5] have conducted studies and/or held conferences about selecting and applying the core concepts of nursing. The implication of such studies is that nursing does have a common core or content unity regardless of the medical diagnosis or agency affiliation of the patient-client. On the other hand, the National League for Nursing test pool for state licensure recognizes five nursing clinical specialization areas. These areas follow the classical specialization pattern of hospital patient classification, that is, medical nursing, surgical nursing, pediatric nursing, obstetrical nursing, and psychiatric nursing. This pattern of licensing examinations has helped to inhibit the evolution of a concept of holistic nursing. Vested interest groups and nurses genuinely committed to nursing as an articulation of these five basic parts work diligently to preserve the uniqueness and differentiation of the parts. Others believe in the nurse generalist who has knowledge and skills in *nursing* and propose that basic nursing is applicable to all people regardless of diagnosis or environment. Between the poles are those who concede that perhaps there is a commonality between medical and surgical nursing and those who would identify medical-surgical-pediatrics into a nursing of adults and children.[6] Others have sought to integrate psychiatric or mental health concepts into all facets of nursing.[7] The National Institute of Mental Health has spent many years supporting grants to schools for psychiatric and mental health integration. Whether or not paper commitments to nursing as a holistic process are made, most often nursing practice and nursing education are carried out in the context of nursing specialization. As nursing matures and evolves, there will be less and less difficulty with this difference of opinion, and nursing will emerge as a holistic process with little emphasis on the classical medical model. Between the vision of the future and the reality of the present is a dichotomy of stated intent and belief and implementation in practice. Curriculum-building faculties must negotiate compromises that reduce the conflict between stated beliefs about nursing and curriculum implementation of fractured parts for philosophical and reality implementation congruence to exist.

3. *Nursing skills are central and pervasive in all levels and all types of nursing practice.* The centrality of nursing skills to all types of nursing is in some dispute, if not openly then through the implications of practice. Most schools of nursing state definitively that direct patient care is one of their primary commitments; yet in actual practice, nonclient contact tasks consume large amounts of time. The very existence of large numbers of nurses who must leave direct patient care to be promoted bespeaks a lack of consonance in philosophy about client-focused skills. This difference of opinion about the place of nursing skills is further illustrated by the extent to which students of nursing are exposed to skills and the kind of activities that are labeled as skills.

Skills are frequently perceived as motor or manual only. Some schools of nursing place primary importance on manual skills and illustrate this by introducing students to manipulative skills early in their education and providing almost daily repetition of the motor skills. An example of this is the student who is required to give a bed bath or morning hygienic care and to change the beds of every client she cares for every time she has a hospitalized client.

Other schools provide little motor skill training and little practice in motor skill perfection. These schools stress the process skills of communication, leadership, decision making, and so on. Often manipulative skills are then viewed only as a communication facilitator, and process skills such as the ones just listed are not labeled skills at all. Status sometimes gets tangled in the issue and further muddles the problem. There is no easy solution for this artificial delineation between types of functions. Perhaps one initial step toward resolving this problem would be to state clearly the definition of nursing skills as those activities (motor and cognitive) necessary to carry out the functions of nursing. This means that faculties will need to view all nursing functions (process and manual) as a tool chest from which the nurse chooses those tools (skills) that most nearly serve the need for any specific task. Regardless of the decision, the role of nursing skills and the desired degree of skill achievement will influence the order, priority, and emphasis of curriculum content. For instance, if the skill of problem solving is deemed the most important skill that the student has to learn, the curriculum must provide as many opportunities for the student to have supervised practice in problem solving (as in bedmaking); furthermore, the student must have learning activities that enable growth in a variety of ways to solve problems and cope with increasingly complex problems.

4. *The democratic mode of operation and the implications of that democratic mode are a keystone of nursing roles, organization, and structure.* The democratic processes such as authority by mutual consent, individual accountability for group activities, and the ability of each group member to contribute to his potential regardless of hierarchic rank or group member role are often stated as essential to the optimal functioning of a nursing group. However, the authoritarian structure of traditional nursing is in conflict with the democratic statements generally found in nursing education philosophies. Place, rank, and authority within the traditional order of nursing hierarchy have long been in evidence. A move toward congruence between behavior and stated belief in the democratic process has brought to the surface the conflicting opinions about various forms of organizational relationships, relationships with students, and all of the other implications of "democratic"

ideals. A democratic system that favors only the faculty and not the students (democratic political systems that favor a selected group) and democratic ideals that support a democratic political system for local and national government but not for nursing schools or departments are incongruent. One teaches best by modeling, and the true test of any belief is the extent to which it is practiced in every phase of life.

The issue in this debate can be made clearer if the panacean statements about the democratic processes are reduced to the issues at stake and discussed and resolved one at a time: When discussing the whole question the issues become lost in generalities. Some of the issues raised by the democratic as opposed to the autocratic organizational format are as follows:

a. Who makes the decisions? A small group, an individual, or the whole group?

b. Is the decision maker elected by the faculty? Appointed by administration?

c. What decision-making powers are inherent in a job and what reserved for the faculty and students?

d. Who has the opportunity to participate in change? Faculty, tenured faculty only, or students and faculty?

e. Are students members of school committees? Only committees that have to do with student activities? All active committees and task groups?

f. What provisions are there for students to participate in the retention and promotion of faculty? By evaluations, by vote, or by committee membership?

g. How are committee and task group assignments made? By fitness for the task, knowledge and skill, tenure and rank?

Resolution of these vital issues is requisite to organizing for change in curriculum structure or carrying on school business, since organizational structure and guidelines reach to the very relationships that exist between and among all the people in a curriculum: students, teachers, administrators, agency personnel, and clients.

A clear statement of organizational (political) commitments must be included in the conceptual framework. If conflict between practice and principle exists, curriculum-building faculty must alter the practice to conform to the philosophy or alter the philosophy to conform to the practice.

5. *Nursing is a profession, and nursing practice and nursing education must reflect professionalism.* No nursing philosophy is ever forged by any faculty without a discussion over this issue. Often arbitrators try to alter the intensity of the debate by qualifying the term "professional" with "a young profession," "a budding profession," or a "semi-profession." It is difficult to find any intrinsic value in the debate or its resolution. One way to sort the issues inherent in the discussion is to explore what the "payoff" would be were the problem solved. Will the decision about whether nursing is a profession alter (a) nursing care quality, (b) nursing care delivery systems, (c) nursing educational practices, (d) nursing research progress, (e) nursing salaries, (f) nursing influence over health legislation, or (g) the quality of nursing literature? The obvious answer is no.

It seems that the only value in being labeled a profession would be to bolster artificially the self-concept of those in nursing who feel that the "professional" tag is necessary to a sense of worthiness. Energy used in this debate would be better spent in other ways. Continuation of discussions on this issue is probably useful to the participants in ways that have nothing to do with the problem of "professionalism" itself.

Dress codes for faculty, staff, and students have a way of getting mixed in with the "professional" image. Professionalism is often measured in the "neat, clean, and well-poised" description that is frequently remarked on in evaluations of student progress. The classical stance of the clean, white, starched, slightly aloof nurse as the picture of professionalism clashes openly with pastel pants suits, long hair, crying with the patient, or playing a guitar quietly to calm a disturbed patient. Nursing's traditional dress code was originally more closely aligned with the attempt to fight the spread of infectious disease and to retain the picture of virtuous womanhood than to convey professionalism. If faculties deem professionalism an important point that requires compromise, simplification of the issue can be achieved by separation of the various problems. Dress and client-nurse behavior patterns are different from behaviors that provide cues to "professional" development.

6. *Nursing roles in order of priority are: protective, nurtrative, and generative.* The priority of roles[8] is probably one of the key philosophical points that must be settled prior to any major curricular changes. The American Nurses' Association states that the professional nursing roles are care, cure, and coordination.[9] Prevention of disease and maintenance of health are listed in this document as a coordination role. Other roles attributed to nurses are the roles of health educator, group leader, and decision maker.[10] Regardless of the nomenclature, the list of nursing functions can become long and detailed, and each faculty member feels strongly about the relative importance of each role. An agreement about the commitment of nursing to emphasize one or more of the roles is important, since it dictates the order of priority of curriculum content. For example, faculties committed to the preventive role with its concomitant teaching and group leadership functions will place emphasis on teaching-learning skills, the utilization of community resources, skills, and the use of pathophysiological knowledge for the prevention of disease and the promotion of health. For a large proportion of their experience, students will be placed in agencies and areas where preventive activities in the practice of nursing are readily available. Faculties committed to the nurtrative role will emphasize

skills that enable nurses to care for people who are sick (that is, have diseases and need care) and the curative, supportive, and other healing and comfortive types of nursing activities.

7. *The loyalty and commitment of the nurse in any role is given unreservedly to nursing above personal loyalty to an educational institution, health agency, employer, or administrator.* Developments in government and foundation-sponsored nursing curriculum projects, research grants, and training grants have helped somewhat to diminish the feeling of proprietary interest in resources, ideas, methods, and materials. The increased numbers of people in nursing with advanced degrees have also partially alleviated the possessive feelings that individuals and groups have toward ideas. One of the true marks of professionalism is the commitment of professional people to the profession and not to a local group, school, or hospital. Commitment to *nursing* demands an attitude of sharing with one's colleagues individually and collectively, that is, other faculties and service groups. Sharing often causes anxiety that others will publish ideas, research data, or methods before the originators. Professional ethics dictates respect for crediting sources, and the need for up-to-date information is so pressing that most people welcome any form of sharing regardless of whether the data are in publishable form or not. The era of policies that forbid the sending out of course outlines, teaching tools, theoretical data, and so forth is rapidly coming to an end. There remains, however, some dispute about the value and usefulness of a more generous attitude.

PRESENTING A PHILOSOPHY OF NURSING

In summary, a philosophy of nursing for a given school should contain guidelines for both the practice of nursing and the teaching of nursing. It needs to be tailored to the individual school of nursing for which it is devised and can be included in the conceptual framework. It needs to be stated in clear, concise terms and be directly related to curriculum practices. Topically, it should contain the following elements:

1. Statements about the values on which the nursing education is based
   a. The future of nursing practice as viewed by the faculty
   b. The moral, ethical, or religious context of the school, if appropriate
   c. The scope and limits of the education provided
   d. The characteristics of people in a democratic society and the implications of these beliefs in the practice of nursing as well as in curriculum
2. Statements about the nature of nursing, its origins, its processes, and its practice roles
3. Statements about the nature of clients, their problems and needs
4. Statements about health—wellness and illness and their relationship to nursing

Initially, to formulate conceptual frameworks for practice, all nurses must decide individually what philosophical base applies to them, how much asceticism, pragmatism, romanticism, and humanistic existentialism or other philosophies are in their particular philosophy, and which of these ingredients have the most influence over their decision making. When these issues are examined and answers found, nurses can formulate their collective conceptual frameworks for practice.

To present a philosophy that truly represents the faculty's philosophical stance, differences and similarities must be raised and resolved. Most faculties will find more commonalities than differences, even though their first impression is of vast differences and irreconcilable conflicts. Techniques for discussion, elaboration, and compromise diminish differences and change the concept of polarity so that commonalities are more readily identifiable.

HEURISTIC

Philosophy—statements of belief about the nature of things—is a composite of the beliefs about life and nursing that an individual or group accepts as valid and propositions taken on "faith." A synthesis of these two elements emerges as "philosophy." Statements of a philosophy of a group must indeed reflect the thinking of the group. However, they must also reflect the theories accepted by the group. The device suggested below is a simple mechanism for promoting exploration of the philosophical base of the curriculum.

Heuristic: *Articulating the philosophy of the school of nursing*

Activity. Several general topics are provided. The participants are asked to state in any way they wish their thoughts and feelings about the area listed. There is a place at the end for other areas that the participant believes are important that are not covered elsewhere. A task group performs three tasks: (1) Compiles all data unedited, duplicates it, and distributes it to all faculty. This allows people to identify commonalities and differences and provides ground-work for subsequent discussions. (2) Sorts the responses into categories and groupings suggested by the data. (3) Provides the faculty with statements that need discussion, compromise, or synthesizing for common agreement.

Materials
1. A set of directions and a form
2. A task group for compilation and sorting data
3. Discussion time

Procedure
1. Distribute directions and questionnaire forms.
2. Set date for collecting forms.
3. Establish a task group and provide it with explicit directions and time limits.
4. Collect the forms on the designated date.
5. Task group compiles responses and distributes unedited to all participants.
6. Task group sorts responses into categories that arise from the data.
7. Task group arranges statements of philosophy that need faculty discussion and consensus.
8. Conduct a discussion of philosophy around the prepared statements.
9. Prepare a statement of philosophy from the data and discussion.
10. Submit philosophy to faculty in written form

Example

> To: Faculty
> From: Steering Committee
> *Directions:*
> This form is devised to help us come to a consensus about our philosophical viewpoint. Much of what we have already completed in the conceptual framework is basic to our philosophy. The purpose of this activity is to help us make explicit the philosophical tenets for our curriculum. When responding to the areas below, use any sources you like. You may quote books, papers, friends, or just respond from your own knowledge and beliefs. You will receive a compilation of every participant's responses so you can see the philosophical statements of each member. A task group will try to categorize and sort the responses and provide us with some statements that we need to consider for consensus. Please return these forms by _____ (date). Try to respond in each of the categories; however, feel free to omit a category if you like.
>
> 1. What values do you perceive as the base for nursing education (include moral, ethical, or religious values, scope and limits of educational responsibility, characteristics of practitioners)?
> 2. What do you believe about open curriculum, career mobility, one's admissions?
> 3. What do you believe about nursing—its origins, its processes, its roles and/or functions?
> 4. Do you identify any practice areas of nursing that are basic or prerequisite to any other practice areas? If so, what and why?
> 5. What do you think is most important about nursing care delivery?
> 6. What are the most essential ingredients in nursing practice?
> 7. What do you believe are the most important and/or desirable outcomes for graduates of this program?
> 8. How would you define health?
> 9. Describe what you believe about the nature of man and the way humans are perceived as clients of nursing.
> 10. How and under what conditions do nursing and the social system intersect?
> 11. Open category. Respond at will.

and ask for comments to be written in the large margins provided.

11. Based on feedback, alter philosophy if necessary.
12. Submit philosophy for tentative consensus.

Puissance

1. Enables the participants to see their own contribution in relation to others.
2. Helps groups to recognize commonalities and differences and thereby forces discussion.
3. By discussion broadens frame of reference for individuals and is therefore educational for the group.
4. Can decrease the time spent over identified differences and provide data for synthesis of ideas.
5. Draws together the philosophies of the group.
6. Produces a document useful for the subsequent tasks of curriculum development.

Contingencies

1. Requires time commitment from faculty.
2. Can solidify differences if resolution is not facilitated.
3. Can be perceived as not germane to the main tasks of curriculum formulation and therefore receives low energy commitment from faculty.
4. Can lack reality unless explicit in the implementation commitments.
5. Can be perceived as a "final document" and not subject to change and revision as testing occurs.

NOTES

1. Durant, Will: The story of philosophy, Garden City, N.Y., 1938, Garden City Publishing Co., p. 3.
2. American Nurses' Association: Educational preparation for nurse practitioners and assistants to nursing: a position paper, New York, 1965, The Association, p. 10.
3. Ibid., p. 6.
4. Smith, Juereta: Improvement of curricula in schools of nursing through selection and application of core concepts of nursing, Boulder, Colo., 1970, Western Interstate Commission for Higher Education.
5. Southern Regional Education Board: Defining Clinical Content, Atlanta, 1965.
6. Dufour, Honor B., and Smith, Juanita R.: A single course in nursing adults and children, Nursing Outlook **11:**516-518, 1963.
7. Schmahl, Jane A.: Experiment in change: an interdisciplinary approach to the integration of psychiatric content in baccalaureate nursing education, New York, 1966, The Macmillan Co.
8. "Nursing roles" is here used to include the functions or activities of nursing, since functions and activities are viewed as the implementation of a role.
9. American Nurses' Association, pp. 5-6.
10. Harms, Mary T., and McDonald, Frederick J.: A new curriculum design, Nursing Outlook **14:**50-53, Sept., 1966.

BIBLIOGRAPHY

Encyclopedia Britannica, Chicago, 1966, Encyclopedia Britannica, Inc., William Benton, Publishers, vol. 1, pp. 946-965; vol. 18, pp. 424-425.

Isiah Berlin, Aikin, Henry D., and White, Morton: The great ages of western philosophy, vol. 2, Boston, 1962, Houghton Mifflin Co., pp. 568-569.

Durant, Will: The story of philosophy, Garden City, N.Y., 1938, Garden City Publishing Co., Inc.

Gardner, John: In time of change no nation is an island, Christian Science Monitor Service, Honolulu Advertiser, May 31, 1976.

Johnson, Dorothy: A philosophy of nursing. In Bullough, B., and Bullough, V. L.: Issues in nursing, New York, 1966, Springer Publishing Co., pp. 145-151.

Treece, Eleanor W.: The philosophical basis for nursing education, International Nursing Review **21:**13-15, Jan.-Feb., 1974.

3

CONCEPTUAL FRAMEWORK: THE SETTING

ELEMENTS FOR A CONCEPTUAL FRAMEWORK FOR NURSING PRACTICE

As stated in Chapter 1, a conceptual framework for nursing education must contain conceptual constructs from three areas to assure its relevance. According to Chater[1] the three areas are setting, student, and knowledge. These three elements are of equal importance, have overlapping areas, and provide the conceptual structure for nursing education practice. Chater visualizes the categories as overlapping circles. (See Fig. 3-1.) Concepts from each of the elements influence the utilization of concepts from the other two elements, and curriculum decisions are made relevant to the extent, pervasiveness, and gravity of the needs and problems being approached in each of the categories represented by the circles.

The structural components of the curriculum conceptual framework are the context or setting of the school of nursing and are those factors that provide it with realistic guidelines for curriculum decisions. These structural or setting components act as both enablers and constrainers and help to provide background for and give meaning to the curriculum. Setting components gives a curriculum a specific time in a specific place. Anything within a setting or environment that influences the behavior of nurse or client, interactions, delivery of nursing services, or health problems is appropriate subject matter

for concepts and conceptual constructs for nursing practice. The curriculum builder or developer has little control over setting factors, and yet these are the factors that provide the basic "set" or "direction" for curriculum revision or development. Some of the structural components of the conceptual framework are factors such as the following:

1. The present and projected health problems and their probable solution viewed within the context of the life conditions that will exist during the working life of the graduate (five to twenty years)
2. The demography of the community in which the school resides; the characteristics, ethnicity, and needs of the population and the services and agencies available to meet those needs
3. The purposes, philosophy, and organizational structure of the institution that sponsors the school of nursing
4. The legal and professional standards and guidelines (nurse practice acts, state boards of nursing, and National League for Nursing accreditation criteria)

The preceding factors are the "materials on hand." Until these materials are inventoried, the faculty cannot determine what additional materials will be needed or how the materials on hand can best be utilized. The preceding factors are the "givens" of any curriculum, and assessing the givens

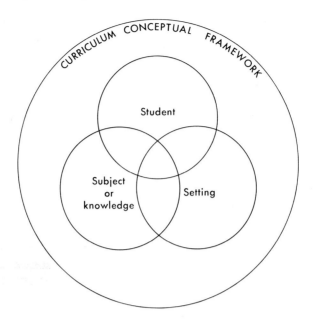

Fig. 3-1. Conceptual framework for curriculum decisions.

or delineating the structural perimeters or boundaries is the starting point in curriculum development or revision process.

The structural components of the conceptual framework are concerned only with descriptions of things as they are and things as they are likely to evolve. Value judgments about the components can be useful in that the value judgments may indicate targets for change, but the basic intent of the assessment is to identify the elements that make explicit the perimeters of the developing curriculum.

PRESENT AND PROJECTED HEALTH PROBLEMS AND THEIR PROBABLE SOLUTION IN GEOGRAPHICAL AREA SERVED, VIEWED WITHIN CONTEXT OF LIFE CONDITIONS THAT WILL EXIST DURING WORKING LIFE OF THE GRADUATE

Change, by its very nature, suggests turning "from" something "to" something. Determining what one wishes to change "from" and what one wishes to change "to" is one of the first problems in the curriculum building process. Forecasting the future is not a matter of second sight or dreaming of things as they ought to be; it is a well-balanced combination of historical perspective, analysis of the present, and anticipation of the future in a reality frame of reference. The term "reality frame of reference" is intended to convey objectivity, that is, avoiding (1) harsh judgments of the past, (2) refutation of the present, and (3) millennial views of the future or wishful thinking.

There are three areas of study suggested above: (1) historical perspectives, (2) analysis of the present, and (3) anticipation of the future. Nursing curricula are built for the express purpose of educating people who can promote optimal health and are therefore organized around central health problems and goals. A thorough grasp of those problems in the world that jeopardize health and a vision of the *possible* solutions to those problems provide a major curriculum decision-making guide. *Education* in its true sense, after all pedagogical dialogue is finished, *is the art of the possible.* The curriculum builder starts with historical, present, and future health problems and finishes with the possible solutions to present and future problems.

Traditionally, nursing has been concerned with the study of itself. With some exceptions[2] large studies in the first half of the twentieth century dealt with nursing, its problems, its shortcomings, its need for identity, professionalism, and its own intradisciplinary problems.

The classical curriculum references for nursing[3] gave content organization outlines patterned directly on the organization of the medical profession and on conventional acute hospital ward patient classifications. Major disease problems or causes of death were often used as criteria for selecting nursing content. The remarkable thing about a review of the 1937 *Curriculum Guide for Schools of Nursing* is how very little nursing curricula today have departed from this guideline. The danger in this is that nursing can become a ritual instead of a process.[4]

Even a cursory examination of that volume gives one insight into its profound strengths and its remarkably few weaknesses. Had nursing educators read more carefully the introductory chapters and followed less closely the chapters on content, the book would have been used more as the guide it was intended to be and less as a mandate for content outlines: Change would have been more an ongoing process and less a response to crisis. The first chapter of the National League of Nursing Education's *Curriculum Guide for Schools of Nursing* suggests:

The concept of a dynamic and progressive as opposed to a static curriculum for nursing schools has been accepted from the very beginning and is continued in this revision. Changes are recognized as desirable and necessary in view of the changed conditions and needs of life. Such changes should be in keeping with the newer developments in educational, social and scientific knowledge. At the same time it is important that the best of the old should be preserved and incorporated into the new. The whole structure should be constructed on flexible lines so that adjustments may be made as needed.[5]

This sound basis for curriculum development suggested by the committee was minimally used by new or developing nursing programs, probably because nursing was struggling to stabilize its shifting base from service apprenticeship to educationally sound programs of specified quality. In a few short years the three editions of the *Curriculum Guide for Schools of Nursing* helped nursing achieve what Flexner had helped medicine achieve earlier: quality preparation for practitioners.

The impact of this volume on nursing education is not surprising when one peruses the list of those who contributed their wisdom, experience, learning, and imagination on a variety of committees and individual assignments. Never before nor since have so many of nursing's great people collaborated in a single effort to produce a document. Despite the clear plea within the first chapter for an ongoing, changing curriculum, a volume giving a clear and definitive prediction of the future as a context for nursing education was not available until 1948, when *Nursing for the Future* was published. Brown's study foresaw developments, predicted trends, and articulated legitimate goals for nursing. Her clear and uncluttered approach to the problems that nursing faced helped nursing grow in response to social needs rather than professional vested interest groups. In the thirty years since the publication of *Nursing for the Future,* many of Brown's predications have become reality, and nursing education routinely studies trends and predicts future developments in health as a basis for curriculum planning. The wheels of change have ground forward to the tune of Ginzberg, Wolf, Bridgman, Sand, Montag, and a host of others.[6] Recently, Lysaught's[7] study recommends definitive directions for change.

Present health problems have too much popular press coverage to be explained at any length again here: the emptying of large mental hospitals of patients in need of nursing services, and nursing agencies poorly prepared to render these services;

water resources drying up; population increasing logarithmically; crowded cities with suicide rates going up and drug abuse growing; insecticide poisoning, rendering lifeless large natural reservoirs such as lakes and streams; alarming maternal and infant death rates in the "civilized and clean" United States; malaria, tuberculosis, and malnutrition still predominate as world health problems despite years of effort to eradicate them; poorly organized and inefficient health agencies unable to respond adequately to the people's health needs; mushrooming types of health care workers with ill-defined roles; exorbitant cost of health care; maldistribution of health care; and finally the uneven availability of health care workers to clients. To read the list of ills sounds like a dirge, but viewed in perspective the health care needs portend the changes in the system of health care that face nursing educators. These current health problems, when viewed with predicted changes in society and predicted changes in society's way of coping, provide a basis for choosing curriculum content.

An example of some of the trends in the next twenty years that will influence curriculum decisions follows. A faculty involved in the process of curriculum building will evolve its own more complete and situationally specific list. The temporal nature of any such list makes obsolescence imminent.

I. Social factors
  A. Revitalized maintenance of individual ethnic identity while continuing the process of integration
  B. Revolution in values
    1. Emphasis on health and health care as an inalienable human right
    2. Equal and comprehensive care and treatment for all people
    3. Resolution of conflict between national production growth and environmental damage
    4. Changing materialistic emphasis
    5. Greater tolerance for individual differences
    6. Changing standards of communication
    7. Changing views of morality

  C. Changing family structure
    1. Meaning of marriage changing, with emphasis on legalizing marriage relationship as a formalization of a permanent contract to establish a family
    2. Family unit changes
    3. Family member role changes (role blurring taking place)
  D. Education level
    1. Increase in educational level of the population
    2. Decrease in social and educational deprivation
    3. Increase in equal educational opportunity for all people
    4. More efficient use of human resources
    5. Decline in basic reading and writing skills of the average high school graduate
    6. Decreased emphasis on college education
  E. Work and productivity
    1. Decrease in number of hours of work per week
    2. More leisure time
    3. Earlier retirement or change of occupation
    4. Higher standard of living
    5. Change from the dole to the job opportunity with a guaranteed minimal income
II. Political factors
  A. Increasing governmental control over all aspects of life
    1. Industry and business
    2. Regulation of individual activity
    3. More responsibility for chronically disabled family members (day care centers, etc.)
    4. Support of health and health agencies and corresponding control, for example, prepaid insurance coverage of all segments of the population, control over standards of health care, education and training of health workers, larger and more efficient health care systems with more flexible and mobile subsystems
  B. Increasingly organized citizens' groups
    1. Exertion of pressure by power groups to effect changes
    2. Increased involvement of public in social, health, and political issues
  C. Increased interest in exercising the franchise, with a larger segment of the population assuming a voice in government
    1. Mechanisms being developed to respond more quickly to public demands
    2. Women becoming an organized and powerful political force
III. Environmental factors
  A. Continued increase in attempts to legislate

for preservation and restoration of environment

B. Growing body of scientific knowledge about the ecological balance and health

C. Continuation of increasing population density with its concomitant problems: crowding, waste disposal, decreased world food stores and food production capacity, decreasing water supply
   1. Increased incidence of psychiatric problems caused by crowding such as thought and behavior disorders, suicide, battered children, alcoholism, drug abuse
   2. Rising pollution-connected health problems, water contamination, communicable diseases, etc.
   3. Population shifts to new, less crowded urban centers, retirement areas, and clean air areas

IV. Technological factors

A. More sophisticated use of computers as information banks
   1. Health records centrally banked with all Department of Health, Education, and Welfare agency records using social security number for instant record retrieval
   2. Scientific information at fingertips, available at every health center and clinic for health personnel
   3. Complete programming of nursing curricula in multiplicity of media with portable study carrels available for home or agency use and instant instruction available through national hookups
   4. Decreased availability of oil-based energy and industry (affecting transportation patterns, plastic production, etc.)

B. Use of more and more sophisticated technology for diagnosis and treatment of health problems
   1. Tiny television cameras enabling internal visualization of patients
   2. Computerized intensive care units for monitoring patients
   3. Automation of hospital rooms with fingertip patient control of environment
   4. Increasing successes in organ transplants, mechanical prostheses, immunization techniques for cancer, preventive measures for heart and other cardiovascular diseases
      a. Prolongation of life concomitant with human aging problems
   5. Falling birth rates to population growth zero—an older population
   6. Mechanization depersonalizing health services, making personal nurse-patient contact difficult to establish and maintain
   7. Continuation of transfer of functions from physician to nurse, extending and blurring nurse's role
   8. Increased place for nurse–clinical specialist, nurse practitioner, and other role diversification with standards and criteria set by the American Nurses' Association
   9. Extended care and satellite facilities in residential areas (changing pattern of care)
   10. Greater emphasis on prevention and on taking nursing care to the people
   11. More widespread and effective home nursing services
   12. Mobile health clinics and other health care delivery services
   13. Change from public health nursing services delivery system to the neighborhood nurse who is responsible for health care of a small neighborhood—functioning as primary care agent, as well as screening, referring, and teaching
   14. Better definition of nursing phenomena and increased clarity about nursing's domain of practice
   15. Increase in chronic illness
   16. Decrease in institutionalization of clients

The foregoing sample list of factors that are in the process of occurring or will occur within the working life span of the nursing students of today has definitive implications for curriculum content. Each factor previously listed can be examined separately and the nursing education implications articulated. For each factor isolated the curriculum builder needs to answer three questions:

1. What are the nursing curriculum commitment implications of this factor?
2. What are the nursing behaviors that will be necessary for the nurse to function within the ramifications of this factor?
3. What are the processes and information (content) that will enable the nurse to develop the desired behaviors?

The answers to these questions provide the nursing educator with three things: (1) one set of conceptual curriculum framework implications, (2) terminal behaviors, and (3) essential content that will be a source of reference for a curriculum check-list or content criteria list for structuring courses. Similar framework commitments, behaviors, and content will tend to appear repeatedly within the list, providing some frequency indicators for establishing priorities.

In summary, an analysis of the present and future life components, problems, and possible or forecasted solutions provides specific data that become part of the system of premises on which a nursing curriculum is based.

Community in which the school resides

The United States is noted for the variety of the people living within its borders. One has only to travel from the Elizabethan English atmosphere of the Outer Banks of North Carolina, through the Amish villages of Pennsylvania, and into communities in New Mexico and Arizona, where the stamp of native and Mexican-American culture is obvious, to see the remarkable variety of communities and peoples. If, in this same cross-country trek, one continues on to the coastal area of California, from Los Angeles to San Francisco, one crosses into a world vastly different from the ones just mentioned, and one where the health problems and solutions are different from those of the Outer Banks, the Amish villages, and the native-American reservations. The curriculum implications for these differences in communities, peoples, and their needs are basic—so basic that when the community setting is ignored, schools situated in those settings may seem to function successfully but actually serve only specific and limited segments of the population.

The community area or state in which the school is situated furnishes some of the population from which the student clientele of the school is drawn. The immediate community is the environment in which nursing is learned and frequently is the place where the new graduate practices.

Communities are formed for the purpose of providing people with a way to meet their common needs for protection, sustenance, shelter, education, health, and general welfare. A school of nursing is a community agency organized as a means for meeting specific needs of that community. To respond adequately to those community needs and to provide data for concepts for decision making, the school of nursing must assess the community, state, and nation in which it resides, inventory its factors, and identify its problems and goals. Is the area urban or rural, coastal, mountainous, plains, dry or moist, hot or cold? This is important for many reasons. If the area is urban, what is it like? Is it a sprawling vague community that blurs together without meaning or boundaries, or is it a tightly knit, impacted city like New York or San Francisco?

If the area is crowded and impacted, the setting will have different urban health problems from those in a sprawling city like Los Angeles or Atlanta. Is transportation a problem? Crowding? Housing? Urban centers tend to have more health resources, more agencies, a wider variety of health care workers, greater accessibility, and at least slightly more even distribution of services than rural areas. Urban centers have large clinics, many hospitals, much industry, a largely insured working class, a wide variety of ethnic groups, and a strongly organized and often vocal health consumer group. They tend to have more suicides, higher crime rates, more unemployment, more ghettos, more alcohol and drug abuse, and less human concern for individuals than in rural areas.

Rural areas tend to have fewer health care workers, fewer specialists, fewer facilities, greater distances to health care, fewer financial resources, and higher maternal and infant death rates. Rural areas tend to be more neighborly, more caring, and more humanistic. Nutrition is sometimes not a matter of food availability but of food use. The rural West has a scattered and scanty population, little industry, and an ethnicity composed primarily of white middle-class Americans, native Americans, and Mexican-Americans, and the health consumer is less vocal about health needs, is poorly insured, and is less oriented to health care quality.

Is the setting in the Southeast, the Northeast, the Southwest, the Northwest, the South Central, or the North Central? Location influences climate and literacy, and health statistics often follow geographical lines. The Southwest tends to be dry and warm, with a low incidence of arthritis and high incidence of coccidioidomycosis (San Joaquin Valley Fever). The Southeast has a high maternal and infant mortality rate and a high incidence of all cardiovascular diseases, especially stroke and hypertension. There are many other sectional statistics, but the point is that geographical location influences health problems.

Just as clients from various locations have different health needs and care, so it is true with students. Students coming from these vastly different communities bring to the school of nursing varied experiences, educational backgrounds, and views of life. They learn the same basic processes of nursing, but the reality of their worlds is different; therefore their use of nursing processes is different. For instance, the nurse in Manhattan, New York, deals with a highly competitive client, whereas the nurse in Gallup, New Mexico, deals with a person whose whole cultural set is noncompetitive. Teaching strategies that rely on intergroup competition are highly unsuccessful with members of selected tribes of native Americans.

Nurses look at housing, income statistics, employment and unemployment, crime rates, recreational facilities, and sanitation when assessing a setting to determine appropriate concepts for practice. Housing is usually classified as standard, substandard, and dilapidated. Health problems occur more frequently in families who occupy substandard and dilapidated housing. This may be generally due to

economics. Federal programs provide funds for such things as housing, food, and preventive and maintenance health care. Few programs assist the poor to stay warm, have clean water, and use good garbage and waste disposal. These services are not available equally in all sections of the country.

Is the area industrial, and what are the industries? Do these industries have occupational hazards or diseases? For example, jobs with high dust concentrations produce a high incidence of eye and respiratory diseases; foundries produce a high incidence of burns and other thermal accidents; white collar businesses produce a high incidence of alcoholism and heart disease.

The political structure of an area has importance, since whether or not the voters are liberal or conservative may indicate support or lack of it for innovative health care programs. Who controls funding flows for health care and what are their priorities? Are there strongly organized political groups such as unions, small businessmen, the League of Women Voters, or people's coalitions? These are questions that need answers for the curriculum to include concepts relevant to nurses as client advocates who have an ability to work within the political system of the setting.

There are many ways of assessing communities. Population composition can be gleaned from federal and local statistical offices, school systems, and chambers of commerce. Crime rates, school absenteeism, suicide rates, alcohol and drug abuse statistics, churches, employing firms, unemployment indices, housing quality and quantity, maternal and infant death rates, life expectancy, population age statistics, and many other community characteristics furnish data that taken as a whole are an indication of the nature of the community and its health needs. Simple surveys of health agencies, their roles in health care, and the extent and limitations of their services indicate the extent to which the health needs identified in the community study are being met.

Assessments of the community not only furnish insights into the setting of the school of nursing, providing grist for the content mill, but they also provide data about the health agencies available to the school as laboratories for clinical experiences for nursing students.

New schools of nursing grow out of a larger community need; existing schools of nursing restructure their curricula in response to the changing needs of this larger community. It is the characteristics of the larger community that provide the stimulus to which the school of nursing forms its response—the curriculum. The more clearly and accurately the larger community is assessed, hypothesized, or predicted, the more nearly the school will come to fulfilling the needs of that larger community and the more successfully the student products of the school will be able to address themselves to health problems of the citizens of that community.

Often nursing schools rely heavily on hospitals and official public health agencies as the major resources for student learning experiences. Nursing is a broadly based community affair. Relatively few nursing clients are seen in hospital and public health nursing agenices. To use the health resources properly of a community in which the school of nursing is situated, a comprehensive list of official and non-official health agencies, health services, clubs oriented toward health needs, health centers, and health professional groups is needed.

Educational setting trends

Nursing schools are educational enterprises and as such their natural affinity is for settings that are educationally organized and have as their primary commitment educational endeavors. In 1948 Brown[8] recommended a gradual transfer of nursing education responsibilities from service institutions to institutions of higher learning. She cited successful liaison between some hospital schools and community two-year colleges, and she also cited one associate of arts college that offered a three-year course in nursing. Montag[9] provided the spark that lighted the way for the nationwide development of nursing schools in the educational setting of the associate of arts college, and thus the eventual current trend and outcome of nursing education at two levels, that is, baccalaureate and associate of arts. In 1965 the American Nurses' Association took a definitive and firm stand on the educational preparation for nurse practitioners and assistants to nurses. In a position paper four statements emphasized with heavy print unequivocal support for the position that *education for those who work in nursing should take place in institutions of learning within the general system of education*. These four statements are reproduced for emphasis.

- The education for all those who are licensed to practice nursing should take place in institutions of higher education.
- Minimum preparation for beginning professional nursing practice at the present time should be baccalaureate degree education in nursing.
- Minimum preparation for beginning technical nursing practice at the present time should be associate degree education in nursing.
- Education for assistants in the health service occupations should be short, intensive preservice programs in vocational education institutions rather than on-the-job training programs.[10]

In the words of Jo Eleanor Elliott, President of the American Nurses' Association when the position paper was finally passed, "The position paper recognizes the realities of today and sets directions for the future."[11] The time from Brown's pointing the way, through Montag's illustration of feasibility and means, to the American Nurses' Association's definitive stand was seventeen years. To state that the American Nurses' Association position was a reflection of a fait accompli as well as a prophecy of the future is true. However, the profession cannot devalue the remarkable fact that a body whose members were predominantly educated in hospital schools of nursing took a stand in the interest of society that supported a movement that will culminate in the obsolescence of their own basic nursing preparation. Schools of nursing that are not integral parts of educational institutions are anachronistic remnants of a way of responding to society's nursing needs. The society for which they were organized no longer exists, the needs they met have altered and changed, and more effective answers to today's nursing needs are evolving rapidly.

Today's educational system for nursing is a monument to a former highly successful system of hospital training for nursing, since only successful systems have the capacity for change in response to changed conditions and needs. And although the pace of change has often seemed slow and cumbersome, change has occurred and is occurring.

One of the first tasks of any curriculum development group must be the examination of its setting to determine compliance with the four propositions just cited from the American Nurses' Association position paper. Schools of nursing that do not meet these basic criteria need first to identify ways and means of establishing themselves within the educational system that best fulfill their requirements.

TYPE OF EDUCATIONAL SETTING, PHILOSOPHY, AND OBJECTIVES OF SPONSORING INSTITUTION

The type, character, and important attributes of the agency within which nursing takes place influence the concepts that form the construct for the setting. Every institution that sponsors a school of nursing has a reason for its existence. Hospitals have charters under which they operate, and frequently they have larger sponsoring agencies behind them. For instance, some hospitals are agencies of local or federal government, some are sponsored by churches or religious orders,

some are private and are sponsored by individuals or groups of individuals, and some are branches of colleges or universities. Hospital schools of nursing reflect the explicit or implicit philosophies and purposes of the sponsoring institution, whether or not there is a conscious effort to comply with those philosophies and purposes.

Colleges and universities have affiliations that dictate their philosophy. Associate of arts and baccalaureate colleges are usually sponsored by states, communities, churches, and private groups. Whoever the sponsoring group, whatever its motivation, and whatever its aims, these motivations and aims become those of the school of nursing. Cognizance of the philosophy and purposes of the sponsoring institution is the beginning. Studies indicate that institutions attract faculties and students with characteristics that are congruent with the sponsoring institution, and differences are a matter of degree, not of kind.[12] For instance, some religiously oriented colleges have in their purposes that students hold specified religious beliefs, that graduates be equipped to fight "materialistic hedonism,"[13] and that the students' life patterns be in keeping with the tenets of the religious beliefs of the sponsoring institution. Theological or "Bible" studies are usually a required part of the curriculum, and nursing content is often included or excluded on the basis of religious conviction.

Liberal arts colleges that exhibit strong philosophies of humanism require different prerequisite courses and have different aspirations for their graduates than religiously oriented colleges. Social responsibility, classical foundations, and highly developed decision-making capacity tend to be predominant purposes of these colleges. Church-sponsored colleges and proprietary liberal arts colleges often have some area of common philosophy; however, studies indicate that the priorities of emphasis are most often dictated by the philosophical and/or theological set of the sponsoring group.

There are as many guiding philosophies

of education, as many sets of educational objectives, as there are educational institutions. Of importance to the faculty who are developing nursing curricula is a definitive and succinct description of the college's philosophy and purpose and the subsequent development of the philosophy and purposes of the school of nursing congruent with the sponsoring agency. Areas of philosophical incongruence provide the battle lines for curriculum problems, whereas areas of congruence provide the base for continuing development.

Charters, legislated mandates, and boards of governors or trustees are usually established to provide the educational institution with a group that is charged with the sole responsibility of providing for the welfare of the college and ensuring that the college curriculum is congruent with established philosophy and purposes. When change does occur, these boards are responsible for ensuring that changes follow the lines of change occurring in the sponsoring body. Financial responsibility is usually vested in and/or administered by this board. Moneys are provided by churches, private subscription, trust funds, or state or federal budgets. Regardless of where the money flows *from,* it usually flows *through* some group that governs the educational enterprise. The degree to which the governing body uses its authority and financial leverage to influence curriculum varies from institution to institution. However, it is a legitimate (although to teachers often an annoying) responsibility of those governing boards to enforce congruence of curriculum and philosophy.

Organization of the institution

Organizational patterns of educational institutions and hospitals usually follow a hierarchical format. A military model of flow of responsibility provides clear channels of administration. The authority for decision making is not nearly as clear as the diagrams for responsibility would seem to indicate from reading an organizational chart and descriptions of communications

channels. There is no need to repeat here types and formats for organizational patterns and chains of command. The important concepts for the curriculum planners to keep before them is that there are ways to work within the system to muster approval for the curriculum changes desired by the faculty. Some of these concepts are as follows:

1. Find out exactly what channels proposed changes must go through and what committees must approve them.

2. Keep those people or groups informed at every stage of development. The fewer surprises they have the more likely they are to approve the changes. Changes require some incubation to become acceptable.

3. Make a point-by-point, written statement about how the changes are in congruence with philosophy, purposes, and trends in the larger institution. Show definitively what should be changed and why and what needs in the educational system, in the health care system, and in the social system the curriculum changes are designed to meet.

4. Keep changes fluid; that is, make it clear that changes are in progress, that changes are tentative or "on trial" so that subsequent revision based on feedback is possible.

5. Provide people with as much evidence as possible that revisions in curriculum utilize the latest technologies and techniques available for effective and efficient student learning. Programs that appear to increase in per capita yearly cost *because* of curriculum changes are indefensible to budget-minded administrators.

6. Use the educational expertise of members of the academic community, community school system, or available consultants. This not only provides the faculty with additional input but it also provides a broader base of support for the needed changes.

Laws, regulations, constraints, and enablers

A part of each setting is a system of controls designed to ensure minimum standards of quality for educational enterprises. These standards arise from the state laws, professional accreditation and credentialing groups, and sponsoring agency policies and procedures. Budget constraints, as mentioned earlier, are only one lever for imposing compliance with agency, philosophy, and general purpose. Agency policy is the most common and tangible implement used to mold compliance. Once nursing faculties assure congruence between the school of nursing's philosophy, goals, and objectives and the sponsoring agency or college and compliance to agency or college policy, they move immediately to assure compliance with state government rules and regulations.

State boards of nursing examiners, by law or regulation, must be notified of any anticipated or impending changes in the curriculum of a school of nursing. Schools who follow the change ground rule of no surprises for any person or group concerned in the change, notify the state board of nursing that change is being considered, and continue to keep in close communication with the appropriate persons on the board as change progresses tend to have fewer problems when changes are ready to be submitted for board approval. Most board of nursing regulations about curriculum are written in sufficiently general terms that innovation in curriculum development may progress without inhibition by the board if the board is involved at an early enough date. There are, in many states, some board rules and regulations regarding the number of students who can be supervised by a single instructor or how many hours, days, or weeks that students must spend in clinical practice. Knowledge about these rules and regulations will decrease problems in curriculum implementation.

National League for Nursing's accreditation function is carried out with the mission of closely guarding standards of nursing educational programs. Each council has its accreditation criteria, and each set of criteria addresses itself to the minimum educational standards for the level of nurs-

ing involved. Early, careful reading of the criteria for appraisal (accreditation) relevant to the type of educational program being planned will help to avert accreditation problems later. If the curriculum being developed is a revision or alteration of an older accredited program, the appropriate accrediting board needs to be alerted that changes are being considered and planned. If the program is a new curriculum, early contact with the National League for Nursing and early consultation from the league may be helpful in ensuring compliance with accreditation standards.

The state board of nursing test pool examination is one measure of success of the program, and both state boards of nursing and the National League for Nursing accreditation bodies as well as regulating bodies look at state board failure rates as one indicator of program quality. State board test scores are by no means specific for any program nor are they the most important measure of program quality. They are, currently, one of the measures for determining whether or not a person will be permitted to practice nursing. If a program purports to prepare nurses for practice and the people prepared for the program fail to be admitted to practice by any quality control mechanism, then questions must be asked about the program's relevance to minimum practice standards. The issue of state board examinations is complex because people with a multiplicity of educational and experiential backgrounds are allowed to use the test as admission to practice nursing. However, as long as the test is used as one of the main practice criteria, administrators of programs are responsible to see that graduates are admitted to practice.

HEURISTICS

There are two heuristics offered as examples for discovering the structural framework of the curriculum. Many others can be developed and used. The ones presented here are (1) a device for gathering data about the possible future of health problems and solutions and (2) a device for gathering data about community health agencies.

Example. Task-group assignments and directions

To: Faculty
From: Curriculum Change Coordinator
Re: Data necessary for curriculum change

We need to look at the social, political, environmental, and technological factors that will affect the nursing practice of our graduates during their working life. We are taking fifteen to twenty years as a realistic mean employment span. A longer employment span would get us into a time span that is difficult to predict; a shorter span would be relatively useless. Our overall purpose is to try to fantasize what conditions will be like in this time span, what the implications are for nursing educational commitments, what behaviors our graduates will need to cope with this predicted world, and what content will best foster those behaviors. To facilitate getting the job done, task groups have been assigned to definitive portions of the job. When we put all the parts together, we will have a comprehensive document.

Directions:
1. Please read through the task-group assignments to obtain a comprehensive view of the whole job. This will help you see your own part in relation to the whole.
2. The first person listed on each task force will please assume the responsibility for calling the group together.
3. Please do not write on the backs of pages; we will need to cut and paste.
4. Please make every effort to meet your target dates, since the next group of tasks cannot be done until your phase is finished. Lag has a domino effort on all work.

Task-force assignments and target dates*

Task A: Predict the future for the next fifteen to twenty years in the area assigned to you. Try to document. However, use your own expertise and knowledge. Don't be inhibited by lack of documentation—you are all experts in your fields and can make reliable estimates about what may or may not happen.

Target date for completion: October 1

Task Force No. 1-Task: Social factors
  Group: Mary P.
          Jane D.
          Joe B.
Task Force No. 2-Task: Political factors
  Group: Hope L.
          Hortense A.

Task Force No. 3-Task: Environmental factors
  Group: Bill D.
          Susan S.
          Janet N.
          Pris W.
Task Force No. 4-Task: Technological factors
  Group: Irene R.
          Teresa J.
          Linda G.

Task B: Compiling work, deleting redundancies, editing, documenting, and making a topical outline (usually requires one small task force).
  Target date for completion: about 10 days

Task C: Establishing implications of predictions: Using the form and outline provided for each predicted condition, determine what the conceptual framework implications are, what the nursing behaviors will be that will enable nurses to function in the predicted environment, and what content will facilitate the ability to so function.
  Suggestion: Go over the form taking each aspect through all four task assignments to its logical conclusion.

---

*This sample format will be given only once. All phases of the job described in this section require task-group assignments and target dates structured around these same lines.

An example page from completed documents follows. The outline of the future provided the task groups is in the left-hand column, the work the task groups produced for task C is in columns 2, 3, and 4. Task-group assignments follow the format for task A.

Predicted nurse behaviors and content based on factors influencing nursing and conceptual framework commitments

Political factors influencing nursing	Conceptual framework implications	Requisite behaviors	Requisite content
Increasing governmental control over all aspects of life: 1. Industry and business 2. Regulation of individual activity 3. Responsibility for disabled family member 4. Support of health agencies and increased control, e.g., insurance standards of care, education, and training of workers; larger more efficient health care systems with flexible and mobile subsystems	1. Nurses assess health needs of communities and work within political and agency structures, use appropriate channels and valid principles to meet health needs of the people and/or make changes 2. Nurses become involved in activities that influence social and environmental conditions affecting health 3. Through effective participation as a citizen, nurses influence the direction of social change 4. Nurses participate in the delivery of health services in a multiplicity of environments 5. Curriculum changes will meet legal and accreditation requirements	1. Able to identify own role in system and function in that role 2. Interpret law regarding prepaid insurance for patient's use 3. Aware of government regulations and work within them or work within system for changes 4. Use resources for money, consultation, and information 5. Evaluate health care given; make improvements 6. Adapt to a large variety of nursing situations and agency settings 7. Able to innovate in delivering nursing care in a variety of environments	1. Political science 2. Community organizations 3. Channels of authority in administration structures 4. Nature of bureaucracies 5. Health legislation and experience in working for legislative changes 6. Principles of planned change 7. Principles of communication 8. Knowledge of community health resources 9. Types of health insurance and desirable insurance coverage 10. Principles of evaluation and their application to health care

Heuristic 1: *Forecasting the changes in the next twenty years and their influence upon health and nursing education.*

Activity. This activity is one that can be accomplished most efficiently by small task-group assignment. Task groups should consist of not fewer than two nor more than four people and should, if possible, represent a cross section of faculty interest and talents. The activity is completed in three phases. Phase one is the assigning of areas to be predicted and documented; phase two is sorting the collected data, deleting redundancy and forming the collected materials into a narrative document; phase three is deducing the conceptual framework implications, the requisite behaviors for nursing in the predicted environment,

and the requisite content for developing the desired behaviors. This same material can be used further when developing theoretical approaches to nursing, when setting content priorities while developing courses, and when developing program and course objectives. Realistic time limits of approximately one working week should be allowed for each phase of the task.

Materials
1. A task-group organization for the complete task
2. A target date schedule listing dates for completion of each anticipated task
3. Question or topical forms to be distributed to all participants

Example

To: Faculty
From: Curriculum Change Coordinator
Re: Health agency survey

Attached is a list of agencies in this community that are concerned in some way with health. If you know of others, please add them to the list. Be sure the name is correct. Put down anything you know about the agency—especially the telephone number and address. Please return by _____ (date).

List of agencies
 Public Health Department
 Visiting Nurse Association
 Home Health Aids, Inc.
 Goodwill Industries
 Sundown Convalescent Hospital
 Holy Cross Hospital
 Baptist Hospital
 Jerome Halfway House
 Dial Crisis
Blanks for your additions:

 _____
 _____
 _____
 _____

Directions:

Attached you will find 18 community health agencies assigned to you for acquiring the information we need to complete our comprehensive community Health Agency Survey. Attachment No. 2 is a comprehensive list of all community health agencies that we have been able to locate so far. If you know of others or can find out about others, please call the office and ask the secretary to put them on the list.

Please call or visit the agencies on the list. Get the necessary information from someone within the agency who is a reliable source. We would like our information to be as accurate as possible.

There are plenty of blanks; get more from the office if you need more. Please try to have your assignment completed by _____ (date).

AGENCY INFORMATION FORM

1. Type of health service rendered (health screening, psychiatric therapy, physical therapy, rehabilitation, home health services, etc.)
2. Name of agency
3. Address of agency
4. Telephone number of agency
5. Sponsor
6. Person in authority
7. Contact person
8. Narrative description of services rendered and population served
9. Puissance (capabilities, powers, authority, jurisdiction, or domain)
10. Limitations
11. Notes and comments

Make a loose-leaf notebook of agency information.

4. Completed work for distribution to all participants at each stage of completion

Procedure
1. Organize the curriculum change participants into task groups.
2. Write definitive directions for each task phase.
3. Establish target dates for the completion of each task.
4. Distribute all directions and all target date deadlines to every participant so that a comprehensive picture of the work to be done is communicated.
5. Discuss the tasks with the group when the tasks are assigned.
6. Make enough copies of finished products to keep on file for future use and to share with interested people.

Puissance
1. Looking into the future helps the group to begin to formulate a more concrete image of the life factors that graduates will be dealing with during their productive years.
2. Predicting the future problems and solutions helps the group to begin to think in perspective and unlock from present problems and vested interest areas.
3. Predictions provide a base for devising a checklist for conceptual framework commitments consistency and practical implementation.
4. Predictions enable concretization of the behaviors that may be necessary to enable nurses to function adequately in the future reality.
5. Predicting the future provides a reference point for establishing the content necessary to develop the desired behaviors and set the content priorities.
6. Outlining materials in one document enables a visualization of patterns of content so that commonalities can be ascertained and a holistic nursing content can begin to be identified.

Contingencies
1. The job of predicting, deducing the conceptual framework commitments, ascertaining necessary behaviors and outlining content may appear to be overwhelming to the group and can cause group anxiety. Breaking the job into tasks helps to allay some of the anxiety but not all of it.
2. Groups can become too futuristic—the line between sheer fiction and possibility is obscure in the present rapid change system.
3. There can be frank differences of opinion about what may occur. These are natural and will have to be arbitrated.
4. Some faculty members will want to know why this is necessary and will wish to start organizing new courses and proposing changes without the necessary groundwork.

Heuristic 2: *Surveying the agencies that respond to community health needs*

Activity. These data can be accrued in several ways. Many communities have a source book of official and nonofficial agencies from which much of the needed information can be extracted. However, source books become obsolete because communities change rapidly, and they often do not provide all the information needed for curriculum development. If no source books exist, a preliminary survey of agencies can be gathered through the telephone book or by circulating to faculty and known agency personnel a letter asking them to list all the agencies with which they are familiar. This initial list can provide the direction of the survey. Sometimes a group of students can take a community agency survey as a community project. Regardless of how the list is accrued, an initial listing of agencies helps to get this activity started.

Agency surveys lend themselves to individual faculty assignments; for example, a faculty member can be given a stack of blank forms to fill out and a list of agencies. Without the list of agencies faculty members may investigate many of the same agencies and thus waste valuable time.

Materials
1. A list of community agencies with space at the end for others to be added as they are found
2. Enough blank forms to provide each faculty member with sufficient forms for his assignment, for additional agencies found, for errors, and for replacing lost forms
3. An assignment for each participating curriculum change group member

Procedure
1. Provide each faculty member with as complete a list as possible of community agencies.
2. Ask them to add any they know about or can find out about by requesting information from other knowledgeable people.
3. Set a specified time and recall the list.
4. Reissue a revised list leaving space at the end for additions.
5. Assign each participant an equal amount of agencies to survey.
6. Provide the group with agency information forms.
7. Set a one- to two-week target date for completion.
8. Compile the completed forms into a manual of agencies.
9. Cross-reference the manual in ways that seem useful, for example, hospitals, nursing homes, rehabilitation centers, day care centers, mental health centers, psychiatric in-patient units, and home nursing care groups.
10. Make the manual in loose-leaf form so that changes can be made without destroying the

format or making it necessary to redo the entire document.

Puissance
1. Provides information on community resources for educational experiences.
2. Provides a picture of the community's response to health problems.
3. Enables rapid communications with appropriate others involved in health and health care.
4. Provides the information necessary for establishing community participation in curriculum change.
5. Provides the information necessary to determine areas in which the community may need to develop better health programs.

Contingenies
1. The list will be incomplete when first compiled. However, as faculty, students, and interested others stay alert to the continuing nature of this manual, agencies will continue to be added.
2. Addresses, telephone numbers, and persons both in authority and assigned as the school of nursing contact tend to change. Efforts will have to be made to keep the manual up to date. Spaces can be left on each page to accommodate changes.

NOTES

1. Chater, Shirley: A conceptual framework for curriculum development, Nursing Outlook **23**:428-433, July, 1975.
2. The exceptions referred to here are as follows:
    a. Brown, Esther L.: Nursing for the future, New York, 1948, Russell Sage Foundation.
    b. Wolf, Lulu K.: Nursing, New York, 1947, D. Appleton-Century Co., Inc.
3. Committee on Curriculum of the National League of Nursing Education: A curriculum guide for schools of nursing, ed. 3, New York, 1937, The League of Nursing Education.
4. Rituals differ from processes in that processes are dynamic (innovative), whereas rituals are static. Both processes and rituals have purpose and system. The purpose of rituals is sometimes forgotten, sometimes obsolete (they lack the feedback system or do not utilize the available feedback that makes change inevitable), but the system persists repetitiously into infinity. Processes, on the other hand, are always relevant to purposes, which in turn are always relevant to a definitive problem or need; therefore nursing curricula change in an endless variety of ways as needs and problems change.
5. Committee on Curriculum of the National League of Nursing Education, p. 10.
6. The authors referred to here include the following:
    a. Wolf, Sand, O.: Curriculum study in basic

nursing education, New York, 1955, G. P. Putnam's Sons.
    b. Bridgman, Margaret: Collegiate education for nursing, New York, 1953, Russell Sage Foundation.
    c. The Committee on the Function of Nursing: A program for the nursing profession, New York, 1948, The Macmillan Co.
    d. Montag, Mildred: Education of nursing technicians, New York, 1951, G. P. Putnam's Sons.
7. Lysaught, Jerome P., editor: An abstract for action, National Commission for the Study of Nursing and Nursing Education, New York, 1970, McGraw-Hill Book Co.
8. Brown, pp. 116-152.
9. Montag, Op. cit.
10. American Nurses' Association: Educational preparation for nurse practitioners and assistants to nurses: a position paper, New York, 1965, The Association, pp. 5, 6, 8, 9. (Reprinted with permission.)
11. Ibid., p. 1.
12. Chickering, Arthur W.: The best colleges have the least effect, Saturday Review, pp. 48-50, 54, Jan. 16, 1971.
13. Ibid., p. 48.

BIBLIOGRAPHY

American Nurses' Association: American Nurses' Association's first position paper on education for nursing, American Journal of Nursing **65**:106-111, Dec., 1965.

Bridgman, Margaret: Collegiate education for nursing, New York, 1953, Russell Sage Foundation.

Brown, Esther L.: Nursing for the future, New York, 1948, Russell Sage Foundation.

Christy, Teresa E.: Historical perspectives on accountability, In Williamson, Janet A., editor: Current perspectives in nursing education, the changing scene, vol. I, St. Louis, 1976, The C. V. Mosby Co., pp. 1-7.

Coe, Charlotte: One approach to the identification of essential content in baccalaureate programs in nursing, Bouler, Colo., Feb., 1967, Western Interstate Commission on Higher Education.

Committee on Curriculum of the National League of Nursing Education: A curriculum guide for schools of nursing, ed. 3, New York, 1937, The League.

Deloughery, Grace L., and Gebbie, Kristine M.: Political dynamics, impact on nurses and nursing, St. Louis, 1975, The C. V. Mosby Co.

Ettaro, Shirley: Educational accreditation and accountability in nursing. In Williamson, Janet A., editor: Current perspectives in nursing education, the changing scene, vol. I, St. Louis, 1976, The C. V. Mosby Co.

Johnson, Miriam M.: A sociological analysis of the nurse role. In Skipper, J. K., and Leonard, R. C., editors: Social interaction and patient care, Philadelphia, 1965, J. B. Lippincott Co., pp. 29-39.

Jourard, Sidney M.: The transparent self, rev. ed., New York, 1972, Van Nostrand-Reinhold Co.

Lippitt, Ronald, Watson, Jeanne, and Westley, Bruce: The dynamics of planned change, New York, 1958, Harcourt, Brace & World, Inc.

McCord, Arline, and McCord, William: Urban social conflict, St. Louis, 1977, The C. V. Mosby Co.

McCord, William, and McCord, Arline: American social problems, challenges to existence, St. Louis, 1977, The C. V. Mosby Co.

Reinhardt, Adine M., and Quinn, Mildred D., editors: Family-centered community nursing, a Sociocultural framework. Part 2. Culture: its influence upon the nurse, patient, and family, St. Louis, 1973, The C. V. Mosby Co.

Roemer, Milton I.: Rural health care, St. Louis, 1976, The C. V. Mosby Co.

Rogers, Martha E.: Nursing education for professional practice, presented at Alverno College, Milwaukee, Wis., Nov. 3, 1967.

Simms, Laura L.: The hospital staff nurse position as viewed by baccalaureate graduates in nursing, New York, 1963, Columbia University Press.

Smith, Alice L.: Microbiology and pathology, ed. 11, St. Louis, 1976, The C. V. Mosby Co.

Thompson, Daniel C.: Private black colleges at the crossroads, Westport, Conn., 1973, Greenwood Press, Inc.

Thompson, Lida F., Miller, Michael H., and Bigler, Helen F.: Sociology, nurses and their patients in a modern society, St. Louis, 1975, The C. V. Mosby Co.

Weaver, Jerry L.: National health policy and the underserved ethnic minorities, women, and the elderly, St. Louis, 1976, The C. V. Mosby Co.

Western Interstate Commission on Higher Education in Nursing: The graduate of baccalaureate degree nursing programs, Boulder, Colo., April, 1968, The Commission.

Wolf, Lulu K.: Nursing, New York, 1947, D. Appleton-Century Co., Inc.

4
CONCEPTUAL FRAMEWORK: THE STUDENT

Students are the hub around which the educational wheel turns. Almost every philosophy and/or conceptual framework contains some mention of responding to the individual needs of students. More and more programs are working toward a "transcultural" curriculum and are making efforts to utilize data about student ethnicity, personal preferences, characteristics, and demography to establish goals and plan learning programs. Knowledge about students is needed so that plans for student learning can progress along desired lines. For instance, if a school wishes to produce nurses who are professional, and if part of professionalism is accountability and autonomy, one must determine if the students entering nursing programs have as their characteristics assertiveness, autonomy, achievement, and dominance. If students entering a program are high in deference and abasement, training programs and reward systems for assertiveness and autonomy can be planned as integral parts of the curriculum. If the background of some students entering the nursing program is extremely different from the white middle class, programs can be planned that use the dialect, cultural norms and values, and cognitive style that are in keeping with the students' cultural, cognitive, and communication characteristics. Missionaries who enter other cultures study the sociology of the people they wish to serve so that the schools and health programs will be accepted by the

people and be successful. Yet in the United States white middle class ethnicity and cultural norms are often erroneously assumed for everyone. The United States is indeed a great potpourri of cultures, dialects, values, and religions. Each ethnic, social, economic, and religious group affects its members in ways that have significance for educators.

Group norms or subgroup norms give some guidelines to curriculum builders for direction, rewards, and learning structure. However, individual differences within groups are often as great as group differences from each other. One advantage of individually assessing each student entering a program is that it enables educators to modify the "usual" curriculum for individual students so that individual needs can be a bona fide stimulus to the teaching program.

Another aspect of the student category of the conceptual framework is learning theory. Teachers structure their teaching behaviors according to the propositions about learning that they think are congruent with the philosophy appropriate to the situation (setting), the students, and their own beliefs and abilities. Decisions about career mobility, open curriculum, modularization, course structure, content requirements, and teaching and learning strategies all have their decision guidelines in the concepts and theories about learning that faculty accept.

This chapter addresses the two topics

within the student category: student and faculty personality characteristics and demography. Personality characteristics are used here to mean personal preferences, character traits, and personality factors and patterns. Demography means statistical data about an individual's life and environment. Learning theory is also described in this chapter as part of the student category. Since learning theory is adapted and used in response to the needs, characteristics, and personal preferences of learner and teacher, it seems logical that it be placed here.

ASSESSING STUDENT-FACULTY CHARACTERISTICS

Faculty are the purveyors and students are the clients of the educational system. Relevance is measured not only by usefulness to society and the needs and trends of society but in usefulness to the students attending each nursing school. Students with different backgrounds, different experiences, and different characteristics need nursing curricula planned for their special profiles. A study done in the San Francisco Bay Area shows that different types of schools attract students with widely varying student characteristics.[1]

The associate degree program, when compared with either the diploma or the baccalaureate programs, was found to attract the oldest group of students, most of whom were married, who had permanent residence closest to the school, who generally had a lower high school grade average, who had a slightly lower immediate family income, whose parents had less formal schooling, who decided on nursing as a career at an older age, and most of whom intended to go immediately into hospital nursing after graduation.

In contrast, the diploma program attracted students who were the youngest, who predominantly were single, who had permanent residence farthest from the school, who formed the middle group between the associate degree and baccalaureate students in four characteristics—in

high school grade average, fathers' years of formal schooling, immediate family income, and age at which they decided on nursing as a career. Their mothers had slightly more formal education, and more of the students planned to continue schooling after graduation than either the associate degree or baccalaureate student groups.

The baccalaureate students formed the middle group in age, marital status, miles of permanent residence from the school, and mothers' years of formal education. These students had the highest high school grade average, had fathers with the most formal education, had slightly higher immediate family incomes, and had decided on nursing at the youngest age when compared with students from the associate degree and diploma programs.

Not only do students vary from one educational setting to another and from one geographical area to another but they vary from year to year if only in minute ways. Demographic surveys done on nursing majors at San Jose State University show some statistically significant differences in the population from year to year.[2] The findings of demographic surveys provide profiles of characteristics of the learner group that enable the curriculum builders to respond to each group's specific needs. Selecting or formulating an inventory form that can be used yearly to provide data about students for ongoing curriculum changes is one of the early tasks of the faculty. Prior to surveying students there are certain assurances that must be made in writing for the purpose of protecting the students. These ground rules are established within the limits of the law, the regulations of the institution, and within the practices of good research methodology. Some of the factors considered as contractual ground rules between the student and the curriculum building group are as follows:

1. Participation is voluntary, and grades or other factors necessary for continuation in the educational institution or

nursing major are not contingent on cooperation in data-gathering activities.

2. Data gathered for study purposes are confidential, and no data on individual students are released in any form to any person, including nursing school faculty, unless requested in writing by the student.

3. All data are treated as a statistical group.

4. Students' names are changed to code numbers, and the code numbers–name list data are kept in locked confidential files.

Most information is not of a private nature but assurance regarding confidentiality is provided as a general rule. Sometimes students feel highly concerned about giving personal information, and protective contracts increase the percentage of participating students.

Students are often interested in the statistical results of such studies, and data accrued from former classes provide students with familiarity about how the information will be used. Making the results of current and previous surveys available to interested students also increases the amount of participation.

Any survey of student characteristics begins with demography. There are several demographic survey forms on the market, or faculties may wish to compile their own. It is simple to make a list of the information desired and compile it in a way that permits easy keypunching so that computerization of data is simply achieved.

Faculty characteristics can be measured by some of the same tools used to measure student characteristics; however, some of the demographic measures need to be different. Faculty educational preparation, professional experience, special professional interest, and philosophy of education and nursing are areas of useful information that will enable a composite picture to be drawn of the school of nursing faculty.

One fairly common method used in assessing student and faculty characteristics

is the self-report personality inventory. There are a wide variety of these inventories on the market; they are easily administered and easily scored. When choosing an inventory, there are several criteria to be considered, as follows:

1. Ease of administration
2. Ease of scoring (purchasable hand or computer scoring programs)
3. Standardization
4. Availability of research data on use of the inventory with a variety of groups
5. Usefulness as a characteristics inventory, but not as a pathological diagnostic test
6. Clarity of interpretation
7. Economy, both in purchasing and scoring
8. Time of administration—no more than 1 to 1½ hours

For example, the Minnesota Multiphasic Inventory (MMPI) and the Edwards Personal Preference Schedule (EPPS) both meet the criteria of ease of administration, scoring, standardization, availability of research data, economy, and timing. Both, with some ease or little consultation, are readily interpreted.

However, the MMPI is primarily a test designed to assess personality characteristics that are psychopathological,[3] whereas the EPPS is devised to assess the strength of manifest needs. Many different scales for categorizing data from the MMPI have evolved through extensive research. Standardized results yield such data as health, psychosomatic symptoms, neurological disorders, motor disturbances, attitudes about sex, religion, politics, and society, as well as data about educational, marital, occupational, and family issues. Finally, the data will yield profiles related to most common neurotic or psychotic behaviors.[4]

The EPPS gives data about the strength of manifest needs. Achievement, deference, order, exhibition, autonomy, affiliation, intraception, succorance, dominance, abasement, nurturance, change, endurance, heterosexuality, and aggression are needs assessed by this instrument. The strength of needs is determined through a forced choice technique.[5] These characteristics are of great interest to nursing curriculum builders, whose curricular goals include developing behaviors of initiative, leadership, nurturance, and so forth. For example, a strong need to analyze the motives and feelings of self and others (intraception) becomes an important characteristic to which the curriculum can respond. Clearly the EPPS provides more useful data about student and/or faculty populations than does the MMPI.

The Personal Orientation Inventory (POI) is designed to measure the values and behaviors that are essential to the development of self-actualization. The POI has twelve scales: time competence, inner support, self-actualizing value, existentiality, feeling reactivity, spontaneity, self-regard, self-acceptance, nature of man, synergy, acceptance of aggression, and capacity for intimate contact. These scales are viewed as useful in assessing mental health and offering positive guides for growth during therapy. The POI is successfully used as a means for studying the level of self-actualization of individuals. It is based on the theoretical formulations of humanistic psychologists such as Maslow, Reisman, Rogers, and Perls. Nursing programs that base any of their conceptual frameworks on the works of humanistic psychologists may wish to consider the usefulness of this tool in assessing their students.

Personality assessments can provide a basis for building a curriculum to fit the needs of students and facilitate the development of nursing abilities that fulfill or channel their needs. Curricula may also be designed with the intent of strengthening or weakening manifested needs. Thus an assessment of personal characteristics can become a yardstick measurement by pretest and posttest comparison techniques.

Some other instruments available to the curriculum developer are the California Psychological Inventory, the Gordon Personal Inventory, the Gordon Personal Profile, the Eysenck Personality Inventory, and many more. The curriculum developer will need to determine what information is needed about students and faculty, survey the field of available instruments, and select those that meet the established criteria. The advice and counsel of testing specialists will be more valuable if the curriculum developer has definitive ideas about the data needed. Any good book on tests and measurements or psychological testing will give descriptive material about tests.

THINKING AND LEARNING

"Thinking" has as many meanings and as many definitions as "love." Thinking can vary from Walter Mitty daydreams to Newtonian insights. Both "thinking before you louse something up" and "keeping your head when all about you are losing theirs" are thinking. In other words, everything from inspiration to meditation has been commonly referred to as thinking. It has been construed to cover anything that occurs in one's head except, perhaps, headaches.

Thinking processes, or the cognitive processes, imply something else entirely: The simple expedient of linking the word "thinking" with the word "processes" gives the phrase another dimension. Thinking thus acquires the three characteristics of all processes: (1) thinking purposefully, (2) thinking systematically, and (3) thinking dynamically or creatively. In other words, the cognitive processes are goal oriented, have system and organization, and are always growing and changing.

Learning, on the other hand, is always used in connection with behavior. In nursing, because nursing is a practice discipline, the cognitive processes of thinking are inseparably linked, for all practical purposes, with doing. The cognitive processes of nursing are part and parcel of all practice skills. So for nursing the cognitive processes, thinking and the development of practice skills, are all covered under the general heading of learning. As with all processes, the more that can be discovered about the organization and system of the learning process the more educators will be able to help students use these processes efficiently.

The learning theory components of the conceptual framework are those components which influence the "thinking processes" used in the construction of the curriculum. Only a few of the cognitive theories inherent in nursing will be reviewed here; the interested reader will pursue the study of contributing theories in the fields of psychology, education, sociology, and physiology. This section deals with theories of learning and postulates from which course structure, content selection, and teaching strategies are generated.

THEORIES OF LEARNING

How people learn is of basic interest to curriculum builders, primarily because these theories help to dictate the selection, organization, and presentation of content. Learning theories help to determine how material is ordered and can dictate the types and kinds of courses. For instance, if one believes with Carl Rogers that truth is personal and only has significance for each person as it is self-discovered and self-experienced,[6] courses will be established that make it necessary for the learner to experience the content in either real or contrived situations. If one believes with Skinner that learning is largely a stimulus-response-reinforcement sequence,[7] courses will reflect that commitment by providing a stimulus, eliciting responses, and selectively rewarding the desired responses.

Definition of learning

Learning is a change in behavior, perception, insights, attitude, or a combination of these that can be repeated when the need is aroused.[8,9] This definition deletes changes of behavior that are a result of physical or emotional maturation and behaviors that are changes due to random

activity, sickness, or other temporary circumstances. It does not eliminate changes of behavior acquired through trial and accidental success, since the success acts as a reinforcer and causes the learner to repeat the activity (practice) and to be able to use the activity as necessary (permanence).

The change in behavior may or may not be directly observable; however, the effects of learning are always observable. For instance, Mary Jane learns that assessment is an essential part of the problem-solving process. The teacher cannot observe the actual ordering, categorizing, relating, and other cognitive activities involved in Mary Jane's cognition. But the teacher can see the effect of this "learning"; that is, Mary Jane can be observed as she visits her patient's room and assesses what equipment will be necessary to give morning care. Mary Jane can be seen asking questions and observing prior to making an assumption about the nature of a nursing problem. In short, in a increasing variety of situations, Mary Jane exhibits assessing behaviors, and as the *practice* of assessments "pays off" in more accurate problem solving, the success feedback acts as a reinforcer and the behavior is carried over into an increasing number of situations. The definition applies to information that may never be used in practice. Mary Jane can read in the newspaper that armadillos produce their young as identical quadruplets. She thinks that this is an interesting piece of information and she remembers it and can recall it. *The change of behavior* is that she does remember it; the observable change of behavior is that she can recall and relate it to another person. Since this is not information for which Mary Jane is likely to have much actual practical application, the behavior will not be observable unless she communicates it. Of course, it could be a useful non sequitur for dull parties. The *practice* is the repetition, the interest, the effort, or associations it took for Mary Jane to remember it, and the relative permanence of the learning is the fact that she can repeat this ephemeral memory gem when the need arises.

Structure of learning

Learning has three identifiable aspects, which exist regardless of the learning theory adopted. Learning has (1) an input aspect, (2) an operation aspect, and (3) a feedback aspect.[10] These aspects are variously called sequences or phases, but since both sequence and phase imply a serial order, "aspects" are preferable, since aspects can occur simultaneously. Graphically, learning is like a triangle with one side each for input, operation, and feedback (Fig. 4-1).

Input is the acquisition of information and the organization of the information into action hypotheses. These activities may be assessments, content information, instructions, recognition that a response is appropriate, or any of the cognitive activities associated with acquiring input.

Operation is the activity phase. It can be directly observable behavior, responses to the input, and/or interactions. It is practice. In memorization it is repetition (either oral, written, or cognitive); in discovery learning it is testing out ideas, either by putting them into action or by interacting with another person. The operation aspect of learning is *response*.

Feedback is the result of the operational test or the results of evaluation. The feed-

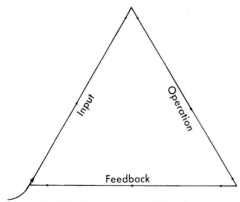

Fig. 4-1. Three aspects of learning.

back becomes input that confirms, alters, changes, or refutes the cognitive phase or input.

Two basic theories of learning

Most sources reduce theories of learning to two schools of thought[11]: (1) stimulus-response associations and (2) gestalt-field theories.

Stimulus-response associationism is most commonly associated with Pavlov and his salivating dog. Pavlov experimented with classical conditioning, or conditioning of existing autonomic responses to occur when elicited by a signal not normally responsible for the reaction. Pavlov taught his dog to salivate when a tuning fork was struck by pairing the striking of the tuning fork with the presentation of meat powder to the mouth of the dog. Soon the dog was salivating on hearing the tuning fork without the meat powder being presented.

Stimulus-response associationism has progressed far from Pavlov's early work, but the basic principle is derived from these experiments. Whereas classical conditioning deals with responses that are inevitable, or reflex responses, operant conditioning, instrumental conditioning, behavior modification, and other types of stimulus-response associationism or behaviorist learning theories deal with voluntary behavior. When the desired response occurs, whether accidental or guided, a reward which is meaningful to the learner is provided so that the probability of the desired response recurring is increased.

Basically, operant conditioning states that *any act may be altered in the frequency in which the act occurs by the consequences of the act.* Consequences are seen as reinforcing or punishing or as positive and negative reinforcements. Reinforcements may be in the form of social reinforcements, for example, status, approval, worthiness; physical reinforcements, for example, warmth, food, creature comforts; value reinforcements, for example, money, valued or desired objects; or internal reinforcements, for example, self-satisfaction and sense of accomplishment. The types of reinforcement may take any form and be classified in many ways.

Experiments demonstrate that spaced reinforcement tends to make the behavior more permanent than does total reinforcement. Behaviors taught through 100 percent reinforcement tend to be extinguished rather quickly if the reward is not presented consistently. Behaviors taught through the use of spaced reinforcement seem to be very difficult to extinguish.

Stimulus-response associationism theories deemphasize the role of the learner "comprehending" the total picture of the learning area, his insight into the learning situation, or his insight into his own behavior. Some theorists maintain that insight, mental discipline, and other forms of higher cognition enable the learner to be conditioned more rapidly but are unnecessary to behavioral engineering. Stimulus-response associationism treats each individual element of behavior separately, relating behaviors to each other, one link at a time, until the learner behaves as desired.

The Yale Learning Theory,[12] sometimes called the Hull-Dollard Theory of Learning, draws forth much of the behaviorist learning psychology. Keesing's[13] verbal description of the Yale theory is one of the clearest and most concise to be found in the literature. In summary, he states that learning behaviors are results of a drive or need to attain a goal or solve a problem. Anxiety rises when goals are established and are translated into action as a result of cues or stimuli. When the goal-response meets with reward, tension is reduced. The reduction of tension is a reinforcement that can "fix" the behavior into a habit. If the goal-response results in punishment (deprivation, failure, increase in tension), the response may either be discontinued or result in frustrations that can be translated into aggression or other compensatory outlets, for example, avoidance. Established behavior patterns (habits) will break down if they cease to bring reward. This opens the way to changes through any of the response guides—imitation of a model, random behavior, or cues from other available sources.

Gestalt-field theory is a theory of learning closely aligned with holism and process philosophy. It has as its salient feature man in his environment as a unit participating in what is called a *simultaneous mutual interaction*. This pnilosophy of learning conceives of perception as all the different ways one becomes familiar with his environment and not mere consciousness of his environment. Things and people are perceived differently by different individuals because their perception depends on the sum total of their life experiences and on how they perceive other things in their life space concomitantly. Whereas stimulus-response associationism emphasizes single units (one organism [human being], one stimulus, and one response and an effective reinforcer), cognitive field theory deals with the concept of *person* (meaning the individual) within his whole field (meaning total environment). Cognitive field theory proposes that hypotheses which help to determine causal interrelationships and organize facts to provide direction and predictability are the heart of a science. Lewin,[14] a major proponent and classical developer of cognitive field theory, states that reality for any one person is what that individual perceives and experiences it to be for himself. Nothing exists in and of itself to people; it exists as relative to a person's total experience. Disney portrayed this concept well when he had Bambi perceive the skunk as a black and white striped "live" flower because he saw the skunk in a field of flowers. Forever after, if you remember, the skunk was named "Flower." The only reality that any human being can ever know is that which he interprets reality to be. Each individual "sizes up" things and situations so that "what do you make of that?" becomes indeed a query of "what is your reality in this situation?" Cognitive field theory maintains that learning is a matter of understanding relationships within a total "field" or area. A thing is what it is because it exists in relationship to other things. For instance, the state of "sickness" does not exist except by comparison or in relation to the state of "health." To understand the concept of sickness, one must see it in the context of health. Learning, to the gestalt-field theorist, takes place when data harmonize, or "add up," when all pertinent facts are taken into consideration and insight is achieved. Wholeness is important to these theorists, and although deemphasized by stimulus-response associationists, the cognitive processes (that is, insight, ordering, relating, predicting, and producing situations) are of great importance. Understanding and using these cognitive processes steers human actions.

In gestalt psychology, behavior is purposive or intelligent. Humans can pursue long-term and short-term goals (fulfill needs); therefore, behaviors or interactions within an individual's field occur in expectation of goal fulfillment. This expectation does not mean realization of goal fulfillment but simply that that interaction will in some way contribute to the attainment of a long-term or short-term goal. Success is attained by those who perceive of and interact with things in their environment appropriate to goal attainment.

The concept of "self" is important to cognitive-field theory. Self is an emerging, becoming concept that is *always* in the making. Thus growth and development are important aspects of this learning theory, which perceives four ways in which the self is always under construction.[15]

1. Goal realization through one's own efforts, responsibility for one's own acts, pride in one's accomplishments, and self-blame for one's failures
2. Values and goals realized and enacted, affirmed and revised, in one's transactions with other people and within one's life space or field
3. Formation of an "ideal self" against which self-measurements and eval-

uations can be made (much like the development of conscience)
4. Prominence of one's "self" in memories of the past and in fantasies and anticipations of the future

A learning theory synthesis for nursing education

The application of learning theories to the practice of nursing and to the teaching of the practice of nursing makes nursing educators acutely aware of the inadequacy of either extreme of the two basic schools of thought about learning. Both theories have a sound basis in logic and experimentation and a high rate of success when used in educational practice. Most nursing teachers are not purists but pragmatists, appropriating the parts of theories that seem reasonable and satisfactory and discarding those that are inconclusive, incomplete, or impractical at any given time. Thus, by necessity, most nursing educators are educational eclectics, and they attempt to choose from both schools of thought those parts that seem most reliable. There are some agreements among educators about how learning takes place that are found in both schools of thought.

Several sources have organized postulates about learning that appear to have value for the teacher and are synthesized from both learning theories. Watson[16] compiled such a list, as did Gagné.[12] Hilgard[18] listed fourteen points on which all learning theorists agree. Bigge[19] has written a chapter entitled "What Principles of Learning Are Commonly Accepted by Psychologists?" that is very useful to nursing faculties involved in curriculum building. Below is a list taken from these and other sources that will be particularly useful to the nursing educator.

LEARNING PROPOSITIONS, ECLECTICALLY SELECTED AND ORDERED IN OPERATIONAL SEQUENCE

1. *People learn when they encounter a problem or need. This need creates anxiety, which in turn produces drive and motiva-*

tion. Watson said that "The superiority of man over calculating machines is more evident in the formation of questions than in the working out of answers."[20] Questions do not occur until there is some reason for them to occur. This reason for thinking is an obstacle or difficulty in reaching a goal, a puzzle or challenge or a basic interest, all of which are here classified as "problems."

The extent or limits of the felt need to learn or the perception of the problem is influenced by the student's ability to perceive the problem and establish realistic goals. Sometimes this ability is called readiness to learn; sometimes it is called ability, capacity, or individual learner history. Each learner is different. Capacity for learning is largely a matter of (a) maturation or developmental level, (b) physical ability and disability (including both neuromuscular and intellectual capacity), (c) learner personal characteristics (that is, perseverance, values, self-image, imagination, competitiveness, ethnicity, and so forth), and (d) previous learning, or the attaining of concepts and principles basic to the recognition and articulation of the problem and goal.

Goal setting is inherent in learning. Problems and goals are opposite sides of the same coin. A goal is what one desires to achieve; a problem is what inhibits the goal achievement. Turning that statement around, a goal is the removal or absence of the problem. Goal achievement and insoluble obstacles are incompatible, so to set a goal greater than can ever be achieved does not keep one striving, as is commonly thought; instead, it defeats, frustrates, and reduces ambition or motivation. Goals that are *possible* are desirable goals and are derived from problems that have a solution. As knowledge and skills mature, more and more "problems" have *possible* solutions, and, as stated earlier, education or learning is the art of the "possible."

In any activity of nursing practice, if the goal or purpose of the activity is clearly identified and articulated, when interrup-

tions or inhibitions to goal achievement occur, the problem is more easily identified. Learning goals expressed in desired behaviors provide both the learner and the teacher with criteria for determining success and with material for identifying problems or inhibitors to the attainment of the goal.[21]

Motivation is a product of mild or moderate anxiety. (Panic or acute anxiety paralyzes, narrows, or distorts perception and response so that motivation is displaced by more pressing needs.[22])

Anxiety states that correlate with intense motivation may reduce the rate of progress toward goal achievement by channeling learning energy into the anxiety system so that activity is focused on emergency coping mechanisms for the anxiety rather than for progress toward the goal or solution of the underlying problem. At this point the teacher activities are centered around anxiety reduction and strengthening coping mechanisms so that the learner can refocus his energy on goal attainment.

On the other hand, crisis—a state of extremely high anxiety and acute problems—provides a fertile field for learning. The person in crisis needs solutions so desperately that he is highly receptive to cues and models. The preceptor who can take the person in crisis through the activities necessary to resolve the crisis has capitalized on a state of readiness to learn and provided the learner with a real situation in which learned behaviors are instantly useful and for which the payoff is immediate and large.

Although anxiety may result from encountering a problem, sometimes the anxiety is so mild that it is not readily observable or it may or may not be within the level of awareness of the learner. Encountering a problem, or recognizing a goal, is always accompanied by an internal "toning up," a sharpening of wits, an increase in alertness that is called anxiety. McDonald calls this anxiety state an "intrapersonal energy change."[23]

Anxiety is the precursor to motivation.

McDonald[24] characterizes motivation as a condition necessary for learning but not sufficient to make learning occur. He defines motivation as having three characteristics: (a) an intrapersonal energy change, (b) affective arousal, and (c) anticipatory goal reaction. The energy change may be caused by autonomic response mechanisms (as with fear), basic life support needs, or the exact nature of the causal sequence of the energy change may be, and usually is, unknown. The "affective arousal" is a feeling, state, or emotion. This state may not be conscious, it may not be strong, or it may be exceedingly intense and be well within the level of awareness. The "anticipatory goal reaction" is the purposefulness of motivation. Motivation is goal oriented, since it is through movement toward the goal that anxiety is reduced and satisfaction or pleasure is achieved. The consequence is that goal achievement returns the arousal state to normal and reduces the energy change to its prior level.

Motivation is extrinsic or intrinsic. Extrinsic motivation is aroused by someone else; intrinsic motivation arises from a self-felt need. For example, using the threat of a test is a teacher-imposed motivation device and is therefore extrinsic; arranging the learning environment so that the learner encounters a challenging problem produces intrinsic motivation. Whether or not the motivation is intrinsic or extrinsic, the three characteristics just listed adequately describe the state called motivation.

Motivation is closely aligned with self-image. The learner who sees himself as able to attain a goal (solve a problem) is free (unafraid) to respond to the energy change and need arousal. Learners who are perceived by their meaningful others as unable to achieve goals will adopt that self-image. Teachers and peers tend to be meaningful others. Religious, racial, and ethnic minority groups tend to be perceived by majority group members as "different" learners, therefore "slower" learners. Thus this view is internalized and becomes a

self-evaluation, and learning motivation is critically damaged.[25]

Success, rewards, and other reinforcement mechanisms, even though they occur after a move toward the goal has occurred, provide a boost for further motivation. Reinforcement, in whatever form it occurs, feeds back into the energy system of learning and makes learning motivation self-renewing. Failure works in an opposing manner.[22] Repeated failure reduces motivation, and in the failure-conscious individual the threat of failure is, in itself, a deterrent to motivation and conflicts with the "need arousal" component of motivation.

Proposition 1 describes four consecutive events, each contiguous and contingent on the next. These four conditions or behaviors necessary to learning are illustrated as follows with an elaboration of the nature of motivation:

PROBLEM → NEED → ANXIETY → MOTIVATION

Intrapersonal energy change	Affective arousal	Anticipatory goal reaction

2. *Motivation and drive produce a learner need for information, cues, models, or opportunity to discover (experiment) that enables progression toward goals or problem solutions.* Motivation, the state of affective arousal and goal anticipation, leads to activities that the learner thinks will enable progress toward the goal or solution to the problem. These activities are the ways people seek to solve problems or "learn." Some of the learning activities that may lead to goal attainment are (a) information that can be translated by the learner into predictive principles or hypotheses about goal attainment and thus provide him with alternatives for action; (b) cues or some message that will make him select one solution rather than an alternative (cues are hints or stimuli that provoke associations so that the learner thinks of possible solutions to his problems); (c) models that will provide a pattern or behavioral guide for the problem solution (models, whether they be living, replica, or

symbolic, provide a basis for "monkey see, monkey do" or "map following" problem solving, which, if rewarded by success or valued gains, becomes a learned behavior); and (d) opportunity to discover ways in which a problem may be solved (discovery or experimentation is the trial of a variety of alternatives that the learner thinks provide possible solutions to the problem).

Motivation is goal oriented. The activities through which the goal is hoped to be achieved may take many forms. These are goal-seeking activities. *The "content of learning" takes place between the motivation aspect of learning and the arrival at the effective solution.* Problems are seldom solved in one giant step. Each learner movement toward the goal is a learning stage.

3. *Progression toward goal achievement is promoted by moving from the familiar to the unfamiliar and actively involving the learner in the learning activities.* Gestalt-field theorists support the position that progress toward goals is achieved when the learner can attain insight or perceive new patterns in ideas that provide a pathway to a solution. For this to happen, there must be sufficient background and preparation so that the concepts necessary to the problem solution have been mastered. Additionally, the relationships operative among the concepts germane to the whole situation must be available. These two provisions enable the learner to arrange the key elements in the problem into new elements that are alternatives for solving the problem. In other words, the learner must have the background knowledge or primary concepts, have available all the relevant facts, theories, and principles, and be able to use this knowledge to hypothesize about solutions to the problem. Stimulus-response associationists take the position that if each movement which is toward goal achievement is rewarded, the goal will be attained. The commonality between the positions is that learning best progresses from simple learning tasks to more complex learning tasks. "Simple" is

a relevant term and depends on the level of complexity on which the learner is operating when the problem is encountered. To the learner the "known" or "familiar" is usually the simple and the "unknown" or "unfamiliar" is the complex. But whether or not the simple or known is a mastered task, an insight or concept attained, progression toward the goal is from the simple-familiar to the complex-unfamiliar.

Learning theorists dwell at length on the learner's previous experiences because they determine the learner's prior conditioning or his prior concept formation. Previous experience provides the foundation for current learning by dictating what is familiar, what is already achieved, and therefore what the learner is ready to achieve. It includes not only previous learning experience but also previous living, that is, cultural conditioning values, self-image, conceptualizing, and other theory-building stages of all kinds.

Active involvement in learning activities is fundamental to learning regardless of the theoretical position. However, the definition of "active involvement" differs from theorist to theorist. Both schools of thought accept the idea that the learner cannot learn optimally by sitting passively and absorbing material presented in lectures, books, movies, and tape recordings. The learner who can engage in activities other than passive ones will learn more, faster, and better. Some possible examples of activities (depending on the school of learning theory subscribed to) are (a) participating in goal setting, (b) arranging known concepts into new patterns or hypothesizing, (c) trying out a variety of possible problem solutions, (d) devising ways a concept can be used in a variety of life situations, and (e) participating with a group in solving simulated problems by exchanging information, devising predictive principles, innovating possible alternatives, and weighing and choosing courses of action.

Some people believe that active involvement is primarily a motivation booster. Active involvement in learning is more than that; it is a learning "fixative" that enables the learner to experience the behaviors personally rather than vicariously and thus to make his own judgment about their usefulness, applicability, and durability. The reward system becomes his own, and the satisfaction, pleasure, or anxiety reduction that comes with goal achievement is self-experienced. A variety of active learning techniques expands both the variety and degree of new concept formation and the many applications of those concepts. The question of whether real or contrived learning situations are better is moot. Both have value, and the choice is determined by the needs of the learner and the conditions of the material to be learned.

4. *Reinforcement of desired behaviors increases movement toward the goal; conversely, absence of feedback of any kind prevents progress, and consistently negative feedback (punishment), deliberate or accidental, leads to frustration, aggression, and avoidance. Progress then halts, and problems are not solved.*

Feedback is information perceived by the learner during and after some act of the operational phase of learning. This information may be interpreted by the learner as positive, negative, neutral, or additive. If it is additive, it provides the learner with more information useful in progressing toward the goal. If the feedback is interpreted by the learner as positive, the feedback will have reward effects. If it is negatively interpreted, it will have punitive effects. Feedback may be extrinsic in that it originates from others, from machines, or from other sources outside the learner, or it may be intrinsic, arising from within the learner. If there is no feedback of any kind, there will be no learning.

Reinforcement is attained when the learner achieves something of value to him. The private nature of reinforcement is never more obvious than when an individual pursues something of interest only to him

in social isolation and enjoys achieving a goal. Every worker of crossword puzzles has his ability to work crossword puzzles improved by the correct completion of a puzzle. Insight and the recognition of relationships and patterns can be very reinforcing. Reinforcement to one individual may not be reinforcement to another. Because of the commonality of human needs, some reinforcements are more or less universal; however, others are rewards only to persons of specific cultures or are completely individual in nature. For instance, reward with a better grade than one's peers is often a reinforcing attainment in the majority American group, but to the Navajo Indian, whose culture does not develop a value for competition, attaining a grade better than one's peers has no reinforcing value—quite the opposite, it can be a matter for shame. Social reinforcement, through attaining prestige, recognition, or position, or through attaining approval from someone who is meaningful, is the most common reinforcer in learning situations. Tangible reinforcers, such as tokens, candy, food, or money, provide concrete ways of fixing desired behavior. Some general guidelines for reinforcements are as follows:

a. Success that is recognized by the learner as success is reinforcing. Goal attainment reduces anxiety and brings about a state of satisfaction. This state of satisfaction is rewarding and is thus a reinforcing phenomenon.

b. Rewards that closely follow the desired behavior or movement toward the goal are more reinforcing than rewards that are removed in time from the behavior.

c. Rewards desired by the learner are more reinforcing than general, or routine, rewards.

d. Rewards or punishments are consequences of behaviors, and the clearer the causal connection or correlation the greater the effect on the behavior.

e. Behaviors learned with spaced or intermittent reinforcement are more difficult to eradicate than behaviors learned with consistent and regular reinforcement.[26]

f. Behaviors that receive no reinforcement decrease in frequency and finally cease.

g. Punishment is a behavioral consequence and can be deliberately imposed (as spanking or privilege withdrawal), accidental (falls, automobile crashes from a careless moment), or a natural consequence of a poor choice (eating hot food before it has been allowed to cool properly).

h. Punishment is a behavior reinforcer. It may reinforce avoidance of similar situations, avoidance of the punishing mechanism or person, aggression (attack on or destruction of the punishing mechanism—as when an individual hurts himself on a door and then kicks it), or the person may retreat or withdraw from learning situations.

i. Punishment may or may not eradicate undesirable behaviors, but punishment *does not* promote movement *toward* goal achievement. Forward movement toward problem solutions is a product of reward.

5. *Repetition with feedback and consequent improvement (practice) accompanied by reinforcement develops behavior habits and patterns.* Repetition is an important aspect of learning, especially in the learning of skills. Overlearning to instill a habit has been the bane of every nursing student's existence. The problem in nursing is not how to provide for repetition and overlearning but when, where, and how to control repetition. A student need not give morning care every morning for several years to attain mastery of the skills involved in basic hygienic care. Still, the nursing care motor skill aspect of nursing is best translated into behavior habits if repetition with reinforcements is provided.

Long-term repetition of the same materials has little value for learning beyond habit fixation. To be valuable, repetition must have an improvement aspect. When repetition contains an improvement aspect, it becomes practice. Each repetition of the behavior that is accompanied by a feedback and correction cycle enables the learner to improve, if only slightly, each time he performs the behavior.[27]

6. *Spaced or distributed recall or more and varied opportunities for application enable the learner to identify central concepts, verify principles, make generalizations and discriminations, and retain learned behaviors.* Learning was defined earlier in this chapter as "a change in behavior, perception, insights, attitudes or a combination of these that can be repeated when the need is aroused." Repetition on demand or some degree of permanency in recall is a characteristic of learned behavior. Studies indicate that recall of "facts" decreases at a high rate. At the conclusion of a course that asks primarily that the student learn facts, the learner can remember about three fourths of the material; at the end of a year he can remember about one half of the material; and at the end of two years he can remember about one fourth of the material.[28] Studies on retention of facts are not conclusive, but one could presume that retention is poor. Conversely, research indicates that the more meaningful the material is the more material is united by clear relationships among facts, and the more behaviors are supported by generalizations, rules, and principles the greater the retention will be. McDonald[29] goes so far as to say that the learning of any kind of organizing principle contributes to retention. Application of learning to new problems provides the student with the opportunity to verify uniting principles and self-appropriate the learning. This "test through application" ensures a high rate of retention.[30]

Recall, and/or application, is the operational phase of learning. It is this facet of learning that results in feedback. Feedback offers the opportunities to make corrections and finer discriminations and to improve skill. Feedback enables the retest of the organizing principles and variations and revisions to accommodate new insights or new theories.

Repetition is most effective if a learned behavior can be duplicated several times when first learned and then repeated intermittently.

7. *Success (achievement of goals) leads to tolerance of failure, realistic self-assessment, realistic goal setting, and continual evaluation.* Success stimulates more success because it enables the learner to develop his learning potential realistically. Recognition that the goal has been achieved necessitates clearly articulated descriptions of goal attainment. The learner who can recognize that he has solved his problem successfully, or performed the necessary behaviors, has access to immediate, meaningful feedback, immediate reinforcement (satisfaction, reduction of anxiety, or pride in accomplishment). The nurse who recognizes that she has met the patient's needs or performed a procedure using good technique is not only a safe nurse but a confident one. Confidence exists only when the learner has experienced enough success to be unafraid to try, knowing that eventually he will succeed. Objective evaluation of one's own problem solving is possible when error or failure is not interpreted as incompetence but simply as a trial or test that indicates some other behavior as more appropriate.

Recognition of success is a product of clearly articulated behavioral objectives or clearly articulated descriptions of desired outcomes.

HEURISTICS

Heuristic 1: *Studying the characteristics of the student (client) of the curriculum*

Activity. This activity requires that some form be created to provide the faculty with information about the student who is the client of the educational system. This form needs to be fairly short, clear, and easily keypunched for computerization and to require little time of the student.

Early in the school year the forms can be given out in class and 10 to 20 minutes provided for filling out the form. A thorough explanation of the use to which the information will be put and how the data will be tabulated helps to assure the students of its usefulness and their anonymity, therefore increasing the number of students willing to provide the data. If there are students who refuse, recontact them in several months to see if they have reconsidered. When charts tabulating data are made, take them along when making explanations to students. This will increase participation.

Materials
1. A dittoed, mimeographed, or printed student characteristics form
2. Twenty minutes of class time
3. Computer

Procedure
1. Create or buy a form that is programmed for keypunching or so that students can put their answers directly on computer data cards.
2. Have several people critique the form to ensure that all the essential information is asked for and no nonessential information is requested.
3. Run a small sample to check the program (do this only if you think it would add to the validity of what you are doing).
4. Have the form duplicated in a quantity that will make the forms available for the number of years you are going to survey the student population.
5. Ask for class time from teachers; 20 minutes should be sufficient.
6. Explain the study to the students. Make the protection of identity explicit, and provide illustration about the use of data and its relevance to curriculum construction.
7. Distribute the forms, allow time to finish, and collect the forms.
8. Computer-tabulate the results and make charts and graphs, as well as descriptive paragraphs, so that the student population characteristics are plainly available for use.
9. Distribute the results to all faculty and interested persons.
10. Repeat for each class of nursing majors as long as data are desired.

Puissance
1. Enables rapid collection of data with little effort.
2. Provides data necessary to make the curriculum relevant to the student population.
3. Enables subsequent studies to be done correlating achievement with specific student characteristics.
4. Provides a baseline from which comparisons in student populations can be made over a number of years.
5. Makes possible comparisons among student populations of different schools of nursing.

Contingencies
1. Some students believe that the required information is encroaching on personal data and will refuse to give it.
2. A higher incidence of ethnic minorities refuse to

Example

Name _____

Code No. _____

STUDENT CHARACTERISTIC FORM*

Information:
1. This questionnaire provides data for School of Nursing Curriculum Development. An ongoing assessment of the people for whom the curriculum is devised (student characteristics and demographic data) forms one of the most essential and basic contextual factors for curriculum change.
2. All data are confidential and will be used for curriculum study purposes only. Your name is code numbered, and individual identity will be masked by statistically treating the data.
3. If you prefer not to participate, simply write "Refuse" and your name. No one except project staff will have knowledge about whether or not you are participating in our study.
4. Thank you for helping in the curriculum study.

Directions:
1. Circle the number of the answer that applies to you.
2. Fill in the blank where blanks are provided in lieu of choices.
3. You may omit any question(s) that you prefer not to answer.
   _____ 1. Student's age: In months (figure to September 15th of the year of entry to nursing courses at this college).
   _____ 2. Ethnicity: (1) Caucasian. (2) Oriental. (3) Afro-American. (4) Filipino. (5) Mexican-American.
   _____ 3. Marital status on Sept. 15: (1) Single. (2) Married. (3) Divorced. (4) Widowed.
   _____ 4. Children: (1) Yes. (2) No.
   _____ 5. Number of children (0+).
   _____ 6. Type of previous education: (1) University. (2) College. (3) Junior College. (4) Mixed.
   _____ 7. Number of years of higher education before taking nursing courses at this college: (1) Two. (2) Three. (3) Four. (4) B.A. (5) Or more.
   _____ 8. Location of previous education: (1) In-state. (2) Out-of-state. (3) Mixed.
   _____ 9. Previous nursing school experience: (1) Yes. (2) No.
   _____10. Previous work in nursing: (1) No experience (this includes anyone who has worked in a hospital, but not with patients in a "caring for" task. Red Cross does not count). (2) Volunteer (any work at all as a nursing volunteer for 6 months during high school or one summer as a Candy Striper, etc.). (3) Volunteer extensive (anything more than above). (4) Salaried nurse's aide work. (5) Work as a licensed vocational nurse. (6) Work as a registered nurse.
   _____11. Previous work experience: (1) No experience. (2) Minor (babysitting, mother's helper, housework, or one full-time, 2-month summer job). (3) Minimum (one full-time summer job and regular hours of work, every week for a year or two). (4) Medium (full-time, or thereabout, summer jobs for at least five summers, and regular hours). (5) Maximum (1 or 2 years' full-time job).
   _____12. Number of siblings (number of children in family *including* student): _____ .
   _____13. Sibling order. Are you the (1) Only child? (2) Youngest? (3) Middle? (4) Oldest? (5) Other?
   _____14. Parents' marital status: (1) Married. (2) Divorced. (3) Widowed.
   _____15. Divorced: (1) No. (2) 5 years or less. (3) 5-10 years. (4) 10-15 years. (5) 16 years or more. (6) No information.
   _____16. Mother living: (1) Yes. (2) Dead 5 years or less. (3) Dead 5-10 years. (4) Dead 10-15 years. (5) Dead 16 years or more. (6) No information.
   _____17. Father living: (1) Yes. (2) Dead 5 years or less. (3) Dead 5-10 years. (4) Dead 10-15 years. (5) Dead 16 years or more. (6) No information.
   _____18. Did the parent with whom you live(d) remarry? (1) Yes. (2) No. (3) Not pertinent.

*Modified from University of California School of Nursing Curriculum Research Project and used with permission of Dr. J. Bailey, February, 1972.

Example—cont'd

_____19. Mother's years of education: (1) Professional training. (2) College graduate. (3) Partial college training. (4) High school plus occupational training. (5) High school graduate. (6) 8-12 years' schooling. (7) Less than 8 years' schooling. (8) No information.

20. Mother's occupation: _____ .

_____21. Mother in medical profession: (1) Nurse's aide or L.V.N. (2) R.N.–Diploma. (3) Baccalaureate nurse. (4) Dental hygienist. (5) Physician. (6) Nutritionist. (7) Other. (8) Mother not in medical profession. (9) No information.

_____22. Mother employed: (1) Never. (2) Employed since student was infant. (3) Employed after student's entry into grammar school. (4) After entry into high school. (5) After high school graduation. (6) Employed during infancy. (7) Employed during grammar school. (8) No information.

_____23. Amount mother employed: (1) Intermittently. (2) Part time. (3) Full time. (4) Not employed. (5) No information.

_____24. Father's years of education: (1) Professional training. (2) College graduate (even though father may have two different degrees, B.A., B.D., so that years count up, he still only gets "college graduate"). (3) Partial college training. (4) High school plus occupational training. (5) High school graduate. (6) 8-12 years' schooling. (7) Less than 8 years' schooling.

25. Father's occupation: _____ .

_____26. Father in medical profession: (1) Physician. (2) Dentist. (3) Pharmacist. (4) Veterinarian. (5) Chiropractor. (6) Optometrist. (7) Other. (8) Father not in medical profession. (9) No information.

_____27. Grade point average on entry to Junior Level Nursing: Drop third number; if 5 or more, add 1 to second number, e.g., 3.24 = 3.2, 3.35 = 3.4.

_____28. Current work hours per week: (1) Under 8 hours. (2) 8-12 hours. (3) 13-16 hours. (4) 17-20 hours. (5) 21-30 hours. (6) 31-39 hours. (7) 40 hours or more.

_____29. Units of credit in which currently enrolled: (1) Under 5. (2) 5-8. (3) 8-10. (4) 10-12. (5) 12-15. (6) 15-17. (7) Over 17. (8) Only nursing courses. (9) Nursing and other courses.

_____30. Source of financial support: (1) Self only. (2) More than 50% self-supporting. (3) Less than 50% self-supporting. (4) 100% supported by other than self.

_____31. Father's yearly income: (1) Under and up to $3,000. (2) $3-5,000. (3) $5-10,000. (4) $10-15,000. (5) $15-20,000. (6) $20-30,000. (7) $30-40,000. (8) $40-50,000. (9) Over $50,000.

_____32. Religion: (1) Catholic. (2) Protestant. (3) Jewish. (4) Buddhist. (5) Islamic. (6) Other.

_____33. Enrolled in work study program? (1) Yes. (2) No.

_____34. Enrolled in educational opportunity program? (1) Yes. (2) No.

give the information than middle-class whites.

3. The accuracy of the data must be taken at face value, since there are no cross-validation techniques.

4. Occupations and religions have proved to be difficult to categorize and program. The question on religion provides no indication of the extent to which the religion is practiced, and "Protestant" is too broad a category to be of much use when speculating on the effect the religion may have had on the values of the individual.

Heuristic 2: _Generating propositions of learning._

This heuristic evolves in several stages with the ultimate goal of selecting learning theories that the faculty believes are workable in their situation. Selecting theories of learning for a curriculum is an educational review, a negotiation, and a compromise situation.

Establishing an acceptable group of learning propositions for any group of nursing educators is difficult for several reasons: (1) Faculty come from a variety of educational backgrounds. (2) Faculty have a wide variety of teaching styles. (3) The implications of various theories of learning require some change in teaching activities for all faculty. (4) The implications of adoption of certain learning theories are seldom completely clear until after the curriculum begins to evolve and teaching strategies are being devised. (5) Teachers seldom have a clear idea about their own philosophy of education and belief in certain aspects of learning theories and therefore find it difficult to be explicit about learning propositions on which they are willing to agree.

Once a skeleton learning theory or series of learning propositions is spelled out, it can be altered and changed as the group grows and becomes clearer on

Example 1. Questionnaire

To: Faculty
From: _____
Re: Learning theories for our conceptual framework

In the space provided below please write your beliefs about teaching and learning. The suggested topical notations are simply a way of steering your thinking into areas; if there are thoughts and beliefs you have that do not seem to fit the categories, place them under "other."

What do you think and/or believe about:
What learning is?

What the role of the teacher is?

What makes learning take place?

What inhibits learning?

What produces skill?

Is there anything about learning that is specifically applicable to learning nursing?

What is the best way to ensure retention?

What is the role of the learner or learning group?

Example 1. Questionnaire—cont'd

What thought do you have about strategies for implementing your philosophy of learning?

What do you believe about motivation?

How do you "teach" creativity?

What are your other thoughts and beliefs?

its theoretical base. This heuristic is devised to facilitate the process of identifying a series of learning propositions on which the faculty can build the nursing courses, devise the learning activities, and plan teaching strategies.

Activity. This activity is designed to enable the group to express their beliefs about learning and teaching, to disseminate information about learning theories, to stimulate discussions about learning theories, and to build a provisional set of learning propositions on which the curriculum can be built. To arrive at a set of learning propositions for the conceptual framework of the curriculum requires several stages and a minimum of two discussion periods.

Materials

1. A copy of the questionnaire in Example 1 for each participant
2. Copies of the compiled responses for each participant
3. A list of propositions for agreement-disagreement discussion for each participant (Example 2)
4. A copy of the propositions to be discussed for each participant (Example 3)
5. A copy of the first draft propositions for each participant (Example 4)
6. A copy of the tentative or provisional learning propositions for the conceptual framework for each participant

Procedure

1. Circulate a questionnaire similar to Example 1.

Ask for thoughts about learning philosophies and theories that faculty members like and use.
2. Provide at least a week for responding.
3. While the faculty is responding to the questionnaire, search the literature for learning propositions that will provide a basis for discussion.
4. Collect the faculty responses.
5. Compile the faculty responses into one document. It is very important that all faculty members get a copy of the compilation without extraneous materials from other sources. This document helps faculty to "touch base" with each other and reinforces the fact that there are more commonalities than differences. So much work will be spent in resolving differences that a reference point for commonalities is important to reduce aloneness.
6. Compile a list of learning propositions from both faculty and other sources, as in Example 2.
7. Ask for responses within a week.
8. Tabulate results.
9. Delete all propositions that have consensual disagreement.
10. Compile in a group all propositions with consensual agreement.
11. List those propositions that need discussion and decision, as described in Example 3.
12. Conduct a discussion along the lines described in Example 3.

Example 2

To: Faculty
From: _____
Re: Developing propositions about learning for our framework

The following statements about teaching-learning are compiled from the literature and from your statements on the distributed questionnaire forms. Numerals at the end of each statement refer to the source from which it was derived, that is, (1) Hilgard, (2) Watson, (3) Faculty questionnaires, and (4) Bigge.

On the left-hand side of each page there are places for you to mark "Agree," "Disagree," and "Discuss." Those propositions about which you have a consensus of agreement will be grouped; those about which you disagree as a group will be dropped entirely; those propositions that you wish to discuss and/or show no consensus about will be negotiated.

Please turn your papers back by _____ (date) so that we can tabulate your responses and produce the document from which we will conduct our discussions on _____ (date).

LEARNING PROPOSITION RESPONSE FORM
(Sample only. There are usually many more propositions to be included.)

Agree	Disagree	Discuss	
_____	_____	_____	1. Absorbing input through reading, lecture, television, audio cassettes, movies, and other information sources is better facilitated through answering questions about the material to be learned than by viewing-listening and reviewing-listening. (2, 4)
_____	_____	_____	2. Active learning—the use of processes and information—is preferable to passive reception of information. (1)
_____	_____	_____	3. Practice (repetition utilizing feedback and improvement in skill each time) is essential to the development of skill, or in memorization of facts. (1)
_____	_____	_____	4. Repetition without reinforcement or improvement does not produce learning of desired behaviors. (2)
_____	_____	_____	5. Students learn from one another. There are, within every student group, a wide variety of knowledges, skills, and resources; most often students can learn more easily from one of their own group than they can from strangers or from a teacher. (2)
_____	_____	_____	6. The size of the student group determines the teaching strategies that are effective. (3)
_____	_____	_____	7. Success is the best reinforcer, and a backlog of successes provides a tolerance for failure so that a "failure pattern" is not established. (1)
_____	_____	_____	8. Learning nursing is independent of clinical area; that is, no clinical area is basic to any other clinical area. (3)
_____	_____	_____	9. Learning concepts are in modules, not units. (3)
_____	_____	_____	10. Some modules are basic to other modules; many are not. (3)
_____	_____	_____	11. Some modules cluster in interrelated groups; some stand alone and can be acquired independently of each other as needed. (3)

REFERENCES FOR QUESTIONNAIRE
1. Hilgard, Ernest R.: Theories of learning, ed. 2, New York, 1956, Appleton-Century-Crofts, pp. 586-587.
2. Watson, Goodwin: "What psychology can we feel sure about?" Teachers College Record **61**:253-257, May, 1960.
3. Faculty statements.
4. Bigge, Morris L.: Learning theories for teachers, ed. 3, New York, 1976, Harper & Row, Publishers.

Example 2—cont'd

Agree	Disagree	Discuss	
———	———	———	12. Personal characteristics (such as aggressiveness, competitiveness, initiative, and strength of felt need to achieve) influence learning. (2)
———	———	———	13. Content can be taught in some intellectual form at any step of development. Simple concepts can therefore be introduced early with further development as the student progresses. (3)
———	———	———	14. Specific content is important in nursing, but only to the extent that it is part of the meaningful context of the whole. (3)
———	———	———	15. The most important learning is the discovery of the organizing principles rather than specific answers to questions or problems. (3)
———	———	———	16. There is selected content that must be taught sequentially to be useful or meaningful to the student. (3)
———	———	———	17. The process of thinking involves designing and testing plausible solutions for the problem as understood by the thinker. (2)
———	———	———	18. Spaced or distributed recalls are more effective for fixing material that is to be long retained than intense repetitive recall. (1)
———	———	———	19. Pupils *think* when they encounter a problem (obstacle, difficulty, puzzle, or challenge) in a course of action that interests them. (2)
———	———	———	20. The teacher is the stimulator of the students' self-growth. (3)
———	———	———	21. The teacher is a facilitator in a student's reach for knowledge. (3)
———	———	———	22. Teachers' behaviors are role models for learners. (3)
———	———	———	23. The role model of democratic group leaders is important. (3)
———	———	———	24. Both teaching and learning are ongoing processes that can take place in any setting but probably do so more quickly in a formalized atmosphere. (3)
———	———	———	25. The teacher promotes an environment of trust and openness in communication. This trust and openness can be threatening, and support needs to be available to teachers in achieving and maintaining such an environment. (3)
———	———	———	26. Teaching must be based on soundly researched theory. (3)
———	———	———	27. Teaching includes encouraging and promoting independent study. (3)
———	———	———	28. Teaching provides freedom for the learner to explore and question. (3)
———	———	———	29. Creativity and flexibility in teaching allow responsiveness to changing student needs. (3)

Example 3

To: Faculty
From: _____
Re: Learning propositions—conceptual framework

Attachment No. 1 is the learning propositions that were consensually agreed on. These seem to need no further discussion. Attachment No. 2 is learning propositions that were designated as needing discussion or on which there was no consensus.* The focus of our discussion today will be to try to reach some conclusion about each learning proposition, and the order of discussion will proceed in the following manner:

1. Read the learning proposition.
2. Decide if it is an important concept to be discussed or if it was covered in one of the propositions on which the group consensually agreed to drop or retain.
3. Decide what it is about the proposition that makes it acceptable to some and unacceptable to others and that makes it need clarification or change. There may be one small change that would alter the whole thing.
4. List the bad things about the learning proposition and the good things about it.
5. Try to select a learning proposition that would provide us with all the good things and none of the bad things.
6. Drop, retain, change, or come up with an alternate proposition.

*No examples will be given of the two attachments—the list will differ from faculty to faculty.

Example 4

Learning theories on which we seem to agree. Please read and be ready to alter and come to a provisional decision on _____ (date). We will then have completed our first draft of our learning theory for our conceptual framework.

1. People learn when they encounter a problem or need. This need creates anxiety, which in turn produces drive and motivation.
2. Drive and motivation produce a learner *need* for *information, cues, models,* or opportunity to *discover* (experiment) that enables progression toward goals or problem solutions.
3. Progression toward goal achievement is promoted by moving from the familiar to the unfamiliar and actively involving the learner in the learning activities.
4. Reinforcement of desired behaviors increases movement toward the goal; conversely, *absence of feedback* of any kind prevents progress, and consistently *negative feedback* (punishment), deliberate or accidental, leads to frustration, aggression, and avoidance; progress then breaks down and problems are not solved.
5. *Repetition with feedback* and consequent improvement (practice) accompanied by reinforcement develops behavior habits and patterns. (Practice is repetition with feedback.)
6. Spaced or distributed recall or more and varied opportunities for application enables the learner to identify central concepts, verify principles, make generalizations and discriminations, and promotes retention.
7. Success (achievement of goals) leads to tolerance of failure, realistic self-assessment, realistic goal setting, and self-perpetrating evaluation.
8. No specific nursing arena provides experiences for learning that are prerequisite to any other specific nursing arena.

13. Compile the agreed-on propositions into a logical sequential whole. If there are propositions that do not seem to fit into the whole, set them aside as conceptual framework agreements. They will probably have a logical place as the conceptual framework evolves.
14. Return the document to the group for critiquing.
15. Alter as necessary.
16. Label the finished document as provisional or tentative to make explicit the evolving nature of all parts of the curriculum framework.

Puissance
1. Begins to draw on the philosophies and knowledge of the teaching group.
2. Enables the participants to see their individual contribution to the conceptual framework.
3. Broadens the discussion to include recognized sources and thereby is education.
4. Helps faculty to recognize commonalities in learning theories.
5. Helps faculty to recognize the extent of common thinking and agreement in the group.
6. Can decrease time spent in debate over identified differences.
7. Produces a document that is the effort of the faculty and gains recognition and commitment to implement.
8. Is excellent for "warming up" task in developing open communication patterns that legitimize the disagreement and argument because subject is "low key" enough to provide material for discussion early in the process of curriculum development.

Contingencies
1. Can be time consuming.
2. Can lock into a win-lose situation if allowed.
3. Can solidify into a document that is difficult to change as the group grows.
4. Can seem to be meaningless to the "real" work of curriculum building, which is sometimes seen as generating new courses without the need to go into conceptual aspects and framework preparation.
5. Can often be difficult for faculty to see the implementation implications.

NOTES

1. Diller, Barbara: A comparative study of reasons for entering three selected types of nursing schools as expressed by graduating students during March, 1971, thesis, San Jose State College, San Jose, Calif., 1972.
2. Bevis, Em O.: Characteristics of nursing majors enrolled in nursing courses, 1969-1971 (unpublished material from data gathered under U.S. Public Health Service, Division of Nursing Training grant).
3. Hathaway, S. R., and McKinley, J. C.: Minnesota Multiphasic Personality Inventory: manual for administration and scoring, New York, 1967, Psychological Corporation, p. 1.
4. Anastasi, Anne: Psychological testing, ed. 3, New York, 1968, The Macmillan Co., pp. 440-441.
5. Ibid., pp. 452-453.
6. Rogers, Carl: Personal thoughts on teaching and learning. In Improving college and university teaching, vol. 6, no. 1, Corvallis, Winter, 1958, Oregon State College, pp. 4-5.
7. Skinner, B. F.: Science and human behavior, New York, 1953, The Macmillan Co.
8. Mednick, Sarnoff A.: Learning, Englewood Cliffs, N.J., 1964, Prentice-Hall, Inc., p. 18.
9. Bigge, Morris L.: Learning theories for teachers, ed. 3, New York, 1976, Harper & Row, Publishers, p. 1.
10. McDonald, Frederick J.: Educational psychology, Belmont, Calif., 1966, Wadsworth Publishing Co., Inc., p. 89.
11. Bigge, pp. 48-77.
12. Dollard, John, and Miller, Neal E.: Personality and psychotherapy, New York, 1950, McGraw-Hill Book Co.
13. Keesing, Felix M.: Cultural anthropology, the science of custom, New York, 1962, Holt, Rinehart & Winston, Inc., pp. 172-173.
14. Lewin, Kurt: Field theory and learning. In Henery, Nelson B., editor: The forty-first yearbook of the National Society for the Study of Education. Part II. The psychology of learning, Chicago, 1942, University of Chicago Press, pp. 215-245.
15. Bigge, pp. 184-245.
16. Watson, Goodwin: What psychology can we feel sure about? Teachers College Record **61:**253-257, May, 1960.
17. Gagné, Robert M.: The conditions of learning, New York, 1965, Holt, Rinehart & Winston, Inc., pp. 58-59.
18. Hilgard, Ernest R.: Theories of learning, ed. 2, New York, 1956, Appleton-Century-Crofts.
19. Bigge, pp. 303-320.
20. Watson, p. 257.
21. Mager, Robert F.: Preparing instructional objectives, Palo Alto, Calif., 1962, Fearon Publishers, pp. 11-12.
22. Hilgard, pp. 86-87.
23. McDonald, p. 112.
24. Ibid., 110-127.
25. Watson, p. 256.
26. Bigge, p. 131.
27. Pressey, Sidney L., and Robinson, Francis P.: Psychology in education, ed. 3, New York, 1959, Harper & Row, Publishers, p. 349.
28. Ibid., pp. 262-263.
29. McDonald, p. 192.
30. Cronbach, Lee J.: Educational psychology, ed. 2, New York, 1963, Harcourt, Brace & World, Inc., pp. 295-296.

BIBLIOGRAPHY

Biehler, Robert F.: Psychology applied to teaching, Boston, 1971, Houghton Mifflin Co.

Bigge, Morris L.: Learning theories for teachers ed. 3, New York, 1976, Harper & Row, Publishers.

Dewey, John: Democracy in education, New York, 1916, The Macmillan Co.

Gagné, Robert M.: The conditions of learning, New York, 1965, Holt, Rinehart & Winston, Inc.

Hall, Calvin S., and Lindzey, Gardner: Theories of personality, New York, 1957, John Wiley & Sons, Inc.

Hilgard, Ernest R.: Theories of learning, ed. 2, New York, 1956, Appleton-Century-Crofts.

Lewin, Kurt: Field theory and learning. In Henery, Nelson B., editor: The forty-first yearbook of the National Society for the Study of Education. Part II. The psychology of learning, Chicago, 1942, University of Chicago Press, pp. 215-245.

McDonald, Frederick: Educational psychology, Belmont, Cal., 1966, Wadsworth Publishing Co.

Mednick, Sarnoff A.: Learning, Englewood Cliffs, N.J., 1964, Prentice-Hall, Inc.

Skinner, B. F.: Science and human behavior, New York, 1953, The Macmillan Co.

Thorndyke, Edward L.: Educational psychology, New York, 1914, Teachers College, Columbia University.

Watson, John B., and McDougall, William: The battle of behaviorism, New York, 1929, W. W. Norton & Co., Inc., Publishers.

Willman, Marilyn D.: Changes in nursing students, In Williamson, Janet A., editor: Current perspectives in nursing education.: the changing scene, vol. I, St. Louis, 1976, The C. V. Mosby Co.

5

CONCEPTUAL FRAMEWORK:
THE KNOWLEDGE COMPONENT

Any profession or practice discipline is an applied science and/or art and, as such, derives much of its theory from other disciplines or the pure sciences. Nursing theory is unique partly in its specificity of application; that is, the special way nurses eclectically choose and combine appropriate theory components and use them in solving nursing problems. To illustrate the place of nursing theory in curriculum innovation, this chapter defines nursing and proposes a theory of nursing that operationalizes the definition and becomes a component of the conceptual framework. The theories and concepts that contribute to or are inherent in the proposed theory of nursing are briefly elaborated.

Nursing has operated fairly successfully for many years without articulated theories of nursing. Many nursing curricula evolve or are developed without attempting to state a theory of nursing. Why, then, is it so important to offer a theory, or a conceptual framework, regarding nursing knowledge as a focal point for the nursing curriculum?

Abdellah and Levine state that "In nursing, a conceptual framework is a theoretical approach to the study of problems that are scientifically based that emphasizes the selection, arrangement, and clarification of its concepts."[1] The nursing theory network developed for the curriculum helps the teacher and the student differentiate between the important and the inconsequential in dealing with nursing problems.[2] Theories of nursing act as pre-

dictive tools, or devices that enable the nurse to determine in advance of nursing activities what the probable results will be. By making nursing theory explicit, the nursing curriculum builder can take implicit facts that are vague or ill defined and sort them into a meaningful way of looking at data. This meaningful way of looking at data (nursing theory or conceptual constructs) includes clear and concise statements about how the facts relevant to nursing behaviors relate to one another.[2] A theory of nursing provides a checklist, guide, or device for seeing nursing holistically and dynamically. It provides guidelines for nursing care that use the appropriate theory components in response to any given nursing problem. In short, theories of nursing provide definitive content-organizing strategies for the curriculum. Furthermore, they provide a content outline or checklist for curriculum and an overview of the curriculum content.

This book elaborates a theory of nursing to illustrate its application in curriculum building for nursing. The theory of nursing discussed here is "a," not "the," theory of nursing. Theories of nursing are in their infancy; only as they evolve and mature will nursing develop a general theory. The following section provides a brief discussion of a theory of nursing and the composition of the theories that contribute to it. It is not possible in this brief volume to provide even a résumé of all the contributing theories. Indeed, the reader must take this general skeleton and fill in the form and shape. Sometimes, only one point of view is provided when obviously other points of view exist and would provide additional choices for the eclectic student. This presentation intends only to illustrate the kind of material that constitutes the continuing data collection for a theory of nursing.

GENERAL STATEMENT OF A NURSING THEORY

A general statement of the theory of nursing proposed in this book was given on pp. 17 to 19. One may call it a conceptual construct or a theory; the similarity and differences between conceptual constructs and theories were discussed in Chapter 1. Adequate definitions of nursing are comprehensive and operational and are statements of one kind of theory. Note that the theory suggested here is in the form of a definition. It is condensed here to provide a reference point:

Nursing is a process: Its purpose is to promote optimal health through protective, nurtrative, and generative activities. These activities are carried out with three client systems: the intrapersonal system, the interpersonal system, and the community system. The tools with which nurses function are the subprocess of communication, caring, problem solving, decision making, managing, and teaching. Nurses are autonomous health care givers, within the limits of employment contracts, collaborating with other members of the health care team for the benefit of clients. They are accountable for their activities, monitor and regulate the quality of the nursing care given, and provide for the education of neophytes. Nurses provide each other with mutual protection, nurturing, and facilitation of growth.

Nursing's protective, nurtrative, and generative activities are a unique synthesis of theories eclectically combined into nursing hypotheses that are validated or refuted in practice.

SYSTEMS THEORY AND THE ORGANIZATION OF THE PROCESS OF NURSING

A system is a device for bringing together parts into meaningful wholes so that the way the parts function together is clear. Processes can be analyzed so that their functions and operations have organization and system, and they are thereby more educationally useful. General systems[3] theory is useful in breaking processes into sequential operations or tasks to ensure goal realization. The number of parts, tasks, or components of the system is totally dependent on what is needed to accomplish the goal. However, there are some components common to any systematized process.

Purpose, goal, or aim is necessary for any process or system. High-level wellness is the attainment of maximal health compatible with individual potential. This is obviously, then, not a static state but a dynamic one, since potential is determined by so many varied factors.[4] Potential varies under different conditions; therefore one's maximal level of health under those changed conditions varies. For example, one's optimal level of functioning or health is different when the environment is free from pollutants than when the environment is polluted. A child who has had proper nutrients and a stimulating home life has a vastly different potential for health than the child who has suffered from malnourishment or deprivation of stimulation. However, as the environment or nutrients change, the child's potential for health alters. Nursing operates both to raise potential and to promote realization of optimal health under the existing conditions. Some limits of potential are set and difficult to alter, but the person's optimal level of health under those limits depends on his ability to develop his potential fully. For instance, physical anomalies, disabilities, or limited intelligence limit potential, but the nurse promotes the development of individual resources so that assets are maximized, limitations are minimized, and potential is realized. Behaviors of the nurse who is required to promote optimal health are classified according to the phase of the health continuum concerned.

In addition, systems are divided into input, throughput, and output. (See Fig. 1-4.) All three aspects of a system are responsive to the frame of reference used. Input is the assessment information of nursing—the problems, the needs, the goals, and the desires of clients and the nurse. The client's nature, for example, individuals, groups, families, agencies, and communities, and data about the nurse and nursing environment, also become part of the input. Dualistic or medical model input is couched in the language of dualism, e.g., diagnosis, physiological, and psychological data. Holistic input is couched in the language of holism, e.g., human processes, goals, and behaviors.

Throughput is the way data are processed or handled, the system it is organized into, and thus it also depends on the frame of reference being used to process the data. If a dualistic framework is used, the organization of the data is into components such as (1) physical: neurological, musculoskeletal, digestive, reproductive, respiratory, cardiovascular, and sensory; and (2) emotional: psychiatric, religious, family, and economic. If the framework is holistic, the organization of data is into components such as communications, problem solving, decision making, learning, stress, maturation, management, change, and caring.

Output is the unique way throughput is synthesized to become a new and different nursing behavior with one or more client systems. Each identified nursing behavior has the potential of being enacted with or in any nursing arena. The nursing behaviors necessary to achieve high-level wellness are (1) protective, (2) nurtrative, and (3) generative. Each of these behaviors is derived from theories that contribute directly to the goal of nursing. The classification of behaviors into protective, nurtrative, and generative is one of convenience. Like any other classification system its purpose is to group by commonality. In this case the commonality concerns the kind of nursing activity involved. Groupings of this type help to provide for efficient cognitive filing and retrieval so that all appropriate and necessary classifications of activities are included in a nursing episode.

Output, the nursing behavioral outcomes of the system, is equivalent to the unique or innovative component of process.

Purpose of nursing

Rogers wrote that "Nursing aims to assist people in achieving their maximum health potential."[5] She elaborates by listing the what, who, and where of nursing. The "what" is maintenance and promotion of health, prevention of disease, nursing diagnosis, intervention, and rehabilitation; the "who" is all people, well and sick, rich and poor, young and old. She lists the "where" as nursing service arenas and states that these arenas are anywhere people are located—at home, school, work, play, in hospitals, nursing homes, clinics—both in this world and in space.

The American Nurses' Association's position paper of 1965 states under "Assumptions" that "Nursing is a helping profession and as such provides services which contribute to the health and well-being of people."[6] Most writers on nursing who mention the subject of purpose at all either intimate or state conclusively that the basic purpose of nursing is to promote optimal health. Elaborations of that basic statement differ, but the essential point remains: Nursing's purpose is to promote optimal health. Purpose is not only the first component of "process" but it is also the beginning of theory. To devise a system for making something meaningful without first trying to ascertain its purpose is to approach the subject from a state of confusion. Once purpose is hypothesized, however, the relationships of other components can be determined in an effort to make sense of the whole. Nursing has a common agreement about its purpose. That, in itself, is a great strength from which to start identifying its common conceptual and theoretical commitment so that the confidence and unity beginning to be exhibited in nursing can mature.

Nursing's purpose is not unique; the fields of medicine, occupational therapy, physical therapy, and other health-related groups are also organized and instituted for the sole purpose of promoting, maintaining, and restoring health. It is not in its purpose, nor in its system, that nursing is unique but in its combining of the many components of nursing process. All components are drawn from allied fields (input) into an innovative synthesis (throughput) that manifests itself in a service that is the unique outcome of nursing process (output). The purveyors of this service function protectively, nurtratively, and generatively in collaboration with individuals, families, groups, and communities to achieve, maintain, or restore health.

Evolution of definitions of health

Because of the nature of nursing, its goal must contain some mention of promoting, maintaining, regaining, or increasing health or wellness. Therefore the nature of health becomes of concern to nursing curriculum builders. The way that health is defined operationalizes itself in the content of nursing programs.

In 1946 the World Health Organization (WHO) defined health as "a state of complete physical, mental, and social well-being, not merely the absence of disease or infirmity." Since this definition uses the word "complete," it makes health an ideal, a goal that can be reached. The WHO definition treated health as an attainable goal, and on that basis WHO mounted massive health programs. Dunn[7] first coined the phrase "high-level wellness," and his contribution to the concept of health and disease as phases or levels of wellness has augmented greatly the theoretical underpinning of the purposes of the health professions.

In 1959 Dunn differentiated between good health and wellness. "Wellness," stated Dunn, "is an ever changing growth toward fulfillment of an individual's potential." Wellness to Dunn has some similarity to Maslow's concept of self-actualization.[8] Wellness and self-actualization are the products of a human being's interacting with his internal and external environments in such a way as to experience growth toward his greatest potentialities. In contrast to his concept of wellness, Dunn defines "good health" as a state of being, a passive adaptability to one's environment. Dunn's definitions become meaningful and workable if one can join him in viewing wellness as a direction that enables progression toward ever higher potentials of functioning. For Dunn,[9] wellness is a dynamic state and is considered individually for each person according to that person's peculiar needs, happiness, hardships, abilities, disabilities, problems, and potentials.

Many other current writers on health and disease, notably Dubos,[10] have expanded Dunn's observations or evolved similar descriptions. Dubos, too, supports health or wellness as a direction. Wellness, being a direction, not a state of being, can be represented by a compass. The compass has wellness-sickness as the north-south axis, with the needle ever swinging, telling the individual his current position and where he is heading, but never when he has reached a destination because there is no fixed destination, just a clear direction toward wellness. (See Fig. 5-1.)

Since wellness and sickness are not states of being but rather are dynamic directional concepts, they are difficult to define and describe. Definitions of dynamic concepts attempt to fix them at a given time, making them seem static and failing to depict their fluid nature. To describe a river without noting its dynamic directional process of flowing toward the sea would omit the essence of the river. Some of the river's water arrives at the sea, but the river itself continues to flow, and one can sit on its banks every day and verify its flowing. Wellness-health-wholeness is a way of living and being for people. There

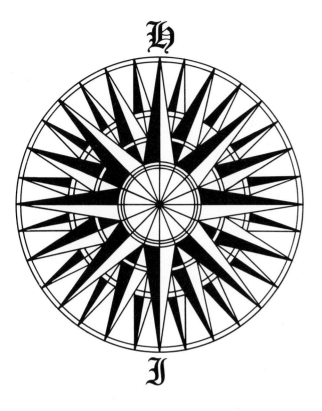

Fig. 5-1. Health-illness compass.

are times when wellness is experienced as having been achieved (Maslow calls this "peak experience"), but these times are transient and short lived. The wellness impetus in people, for the most part, moves, shifts, adapts—changes flowing toward health as relatively defined for each individual.

Health can also be a matter of perspective. Is a person healthy if free from disease? What about people who are clinically disease free but are nagged by low energy levels, vague or even specific aches and pains, or feelings of unrest or depression? Are those people well? What of the person who may clinically have some disease, such as cancer, that has not yet presented symptoms and has not yet been clinically diagnosed? He feels good, produces well, and perceives himself as healthy. Is this person well? In other words, is health an objective state defined by other people (physicians) using test and tools, or is it a subjective state

as perceived by an individual about himself?

Holism and health. Part of Webster's definition of health is "being whole."[11] This idea is gaining respect in modern health care philosophy. Treating a human being as an organized whole, an entire unit, a basic total system interrelating with other systems in his environment provides the perspective for a new mode of care. Traditionally, Western society has treated man as a set of assembled parts (dualistically). In reality, dualism treats man as having two parts—his emotional aspect, called psyche, and his physical aspect, called soma. As modern science became more sophisticated, more scientific, and more highly specialized, the original two parts became many more parts. Man was and continues to be studied in intricate detail in such separate areas as anatomy, sociology, psychology, physiology, biochemistry, neurology, theology, and scores of others. As each field further fragments its wholeness, man becomes an assembly of carefully compartmentalized aspects. Few, if any, sciences study the human being as a unitary system. This dualistic approach gave rise to viewing poor health, disease, and disability in a simplistic manner. Scientists looked at a health problem, described it, and gave it a name and classification. Based on the natural law of cause and effect, a cause was sought and a culprit was found and blamed. Then a carefully planned attack was mounted to eradicate the culprit. The belief in a single etiology for a single disease or single part being affected generated many treatments, all aimed at that identified single cause. This approach has been and is an effective way of controlling disease. Unfortunately, however, it has in many cases provided only for a state of health that was not more than freedom from that single disease. When one has a specific problem, it is life saving to have a specific treatment. However, the error has been that having a specific treatment copes with only a small part of the person's problems.

For health purposes, then, a human being cannot be treated as a group of parts but as an integrated whole, living and interacting with his environment, with the entire suprasystem being in ecological balance progressing toward perfection and wellness for these systems involved. Nursing roles are designed to work with communities, groups, families, and individuals so that prevention and maintenance are valued aspects of health care.

Since health and illness are relative to the individual and not absolute states, they do not exist as pure entities. Every adaptation or coping pattern, whether positive or negative, optimal or not, leads to a relative health position. For convenience, judgments are made about whether the states of being are arbitrarily called health or illness.

Definitions for this book. *Health,* as a holistic definition, is progressively positive adaptive responses to stresses in the internal and external ecological systems.

Health is a positive level of wellness that is cyclic, varying its levels of wellness according to conditions, circumstances, and environmental factors. Another way to phrase it would be to say that *health is continually dynamic, optimal coping with any stress or stresses, internal or external, through adaptations within the client or alterations in the environment. A healthy state is a state of being perceived by the individual and is the ability to mobilize energy to establish goals and make consistent progress toward meeting those goals with a minimum cost in time and energy to self and others. It is doing this while feeling good about oneself and doing positive things to help others in feeling good about themselves or, at the least, producing minimum negative effects on others.*

Wellness is also a self-perceived position on the health-illness cycle and is individual for each person. *Wellness* is the extent that the individual, family, or group can optimally operate in all aspects of living and growing.

Nursing's task is to provide whatever care, counsel, and/or therapy will enable people, individually or in groups, to increase their ability to do the preceding things.

Nursing. From the previous definitions it is evident that nursing has drawn heavily on writing in allied fields for much of its theoretical basis. However, the differing definitions of care and cure are a matter of primary focus. Physicians provide medical therapy. Nurses provide nursing care. Medicine usually focuses on etiology (cause), pathology (results), and therapy (treatment). Nursing focuses on what happens to the client, his family, and his community before, during, and after illness. In addition, nursing concerns itself with well people maintaining their wellness and facilitates attainment of higher and higher levels of wellness. In addition nurses, more than any other group of health providers, are primarily concerned with client advocacy, both on a personal health service basis and on a legislative level.

NURSING: A SYSTEMS MODEL
Input—based on theories of nursing process

All systems begin with input. As stated earlier, input comprises the needs, problems, goals, and desires of the actors in the system, that is, the client and the nurse. What is put into the system depends on the perceptual framework of the nurse curriculum builder. There are several popular ways that nurses view the needs of the nursing process system; these are the dualistic or medical model view, the Maslow hierarchy-of-needs view, the maturational (Erikson) view, the nursing-problems or decision-making view (both Abdellah and nursing process), and the interactional view. Each point of view determines the kind of data that will be put through the system and the kinds of nursing problems that will be addressed.

The importance of this to the curriculum-building process is that the problems to be addressed influence the type of skills and behaviors which nurses will need to solve the problems, thereby influencing the choice of content for the nursing curriculum. Nursing has many curriculum models; only broad categories are presented here, with no attempt to sort all nursing theories into these categories.

Dualistic or medical model. The dualistic model, as stated earlier, states input in terms of diagnosis or pathological, psychological, emotional, and religious assessment and resultant problems. This framework views the client as primarily having a medical diagnosis, and all nursing problems and client needs are centered around that diagnosis and the treatment (medical) and cure goals. Input influences throughput and outcomes so that throughput is geared to the dualistic framework, and information and organization of content is around the physical and psychological processes. Outcome is usually measured in terms of the disease process and

what happened to it, not in terms of the total client and his responses to the health problems.

Problem-solving and human needs frameworks. Problem-solving and human needs frameworks may also be called analytical frameworks. They include nursing process frameworks, research frameworks, and problem-solving frameworks and are closely aligned with the human needs frameworks and the systems theory frameworks.

In the problem-solving framework all input is viewed as problems to be solved by the patient, nurse, or others. The nursing process dictates that assessments lead to the identification of patient needs or nursing problems (not necessarily the same thing) and that all throughput and output of the nursing system is regulated by the "problems of the client."

The human needs framework is much like the problem-solving one except that the problems examined arise through an organized articulation of human needs. Maslow[9] established human needs in order of priority. Abdellah[12] sorted nursing problems into twenty-one categories. Viewing nursing practice through a client needs or problems reference emphasizes the client's needs and not the process of problem solving. Problem solving is used, since it is a pervasive life process and a key methodology for nursing practice. Maslow's hierarchy of needs lists human needs from those which are most important or essential to life to those which are least essential but help to attain what he refers to as self-actualization, in other words, fully attaining one's potential. Abdellah's twenty-one nursing problems are historically significant as one of the earliest attempts to provide a nursing framework and depart from the medical framework which was being used by nurses as a model for practice. Many nursing theory models have evolved from Abdellah's work. All have in common a classification of patient needs by the nursing problems that those needs create.

Most of the time the process for problem

solving/decision making is clearly formulated or systematized so that content becomes the factor that influences decisions. Systems models use systems language and a systems flow of input, throughput, and output as their format.

Interactional framework. In the interactional view, clients are seen as interacting systems and nursing as an interactional discipline. All nursing action, in this framework, is viewed as an interactional process. Peplau[13] was one of the nursing theorists who was a proponent of this approach. The nonnurse theorists contributing immensely to this model are people like Carl Rogers, Eric Berne, Fritz Perls, and B. F. Skinner.[14] Each of these theorists brings to nursing a viewpoint that provides choices of modalities for nursing. Nursing theorists have provided the ways and means by which all of nursing content can be sorted and selected, based on the perspective that nursing problems are interactive in nature and that all nursing roles, functions, and skills revolve around human interaction. Reusch has developed communications theory that provides an umbrella under which other interactive models can be housed.

Maturational or developmental framework. The method of labeling client needs and problems in terms of a maturational or developmental framework is largely based on the work of Erikson and Piaget. Clients are seen as being involved in maturational tasks that influence health. Families, groups, communities, and agencies are viewed as having maturational tasks so that they may continue to mature, grow, and be healthy. The maturational level of all client systems can be assessed and the nursing system input can be labeled according to the maturational tasks and/or problems being faced. Maturational life crises are also seen as part of the input. Situational crises as situational problems are not used here but rather are used in the stress framework. Travelbee[15] drew, in part, on this framework for her Developmental Systems Model for Nursing.

Stress framework. Input into the nursing system is frequently labeled in terms of client system stress.

In this model clients are viewed as having stressors (the wear and tear of life) to which they respond in adaptive or maladaptive ways. There are many different perceptions or forms that this basic model takes. Each one emphasizes a different group of stressors or of client responses (stresses). Some of these models emphasize the conservation of energy, some homodynamics, and some of the stages of stress. Selye[16] did the basic work, whereas others like Riehl and Roy[17] have built on Selye's efforts to evolve nursing theory models that view clients as having a series of developmental or life crises or stresses. Nursing roles and functions are, in this framework, organized around facilitating attainment of developmental tasks. Many other authors use some life-cycle episodes to view people. Usually these are times of crisis or significant events.

Holism as a framework. Holistic input for the nursing system is eclectic input. It avoids the schism of mind and soma and looks at client needs, problems, desires, and goals as arising from the total ecological system, client, nurse, and environment. Category systems are devised that are eclectic and whole. Martha Rogers pioneered holistic frameworks. These categories are used for viewing and assessing the client and labeling the input. Usually there are two basic categories: (1) the client system and (2) the environment. Each category is so mutually inclusive that large parts of each category overlap and include the other. Subcategories of the client system can be such things as maturation, stress, perception, communication and relationships, problem solving, learning, and energy. Subcategories of the environmental system can be such things as housing, economics, geography, the health care system, and so on.

These categories provide the nurse curriculum builder with the ability to provide input to the system which will enable the fulfillment of the needs, problems, desires, and goals of every aspect of life which are important to the client so that the throughput and the output will be responsive to the whole client system. Nursing content and nursing skills, roles, and functions, then, become centered around the organismic nature of the input to the nursing system.

Throughput

The seven processes selected to be discussed as essential to the creative component of nursing process (throughput) are explored only briefly. There is no attempt to review the literature extensively. The purpose is simply to provide a résumé of the type of content essential to the practice of nursing. The seven processes that are discussed here are divided into two groups. Group 1 comprises the tools that nurses use in the practice of nursing, including (1) problem solving/decision making, (2) communication, (3) teaching/learning, (4) management/change, and (5) caring. Group 2 comprises two other conceptual constructs, which are the health-producing tasks of life, for example, (1) adaptation and (2) maturation.[18] The life tasks will be discussed first, followed by the nursing tools.

The processes of learning and the change part of management are discussed in more detail in other parts of the book; therefore only a résumé of propositions is included here.

Life tasks concepts

Stress. For use in this theory of nursing, Engel's[19] theory of stress and strain will be used, and both Engel's and Selye's theories will be condensed and combined. Stress refers to those forces that press in upon or noxiously stimulate the individual. The stress response is always an attempt at adaptation. Maladaptation is a matter of perception, not of the intent of body response. The results of stress are responses that, according to Engel, are called strain. Every reaction to stress may not result in strain that is measurable or observable. However, stress has a cumulative nature,

and the resulting strain may not appear until the number and degree of stresses accrue sufficient weight to cause an observable response. Fig. 5-2 is a paradigm of the dynamics of stress.

Strain expresses itself in symptoms, signs, or behaviors that signal responses. These symptoms, signs, or behaviors may be a result of a strain induced by an infective organism, a decision dilemma, a degenerative process, or any combination of a wide variety of strain-producing factors.

Stress is a process and has the three elements of all processes: purpose, organization, and creativity.

The purpose of stress is to stimulate the organism. Stimulation provides the motivation for growth, reproduction, and death—the basic processes of life. It also provides the motivation for work, love, and friendship—the basic human activities of life. Stress is life's necessary elixir and always results in some response.

Stress is organized into three stages of strain or stress response: excitement, resistance, and exhaustion. Excitement is the flight-fight aspect of strain. The symptoms include heart rate increases, respiratory changes, dilated pupils, and others, all of which are manifestations of the organism's readiness to flee or to fight. A group has a flight-fight stage manifested in rapid consolidation and drawing together, organization for defense or attack, much movement, and involvement of members.

The resistance phase is the attempt of the organism to resist harm from the stress. The resultant strain is often a coping mechanism. The success of the coping may or may not influence the healthiness of the organism's stress response. Selye's[17] "local and general adaptive syndrome" are results of coping behavior on the part of the organism. Sickness, ill health, and health problems manifest themselves first in the second stage of stress responses—resistance. Most nurtrative nursing behaviors commence in this stage of strain.

Exhaustion is the third stage of strain

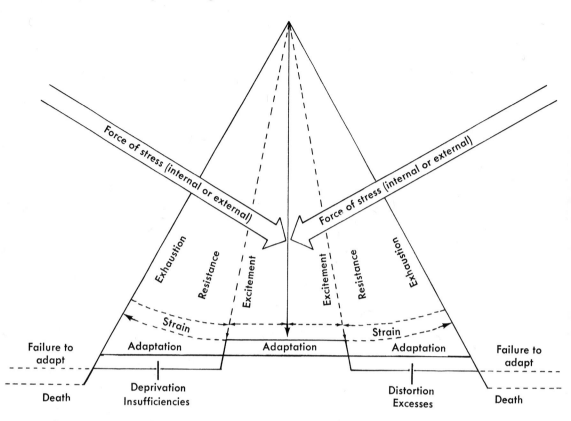

Fig. 5-2. Dynamics of stress and strain—adaptive and maladaptive. (Developed by H. Dufour, D. Siegele, and G. Vanisko.)

or stress response. Exhaustion is simply that the organism—individual, family, group, or community—is worn out and all systems are failing. Individuals who have this happen need almost total nursing care support. They may have respirators, pacemakers, intravenous feeding, catheters, dialysis, and/or any number of support systems to augment or replace exhausted parts. Problems resulting in total withdrawal, the end product of drug overuse, alcoholic inebriation, and other types of slow or quick suicide can be viewed as exhaustion. Unrelieved exhaustion results in death.

The creative element of stress is the ever new and unique way that the strain manifests itself and the organism copes.

A stress-strain theory that is incorporated into a useful theory of nursing needs to have several common elements.

Stressors are stimuli or factors that interfere with the satisfaction of needs or the balance of the human organism's internal or external environment. Selye called them the "wear and tear of living." They are normal in everyday life.

Stress can be evaluated by (1) its virulence, (2) its saturation, density, or dosage, and (3) its persistence or longevity. The virulence of the stress is the importance of the threat to the organism or its ability to cause strain. For instance, in the person who has incipient diabetes, the stress of weight gain is a greater threat than it is to the person who has no propensity to diabetes. Virulence is the strength of the stress as measured by its relationship to the potential resultant strain in any one individual, family, or community. Sudden rises in unemployment can be a virulent community stress.

A second way to evaluate stress is by its saturation or density. Stresses that appear in multiples or groups tend to exert greater threat and elicit greater strain than the sum of the individual stresses would indicate. The proverbial "straw that broke the camel's back" was not one little stress but the accumulation of many stresses at one time. One ant sting is a minor irritant; a thousand may kill the victim. To the incipient diabetic, weight gain alone may not result in diabetes, but add infection, lack of rest, family or work problems, and so on, and the cumulative stress produces the strain response of a reduced ability to metabolize glucose. Saturation, or dosage, of stress can be seen in a community that experiences only a moderate rise in unemployment, but added to conditions of inadequate housing units, substandard recreational facilities, and insufficient health care, the resultant strain might far outweigh the community response to any one of the stresses taken individually.

A third element of consideration with regard to stress is persistence or recurrence, which is the duration of the stress or its frequency of recurrence. Even the strongest of steel beams begins to demonstrate strain with a persistent stress; a marble staircase shows the strain of wear after years of frequent treading of feet, day after day, in a recurring pattern. Response patterns to frequently recurring or persistent stress can be highly developed and stylized because of "practice." Frequent or persistent stress tends to establish a vicious circle of strain response that makes each subsequent presentation of the stress more able to elicit the strain response.

Strain. Strain is a human response that attempts to cope with or adapt to a stress or group of stressors. Strain, according to most theorists, is always adaptive by intent and only results in health threats because the adaptation itself is harmful to the client. For instance, the inflammatory response to a stress of infection is obviously adaptive even though it is painful, edematous, or immobilizing because it is adaptive

in its healing properties. Strains exhibit themselves in symptoms, syndromes, or disorders. The community with the stress of a sudden rise in unemployment may have the resultant strain exhibited in the symptom of a rise in crime rate. As long as the strain is not symptomatic, it is usually unnoticed. There is a delay between the removal of the stress and the disappearance of the strain, since the organism must progress back up through the stages of strain. The lag between stress removal and a return to normal by the human organism is not a simple matter of resilience as one sees in steel beams but is the compilation of many factors. Therefore the resulting strain may be exhibited in a pattern of behavior that persists long after the causative stress has disappeared from the scene. Responses to stress tend to be stored in some type of somatic memory bank so that subsequent stresses stimulate the response more quickly and the strain persists longer.

Timing and circumstances seem to play a major role in strain response. The strain response to measles is generally less severe in a child than in an adult. Conversely, the strain of parental separation is greater in the child than in the mature adult. Healthy patterns of response to stress can become cyclic, as can unhealthy patterns. In healthy responses the integrity of the person is strengthened so that each succeeding stress has less and less ability to cause predominantly unhealthy responses. These individuals generally develop a high resistance to the kinds of stresses to which they have had successful responses. Thus there is the individual who "never gets bad colds" and the one who "never gets stomach pains" when confronted with stressful situations.

Nursing's responsibility is to (1) prevent the occurrence of the stress, (2) promote healthy stress responses, (3) care for patients exhibiting unhealthy responses (strain), (4) renew the phases of stress response, and (5) reestablish and maintain organismic integrity. For instance, if the stress is an infective agent such as measles, the nursing behaviors would be protective in that they would be geared to preventing the disease (strain symptom) from occurring. If measles did occur, the nursing behavior would be primarily nurtrative—taking care of the person while he was ill during the phase of resistance and helping him to recover. Once the strain symptoms began to disappear, the primary responsibility of the nurse would be to help the client reestablish integrity so that resistance to strain is built up and maintained. The three classifications of nursing behaviors, protective, nurtrative, and generative, never occur in the pure state, and during any strain episode the nurse exhibits all three of the behaviors. However, one of the behaviors usually has priority because of the stage of strain response being experienced by the patient.

Maturation process. The process of human development is perhaps one of the more meaningful and central processes to be explored in this age of rapid generalization of knowledge. Freud's psychoanalytical theories produced a chain reaction of investigations into the nature of human behavior. Erikson's[20] study of human development is part of that chain reaction, and his works and life contributions regarding developmental tasks constitute a restatement and evolution of psychoanalytical theory in a way that is eminently useful for the promotion of health. Gesell and others[21] have taken up the task, and a large body of knowledge now exists that provides the student of human behavior with data easily translated into action hypotheses suitable for every nursing situation, that is, any person of any age group in any environment.

Man, as a developing being, moves through life from one changing level to another, with each level progressively differentiated from the other and each integrated with the other at more advanced levels. In nursing practice, nurses give nursing care with full consideration to the developmental status of individuals and groups. Thus developmental status becomes one of the variables that influence nursing care because health-wellness and, consequently, nursing care impinge on, encourage, or inhibit development as it moves from differentiation to integration through progressive phases.

Any conceptual framework for nursing that omits a consideration of the developmental level of the client denies the essential aspect of human nature—that life is a process not totally understood, an orderly series of stages that form a complex, yet integrated, whole. In any encounter with the human being, nursing, because of its nature, thrusts itself into human lives at critical periods and consequently has important impact for the enabling or inhibiting of integration.

For clarity of presentation, human development aspects can be categorized into physical, motor, perception, psychological, cognitive, communication, social, self-awareness, and play development.[22]

The nurse's knowledge of normal growth and development is used both as a reference point for assessment of patients and for determining nursing intervention strategies. Nursing intervention strategies that incorporate concepts appropriate to the client's developmental tasks are more successful than those devised without consideration for this aspect of the life process. For instance, in late adulthood attention span declines. When long television shows have involved plots, the elderly often lose track of the plot and therefore lose interest. Families notice that "grandmother" loses the thread of the story and is afraid she is becoming senile. If the nurse helps the family to plan activities for her that require shorter attention spans, the client will have more successful experiences in following an intellectual activity pattern. Anxiety over the elderly person's mental capacity diminishes because the tasks established for her participation are designed for her present abilities. It seems much easier for families to organize activities around the short attention span of children than it is to do the same for the shortened attention span of the elderly. A declining attention span is more difficult to accept than an increasing one.

It is difficult to locate a developmental framework that is holistic. Man has essentially been studied by breaking him into bits and pieces. Theories of development follow the divisions of science. Each school of nursing which accepts the premise that human developmental levels are part of the context for nursing decisions needs to locate an acceptable framework for operational purposes.

Nursing tools concepts

Problem solving/decision making. Decision making is the acquiring, ordering, and selecting of tools or alternatives for reaching goals or fulfilling needs. Problem solving is the system used to arrive at a place where decisions can be made. Decision making is the end product of problem solving and presupposes that problem solving has taken place.

The subprocess or subsystem of problem solving/decision making involves all of the analytical processes, including nursing process and research processes. Neither nursing process nor research process will be discussed here.

Every thinking human being solves problems from birth to death. The individual who does not solve problems is completely nonresponsive to his environment, since almost all response to stimuli is an attempt to solve some problem, whether the response be reflex or voluntary.

Voluntary problem solving and decision making with a consistently high degree of success have as clear an operational sequence as does reflex response with its neurological pathways, synapses, and reflex arcs. Problem-solving activities in nursing are no different from problem solving in any other field because the end product of any problem solving–decision making process is some activity sequence. Problem solving is the key process in the innovative component of nursing and is pervasive in all other processes and subprocesses.

Problem solving and decision making are processes that have been fairly thoroughly examined. Newell and Simmon[22] were two of the men primarily responsible for bringing about a synthesis of theories and presenting a unified theory of human problem-solving behavior. One of the best and clearest presentations of problem-solving theory can be found in McDonald.[23]

The problem-solving process has an operational sequence that promotes a consistently high-quality decision and has the characteristic of all processes—a fluid feedback system that enables one to flip forward through operations without completing them wholly and kick backward to previous operations when new ideas occur. This fluid feedback system, when implemented, provides for a more thorough use of all the phases or elements in the process so that the decision choices are clearer. There are four facets to problem solving: (1) problem identification; (2) problem data; (3) problem solution alternatives; and (4) decision making.

Visualize problem solving as a *pyramid* at the base of which the three sides or facets are (1) problem identification, (2) relevant data, and (3) alternatives. The stones that make up the sides are the operations within the facet. The pyramid comes to a point at the top, which is decision making (the *many* parts combining to make the *one* new and unique item that is characteristic of all processes). The whole pyramid is built around a feedback matrix that provides for instant shuttling of data throughout the system (Fig. 5-3).

The problem-solving process manifests the characteristics of any process—purpose, system, and creativity. The process components are briefly outlined as follows:

I. *Purpose*

To enable optimal utilization of the environment for the accomplishment of goals.

II. *System*

A. Problem identification sequence (assessment leading to problem identification)

1. Articulate the purpose of the behaviors or activities that are occurring.

2. Classify and sort all elements of the problem situation:

a. Who is involved?

b. What is occurring or not occurring?

c. When is this occurring?

CROSSCUT OF PYRAMID BASE

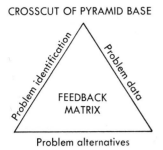

Fig. 5-3. Problem-solving, decision-making process.

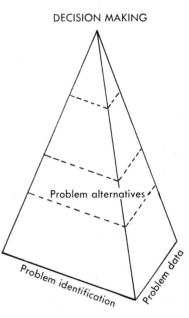

d. Where is this occurring?
e. What information do you have that is relevant to this situation?
3. Isolate the element or elements that are missing.
4. Articulate the missing element(s) in terms of a problem confronting the problem solver.
5. Synthesize the classified and sorted data with missing element(s) and relevant knowledge into an interpretative statement of the problem. State the problem as a goal (optional).
B. Problem data sequence
1. Classify and sort data relevant to the problem.
2. Determine data needed that are not already acquired.
3. Acquire additional relevant data utilizing:
a. Written references.
b. Consultants.
c. Appropriate persons.
d. Observations.
4. Develop predictive principles (predictive hypotheses—promoting and inhibiting theories) from the data.
C. Problem alternative sequence
1. List alternative actions that are possible solutions or movements toward a solution that are direct outgrowths of the predictive principles.
2. For each possible alternative, forecast:
a. The possible consequences if that alternative is implemented.
b. For each possible consequence forecasted, estimate:
(1) The probability that the consequence will occur.
(2) The value for the solution of the problem if it does occur.
(3) The risk involved if it does occur.
D. Decision sequence
1. Determine which consequence is the most

desirable (valuable) and has the least risk.

2. Determine if the alternative action that will promote this consequence has any other undesirably risky concomitant consequences that have a high probability of occurring.

3. Choose the alternative(s) that have a high probability of occurring and have valued or desired consequences that are within the risk range acceptable to the problem solver.

4. Arrange acceptable alternatives in a priority sequence so that the alternative(s) of greatest value has the highest priority and other alternatives are available in declining order.

5. Test the validity of the choices (hence the process) by implementation.[24]

The four operational sequences (or inherent organization) that comprise the system for the problem-solving process deserve further consideration and elucidation. Learning logical, ordered, sequential problem solving requires the same activity sequence as any learning requires: input, operation, and feedback (see p. 71). This means that (1) the input about problem-solving theory must be relevant to a real or simulated problem, that is, requires informational input, cues, models, and other stimuli; (2) the operational activities that provide practice must be activities that are meaningful and relevant; and (3) feedback is necessary for reinforcement, transfer, evaluation, generalization, correction, and the development of skill.

Part of the input sequence of learning problem-solving behavior follows.

PROBLEM IDENTIFICATION SEQUENCE. The problem identification sequence has several operations. The first operation in this sequence is to identify the type of problem situation occurring. The literature identifies four types of problem situations:

1. The goal is obscure (ill defined or poorly identified); therefore the subsequent steps of problem solving cannot be enacted because their relevance cannot be determined.[28]

2. The goal is clear, but there are several alternative pathways for attaining the goal.[29]

3. The goal is clear, but a barrier interferes with goal attainment.[27]

4. More than one goal exists, and the problem solver must make choices between two or more equally attractive goals.[28]

Fig. 5-4 depicts these four types of problems.[26]

Problems are either presented to or discovered by the problem solver. When problems are presented, some "other" person presents or gives the problem to the problem solver. This other person may be the teacher, an employer, supervisor, or colleague. Presented problems have the characteristic of being clearly defined, and the problem solver uses few of the problem identification operations.

Discovered problems require the use of the operations involved in problem identification because the problem solver must discover what the goal is or what is preventing goal realization. The assessing behaviors of problem identification are (1) data gathering, (2) sorting and classifying data, (3) determining validity of data, (4) determining relevance of data, and (5) synthesizing and interpreting data.

Many of these same operations occur after a problem has been identified. These operations are used prior to problem identification to determine the nature of the problem and to establish a goal; they are used subsequent to problem identification to find an acceptable solution to the problem. Thus, although the operations used may be the same, they are done for different reasons and using additional data. For example, data gathering for problem identification will involve sources that can throw light on the problem situation—observations, interviews, and so on. The data gathering that occurs for the purpose of solving the problem (attaining the goal) will involve things that one needs to know to solve the problem. This includes facts, concepts, and all levels of theories that may be helpful in the generation of alternatives, selection of choices, estab-

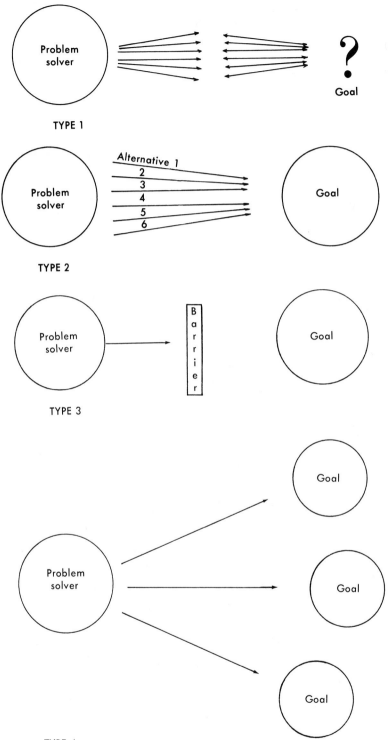

Fig. 5-4. Four types of problems. In Type 1 the goal is obscure; therefore the subsequent steps of problem solving cannot be enacted because their relevance cannot be determined. In Type 2 the goal is clear but there are several alternative pathways to attainment of the goal. In Type 3 the goal is clear, but a barrier interferes with goal attainment. In Type 4 more than one goal exists and the problem solver must make choices between two or more equally attractive goals.

lishment of priorities, and prescription of actions.

Classifying and sorting may be done in any number of categories. One useful category system is Who? What? Where? When? Why? or How?

Determining validity and relevance probably comprises the most important step in problem identification. These skills are most useful to the problem solver. A nonvalid or irrelevant bit of information can become a time-consuming "red herring" that clouds issues and actually sidetracks the process.

Synthesizing and interpreting the data require the most sophisticated skills, involving the putting together of all the data in a meaningful pattern and understanding the importance of the data pattern. All epidemiology is the study of patterns and their meanings. Interpretation requires some knowledge of the content of what is going on as well as the process of assessment. For instance, any person—nurse, parent, or other—who has been around infants with diarrhea or who has studied fluid and electrolyte balance knows that infant diarrhea is a problem requiring immediate attention, whereas adult diarrhea can be allowed to persist for much longer periods of time and with much larger fluid loss. This knowledge will influence the interpretation of problems in that category. However, skill in the process of problem solving does provide the problem solver with the ability to know when inadequate information is preventing him from making proper or adequate interpretations and frees him to consult with those who may have the content knowledge.

PROBLEM DATA SEQUENCE. Problem data sequence is the informational part of the process of problem solving. The more information the problem solver has that is relevant to the subject of the problem the more likely he is to think of all appropriate alternatives for action and to make appropriate choices among them. The problem data sequence is the collection of all facts, theories, concepts, and predictive principles relevant to the subject of the problem.

PROBLEM ALTERNATIVE SEQUENCE. The problem alternative sequence begins the decision-making activity phase of problem solving. In this sequence one determines the solution action alternatives. (The available action alternatives are natural outcomes of the predictive principles, that is, promoting and inhibiting theories or the third level of theory building.) In the problem alternative sequence each alternative must be considered by foreseeing the probable consequences of that alternative, the probability of a consequence occurring, and the value or risk involved if it does occur. For instance, a child falls from a tree. Moving him to the house is one alternative for the first action. (Other alternatives would be to assess his reflexes where he lies, determine whether or not he can move himself, call a physician to the spot, and so forth.)

The one alternative, moving the child to the house (prior to any other action), has several possible consequences, some of which are (1) further injury, (2) no further injury, (3) making him more comfortable (warm, better support, dry, and so on), and (4) causing pain. Each of these possible consequences has a probability of occurrence and a value of risk. The *probability* of occurrence is a subjective judgment based on experience, knowledge of the subject, or "hunch" material. It can be expressed in any code convenient to the problem solver. McDonald[29] uses 0 to 1, expressed in increments of one-tenth, 1.0 being the highest probability and .00 the lowest. The value of the consequence is based on the value system of the problem solver. In other words, if this consequence occurs, will the problem solver achieve something he values? The counterpoint of value is risk. If this consequence occurs, what does the problem solver place in jeopardy? Using the example of the child who fell from a tree, for the alternative of moving him to the house, the first consequence, further injury, is high to medium probability, low value, and high risk. In other words, if this alternative is chosen as a first alternative, the possible conse-

Decision schema using one alternative for child who fell from tree

Alternative	Some possible consequences	Estimates		
		Probability	Value	Risk
Move him to house (prior to any other action)	1. Further injury 2. No further injury 3. Making him more comfortable 4. Causing pain	1. .7 to .5 2. .3 to .5 3. .4 4. .5	Low High High None	High Low Low High

quence of further injury has at least a 70% to 50%, or .7 to .5, chance of occurring, which is a fairly high chance. Furthermore, if it does occur, nothing of value will have been achieved and grave damage could result; hence, this possible consequence of the alternative contributes to that alternative being a low value–high risk choice. For this alternative, because of the high probability of undesirable consequence, the decision would be to *not* choose this action. To make the final decision about the choice of an alternative, each possible consequence of each alternative must be considered for probability of occurrence and value.

Value is whether or not something desired is achieved without risking more than the desired end is worth. Risk and value are opposite sides of the same coin. Consequences of high value are usually of low risk and vice versa. Occasionally an alternative has high risk and high value because one or more of the possible consequences has a high probability of occurring —a high value if it does occur and yet containing a grave risk. If a baby is choking, an alternative of choice is an emergency penknife tracheotomy. This is a high-risk procedure, but if all other conservative actions have been exhausted, it is a high-value procedure and the risk is no greater than the risk of not performing the operation.

The *decision,* the culmination of the problem-solving process, then, is the final weighing and summation of probability, value, and risk, and the choice among the alternatives based on high probability of occurrence of a valued consequence that carries with it a risk no greater than the

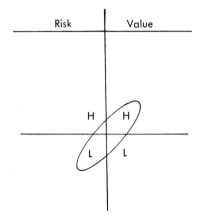

Fig. 5-5. Desirable decision choice.

problem solver is willing to take. Generally, a desirable decision choice is an alternative that is *low* risk–*high* value as illustrated in Fig. 5-5.

USE OF HEURISTIC DEVICES. A heuristic is a tool, a device for gaining an end, a strategy for learning or using a process. There are many heuristics available for every process, and some apply to a large variety of processes. Problem solving is a process— it has distinct definable stages or facets. Everyone performs the act of problem solving, but some problem solvers are better than others. The expertise with which one solves problems is probably related to two factors: (1) the utilization of all of the stages or facets of problem solving and (2) the number of tools or heuristic devices that the problem solver uses skillfully.

Interaction Associates, Inc.[30] compares problem-solving heuristics to a box of carpenter's tools. A competent, expert, and versatile carpenter has at his disposal a great many tools that he knows how to use well. He can then choose the tool most likely to accomplish a given task. Each problem solver needs to inventory his problem-solving tools and begin to add to his repertory. *Strategy Notebook: Tools for Change,* published by Interaction Associates, Inc., describes a large number of heuristics for problem solving. Some examples of heuristics for solving problems are synonyming, brainstorming, comparing and contrasting, defining, working forward, working backward, postponing, dreaming, fantasizing, predicting, and listing.

Some heuristics can be used for approaching problem solving, for innovating alternative actions, and for foreseeing consequences of those alternatives; all are useful for promoting creative solutions to problems. Each heuristic is listed with its powers, its limitations, and an exercise for using the heuristic.

CREATIVITY AND PROBLEM SOLVING. Creativity has been defined by using such phrases as "original behavior," "unusual behavior," or "unique behavior." Whatever the descriptive wording, it is clear that creativity is the ability to think of or to do things in unique ways. McDonald[31] speaks of creative behaviors as being inventive behaviors. Torrance, who has pioneered research in creativity, defines creativity as "the formation and testing of ideas and hypotheses."[32] Torrance[33] and Raigh further state that creativity can be taught by specifically structuring classroom activities that promote the generation of hypotheses and inventing ways to test those hypotheses. However, the ability to think of a wide variety of innovative alternatives or to combine many common elements into one unique idea is infrequently structured into curricula. The use of systematized, problem solving–decision making methodology—training in the use of heuristics that enlarge the number of approaches to problem solving and the probable options or alternative solutions to a problem—increases the creativity of individuals. Thus systematized problem solving provides for more

successful application of knowledge and the achievement of nursing successes.

Communicating process. The communicating process involves a whole series of subprocesses such as becoming self-aware, sensitive, and responsible to oneself and others. Group dynamics, family dynamics, and all the range of human interactions and relationships are subconcepts in this category.

Perception, although not discussed here, is the individual's or group's interpretation of received stimuli and is the keystone of the processes of communicating.

Communication and communicative behavior exist in all humans. Nurses utilize communications and communicative behavior whether or not they utilize it systematically. As in all processes, communicating is improved as the process is more fully analyzed and understood so that communicative behavior may be devised that more nearly approximates the true nature of the process. (See discussion of nature of process, pp. 8 to 11.) The success or failure of communications—intrapersonal, interpersonal, and community (group)—determines the health of the organism, the productivity of the organism, and even the ability of the organism to survive. This is true whether the organism is an individual, two individuals, or a group of individuals.

Communication, according to Ruesch and colleagues,[34] is the ability of one mind to affect another; communication processes are all those procedures by which one mind affects another. This includes all methods for transmitting and receiving messages: pictures, paintings, sculpture, music, dance, signs and signals, and written, vocal, and extrasensory transmission. The communication process is circular in the manner of all devices with built-in feedback systems (Fig. 5-6). There exist in the communication process the following factors:

1. Communication systems with defined limits. These are (a) intrapersonal, (b) interpersonal, and (c) community.

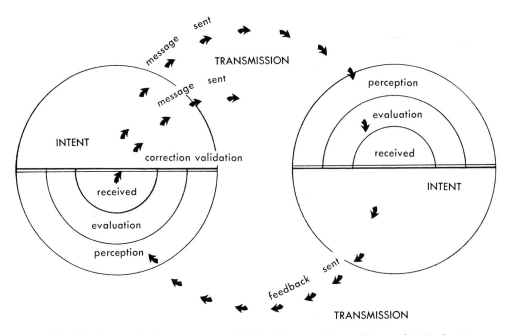

Fig. 5-6. Communication process model. (Used by permission of Mrs. Jackie Dunbar.)

2. Human organism communication apparatus. This includes (a) sensory organs to receive stimuli, (b) motor organs to send messages, and (c) thinking process apparatus that enables labeling, sorting, classifying, remembering, organizing, predicting, and making decisions.
3. The three phases of the communication process itself. These are (a) the purposive transmission of a message, (b) the perception of the message by a receiver, and (c) a signal that a message has been received.
4. For successful communications, some validation device to determine whether or not the message sent is the message received. This subprocess is called "feedback and correction."

These communication components tie together to form communications for the three systems. A cursory elucidation of the communication mechanisms in the three systems follows.

Intrapersonal system. The intrapersonal system comprises the organization of past experiences into patterns such as ideals, images, fantasies, sentiments, concepts, predictive and inhibiting principles, and problem solving. Furthermore, to be "communication," these organized experiences must be transmitted between the various systems of the body. Primarily, intrapersonal communication is commonly referred to as thinking and feeling. Others cannot perceive or understand unless the individual transmits some sign, symptom, or message. Intrapersonal communication can be anything from an increased pulse rate that results from the communication between a fantasy system and the adrenal cortex producing an autonomic response that emits perceivable signs and symptoms, to an organized and well-thought-out idea about the nature of centrifugal force. However, once the message is externalized, it becomes part of another communication system.

Interpersonal system. The interpersonal communication system is the sending of signals by one human being, their perception and interpretation by another human being, and the perception by the sender that the receiver has received the signal. Fig. 5-6 is a model of the interpersonal communication process.

The expressive action on the part of the sender can be, among other things, a result of the work of many persons (as an article by two or more persons), a series of sign language signals (as used by the deaf), a meaningful posture or body language, or a verbal statement by an individual. As long as it is a purposive expression of intrapersonal thoughts or feelings, it is a statement. When that purposive expression of personal thought or feelings has been perceived and interpreted by another individual, it is a message. When that message is acknowledged as received in any way, it becomes interpersonal communication. For the interpersonal communication to be perfected (clarified or corrected) or for any growth and change to occur, *feedback* must take place. Response to the message must be perceivable by the sender. For feedback to be useful, it has to be properly timed, appropriate to the situation, and delivered in a clear, understandable way. Negative and positive feedback play a part in growth and in stabilization of the individual.

Community system. Community communications is referred to as group communications by communication theorists. Group communications can be one individual and a group or two groups sending, receiving, interpreting, and responding to a message or series of messages. One of the characteristics of group or community communications is that in one to many or many to one (an individual and a group of people) and in many to many (group to group), feedback and correction are slow. As a general rule, the more people involved and the more bureaucracy involved in communication situations the more slowly perception, response, and correction occur. It is the ponderous nature of group communications that stimulates some groups to attempt to speed the process by the use of violent communication tactics.

Process organization of communications[35]

1. *Purpose:* To enable collaboration in finding solutions to problems and meeting needs.
2. *System*
   a. Organization of past experiences, needs, problems, fantasies, sentiments, concepts, or theories into a pattern the unit perceives as useful to the goal
   b. Transmission of this message to another unit through a communications apparatus
   c. Reception of message through perception apparatus by one or more units
   d. Signal of received message by perceiving unit
   e. Validation of message sent as message received between sending and receiving units with necessary corrections made
3. *Creativity:* The evolving ability to grow in the ability to communicate more effectively. Each communicative behavior becomes one of the many that add to the unit's ability to have a new communication experience—each different from the previous experience.

Communication breakdown

1. *Overloading the system.* Human communications share a characteristic with animals and machines—overloading will cause a breakdown of the process. A computer will click out on overload; an animal will show signs of purposeless behavior, erratic behavior, motorneuron synaptic failure, or other signs of "nervous breakdown"; a human being will replace normal modes of communication with private modes, restrict communication to the intrapersonal system, or use some other protective device.
2. *Malfunction of the communication apparatus.* This can be from disease or from poor or insufficient mastery of the use of communication apparatus.
3. *Incorrect information.* This is faulty

data or the erroneous perception or interpretation of data. Any time the input is faulty, the response will probably be faulty.

4. *Misuse or no use of strategies and tactics to obtain and utilize feedback that enables correction, growth, and change.* Without correction, growth, and change, misunderstandings and conflict cannot be resolved; thus frustration and its sequelae occur.

   Learning. Theories of learning will not be pursued further here. The process of learning is elaborated in Chapter 4. Briefly, the propositions selected in this book as an eclectic, systematized learning process theory can be summarized in eleven propositions. They are presented here in serial order, following a process pattern of three component parts.

1. *Purpose:* Self-actualization through the utilization of the environment to fulfill individual needs at any given time.
2. *System*
   a. People learn when they encounter a problem or need.
   b. Problems and/or needs create moderate anxiety.
   c. The moderate anxiety manifests itself in motivation and drive toward solutions to the problem or need fulfillment.
   d. Motivation and drive produce a learner need for solution-oriented input such as information, cues, models, or opportunity to discover (experiment).
   e. Input enables progression toward goals or problem solutions.
   f. Progression toward goal achievement is promoted by moving from the familiar to the unfamiliar.
   g. Active involvement of the learner in the learning episode makes learning more meaningful and useful, that is, self-experienced, self-appropriated, immediately rewarding, and relevant to the learner's own goals.
   h. Reinforcement of desired behaviors (including insight) increases move-

ment toward the goal; conversely, absence of feedback of any kind prevents progress, and consistently negative feedback (punishment), deliberate or accidental, leads to frustration, aggression, and avoidance. Progress thus breaks down and problems are not solved.
   i. Repetition with feedback and consequent improvement (practice), accompanied by reinforcement, develops behavior habits and patterns.
   j. Spaced or distributed recall, or more and varied opportunities for application, enables the learner to identify central concepts, verify principles, make generalizations and discriminations, and promotes retention.
   k. Success (achievement of goals) leads to tolerance of failure, realistic self-assessment, realistic goal setting, and self-perpetrating evaluation.

3. *Creativity:* The varied and unique ways that the learner appropriates the many things in his environment for the solution of his problem or the realization of his goals.

   Caring.[36] The process of caring is as central to nursing as problem solving or communicating. It is implied every time "nursing care" is referred to. Instead of *nursing* care the emphasis is on nurse *caring.* The process of caring can be sorted into four levels, or stages, of development, each comprising several sequential tasks. The nurse who is familiar with the process can more readily apply it. For instance, nurses can more easily identify the stage of caring they share with clients and determine how to facilitate forward movement of the relationship. Nurses can select the aspects of a phase in which they wish to participate and those in which they do not. They can assess the client's stage in the caring relationship and understand some of the needs and expectations of clients who are entering into an intensely caring relationship. People who are sick, in crisis, and in need tend more readily to accept rapidly developing caring relationships. In other words, the circumstances under which the relationship is developed may increase the speed at which one attains a given stage of development. Nurses, on the other hand, develop a variety of caring relationships with clients daily and therefore carefully choose the degree of reciprocation that they are willing to give. Furthermore, when caring is divided into its sequential stages of development, activities can be developed that help people to learn caring.

The nurse-caring relationship tends to be a variation of the usual caring relationship in that it generally operates in one direction (clients being the prime recipients of caring). The crisis, need, and generally lowered functional capacity typically experienced by clients during their interaction with nurses facilitate a one-way flow of caring energy. On the other hand, because the relationship is of a caring nature, clients recognize that they receive more than they give and often comment about that aspect. As energy returns and is available for giving to others, clients often attempt to put the caring relationship on a more lasting basis by inviting the nurse into greater participation. This is normal and necessary to the maturation of the caring process. Nurses can choose whether or not to facilitate the development of the relationship because if they know the tasks and stages, certain behaviors are fairly predictable.

The process of caring has the three attributes of any process: purpose, organization, and creativity.

Purpose. The purpose of caring is intimately joined with some health forms of love. Caring impels one to create an environment for loved ones that enables them to fulfill themselves. In this manner the purpose of caring is self-actualization—or more likely, mutual self-actualization. For Fromm,[37] caring helps people overcome separateness, achieve union, and transcend their individual life. Mayeroff states that caring gives "comprehensive meaning and order to one's life."[38] One of the basic

drives of all life forms is the drive to complete oneself, a principle to which even microorganisms hold. In humans it is manifested in the drive to grow, to fulfill, to transcend one's prison of self, one's locked-up inner life. The conditions of caring and the caring process are the conditions which enable that to happen; the drive to completion is the drive of growth; the purpose of caring is growth—mutual self-actualization.

Organization. The organization of caring is the system for achieving growth of self and facilitating growth of the one cared about. It is a system necessitating a relationship between two or more people. The process described here is basically that of a two-person relationship. The process applies whether or not the relationship is one to one, one to several, or several to several.

There are four levels, or stages, to the process of caring. Each stage must be successfully attained before the next can be successfully completed, since each successive stage includes the behaviors of the previous ones. Although the process can be entered at any point in the first two stages, it may be impossible or difficult to enter the process at late Stage III or IV. However, before maturity in any stage can be attained, the behaviors of the previous stage(s) must be achieved.

The four stages of caring are Stage I—attachment, Stage II—assiduity, Stage III—intimacy, and Stage IV—confirmation. Each stage comprises several tasks that are sequential and build toward successful attainment of each stage. Self-revelation, which is the basis for getting to know another person, is a theme that runs throughout the first three stages but takes on different behaviors in each stage. Therefore self-revelation is described as having three steps—one for each of the first three stages of caring. For example, self-revelation in Stage I contains information that is safe and nonthreatening, and individuals choose carefully the information that they are willing to reveal. As one moves through the stages, the information revealed about

Table 3. Four stages of caring and their components in serial order

Stage I Attachment	Stage II Assiduity	Stage III Intimacy	Stage IV Confirmation
Recognition- acknowledgement Self-revelation, step 1 Validation Potency	1. Respect 2. Potentiality 3. Attentiveness 4. Honesty 5. Self-revelation, step 2 6. Responsibility 7. Confidence 8. Courage	1. Probity 2. Self-revelation, step 3 3. Perspicacity 4. Sexuality 5. Inclusiveness	1. Personal validation 2. Augmentation 3. Sustainment 4. Expansiveness

oneself becomes more personal and meaningful. The sorting of tasks into stages does not imply that there is a clear-cut division of the stages. Some tasks may be completed early, and subsequent tasks from another stage may be started long before the major energy force of the caring participants moves into that stage. In other words, there is a great deal of flux and blurring of the tasks in each stage. The sorting into categories is meant to demonstrate where the major focus and activity usually occur.

Table 3 provides an overview of the process and the tasks included in each stage. Only a brief definition and description of the stages and their tasks will be included here.

INTRODUCTION TO STAGE I—ATTACHMENT. Attachment describes the behaviors or tasks in the initial stage of caring. This attachment is accomplished by moving through the four tasks of Stage I—recognition, self-revelation (step 1), validation, and potency. After the initial meeting of another person, one may intuitively recognize him as someone interesting to know.

Stage I is the starting point for getting to know others. The speed at which individuals pass through this stage will depend on their individual needs, former caring experiences, the time given to being together, stress levels, people and contingencies of the situation, and other factors and conditions. The success experienced in sharing and validating information about self and perceptions of the other caring person brings into focus an awareness of the possibilities for the relationship.

At the end of Stage I, preparation for moving into Stage II has been accomplished. The choice to progress or to keep the current status in the relationship is made on the basis of success in Stage I and desire to continue to develop the relationship.

STAGE I

TASK 1—RECOGNITION. Being aware of another's presence is the beginning of getting to know another. This recognition may be made operational in several ways. Ritualistic behaviors that are safe and predictable are generally employed first. Examples are handshaking, smiling, eye contact, firm touching, and typical questions such as "How are you?" Through these behaviors one indicates recognition, notice, and initial awareness of another. Within this awareness there may be the acknowledgment to oneself and to the other that this recognition is potentially meaningful. This is the time when one assesses whether or not he desires to learn more about the other. Task 1, recognition, is acknowledgment that this person may have potential personal significance.

TASK 2—SELF-REVELATION (STEP 1—DATA GATHERING). Self-revelation has three steps—one step in each of the first three stages of caring. The desire to know more about another individual leads to data gathering and self-revelation, step 1. In the beginning of a relationship one generally approaches or reveals areas that are nonthreatening and low risk. Data gathering may consist of vital statistics information, finding things in common, learning likes, dislikes, and hobbies, or sharing low-risk hopes and dreams. Through the sharing of this information, one has started the process of getting to know another person.

TASK 3—VALIDATION. During data gathering and self-revelation, each person begins to identify, examine, and validate positive and possibly negative aspects of the other individual. This validation is shared through giving approval of information shared and behaviors exhibited. Most of the validation probably will occur around positive things because there may be a fear of sharing one's "real self" until more is known about the other individual. This is a fear of not being liked or accepted "if you know what I am really like." Positive validation at this point begins the acceptance of being "OK" individuals within this relationship. There is also identification and validation of liked qualities or qualities desired for oneself within the other individual. Validation increases the desires of the individuals to move forward in the relationship.

TASK 4—POTENCY. Data gathering, self-revelation, and validation may spur the desire to move forward in the relationship or to get to know the other even better. With this realization may come an examining of the capabilities and alternatives for moving forward in the relationship. Potency indicates the will and power to begin moving forward. This may be the beginning of developing expectations indicating how each party will contribute at this point to progress in the relationship. Statements about expectations, desires, and future plans may be shared. An agenda of things to do together may be developed; for example, "I would surely like to go biking with you," or "I want a friend who talks straight with me." Potency also refers to the capacity to fulfill these expectations in the future, including the willingness of the individuals to put forth the energy to bring about the desired caring relationship.

STAGE II—ASSIDUITY. Assiduity is characterized by intense work between the caring parties. In addition to preserving the Stage I tasks accomplishments, there is constant close attention to the business of building the caring relationship and "getting to know" each other. This phase is marked by solicitous, persistent, personal attention. It involves sitting beside, being with, and concern for the welfare of the other person. It engages the constant energetic application of self to the enterprise of caring. This is a selfish phase, and one of the conditions that marks it is its exclusiveness. In Stage II the caring persons limit their attention to each other, tend to be somewhat possessive of each other's time and attention, and give special privileges to each other that exclude others from participation. They impose social restrictions and, for the duration of the early tasks of this phase, wish the undivided whole of the other person's time and energy together. Continuation of these conditions and the behaviors that mark them inhibits the maturing of the caring relationship, but they are typical for Stage II. Exclusiveness, which becomes inclusiveness in Stage III, is short lived and probably only occurs because of the intensity of the work taking place in this phase. If the work proceeds on a more leisurely basis over a long period of time, this degree of exclusiveness may not be an element.

Assiduity, close attention to the building of the relationship, includes the tasks of (1) respect, (2) potentiality, (3) attentiveness, (4) honesty, (5) self-revelation (step 2), (6) responsibility, (7) confidence, and (8) courage.

TASK 1—RESPECT. The first behavior in the assiduity phase of caring is respect. The behaviors of respect are being reverent, being accepted, and being nonjudgmental. Respect is inherent in caring and begins early in the relationship, but it is not until Stage II that it hallmarks the relationship. Respect is first for the humanness of the individual and as such is impersonal. Without respect for one as a human, nurse caring is perfunctory and ritualistic. With respect for humanness comes a reverence for life and acceptance of individuality, separateness, and a nonjudgmental attitude that enable support for the other person in his or her own ethnic, ethical, and behavioral mode. This means an understanding and appreciation of the universality (need, experience, joys, and sorrows) of another. The paradox is that both the universality and the uniqueness of the one cared about are prized and respected. Respect means acknowledging and accepting the wishes, preferences, differences, needs, and desires of another and feeling OK about them.

Admiration is part of respect. Caring relationships begin with a healthy measure of admiration for the one cared about. One may admire the other physically for how he looks, walks, wears his hair, or keeps his nails. For caring to persist and grow, admiration must entail respect for how the person thinks, acts, and behaves in certain situations and what he values.

TASK 2—POTENTIALITY. Potentiality is an awareness of the possibilities for persons individually and together in the relationship. Some drugs, when given together, potentiate each other; they are synergistic, each receiving benefits or hazards of the other, which increases the potency of each. Caring has the same capacity. Potentiality is the effort to realize the richness that is the possibility of caring, the possibility of changing, growing, and becoming, because of the reciprocal relationship. At this stage there is work toward fusion, mutual enhancement without compromising individuality. The intense work of this stage partly depends on the ability of each participant to dream the dream and see the vision of the potential in the relationship. It differs from potency in Stage I in that potency is chiefly establishing primary expectation and choosing to commit time and energy to further develop the relationship. Potential in Stage II, in addition to seeing potential for the relationship, sees how much the relationship can help fulfill individual potential and self-actualization.

In addition to awareness of growth possibilities for each person as with potency in Stage I, there is the possibility that the relationship can progress to the third stage and the choice is there to be made. The decision to move forward may be based on an analysis of the relationship. Caring people in this stage analyze the problems, possibilities, and assets of the relationship and the mutual effect. They continue to analyze what they would like from the relationship and what they are willing to give to it. From this analysis come more implicit or explicit behavioral contracts than were made in Stage I, setting the scene for the third stage.

TASK 3—ATTENTIVENESS. Attentiveness is a behavior necessary to assiduity and comprises heeding, attending, and listening in a discerning manner. It is one of the most important things that a caring person can do for another. It provides a bridge for individuals to reduce aloneness. In a caring relationship one learns to listen to content, the process (the message behind the words), and feeling tones in a conversation. Caring people determine what they are willing to listen to; for example, a person in a caring relationship may not be willing to listen to the other person discount or devalue himself.

Another part of attentiveness is awareness of how one responds to what is said. Allowing another to express ideas, feelings, or thoughts different from one's own requires that one neither discount nor judge the other. Each person is not held to the exact words that are spoken, but intent and meaning are sought so that clarifying is part of the communication process.

If the relationship is to mature and progress, then "You said it; therefore you mean it" is not a part of the communication of caring. Each individual is allowed to have thoughts and words unfold, develop, be retrieved, and be changed as the conversation progresses. In this stage, caring people develop communication patterns that enable them to trust enough to think aloud together. Such thinking aloud occurs in the third stage, but the groundwork and pattern for it are laid here.

TASK 4—HONESTY. In caring, honesty is

present in the behaviors of being open, genuine, and truthful. It includes actively confronting oneself and the other person. Honesty implies congruency among content (words), feeling tones, and behaviors. Honesty does not imply being brutal, tactless, or disregarding the feelings of oneself or others. It can be attained and acted on with gentleness and consideration. Instead of saying, "This is the worst meatloaf I ever ate," one can, if asked, offer ideas about what is missing: "I think more salt and less celery seed would have been better."

Honesty in response is essential to the caring relationship. When asked a direct question, one either answers truthfully or states clearly that one does not wish to talk about the topic. Respect for the wishes of the other, for what they wish to reveal or discuss (task 2), is necessary to honesty. Honesty is practiced within the limits of the self-exposure that the individuals are willing to allow at each stage of the caring process; for example, one need not "tell all." In Stage II, the inquiry, "Have you ever smoked hash?" may receive a dishonest answer or an expressed desire not to discuss the topic because the information requested threatens the individual and trust has not been sufficiently established to support the admission of socially unacceptable or illegal personal data. If lies are told, corrections must be made later or trust can never achieve the level necessary to the mature caring relationship. Honesty is one of the elements that comprise trust, just as trust is an element that enables honesty. The two develop together. Additionally, respect helps the caring person to recognize the limits and potentials and to assess the current status of the relationship clearly so that no more honesty is required than there is trust to support it.

TASK 5—SELF-REVELATION (STEP 2). Self-revelation in this stage goes beyond the data-gathering phase of Stage I into material that is closely aligned with who the person really is. The philosophy by which the person lives is a part of the content, as are formative experiences that contributed to or detracted from the individual's basic sense of self and self-esteem. Early experiences characterize this phase, such as childhood scenes that impacted on the individual's character and personality. The self-expression of this phase is an attempt to explain oneself and to be understood. It is a declaration that "This is what I am all about and what makes me tick." It is often tentative because of fear of what the other may think. There is testing, affirmation, progress, and retesting until the trust level is reached that enables transition into Stage III. Sentences in this task often begin with "I believe . . ." or "I am really commited to. . . ." "I was raised in a foster home until I was 12" would be the kind of formative experiences shared. Socially unacceptable experiences are not usually shared until Stage III. Because of the intensity in the need to share biographical and personal philosophy data, and partly because of the vulnerability that accompanies self-revelation, time alone with the cared one is valued.

TASK 6—RESPONSIBILITY. The responsibility in caring is dual: (1) responsibility for oneself and accountability for one's own behavior, thoughts, feelings, and words; and (2) responsibility to respect the vulnerability of the one cared about.

Responsibility for oneself means owning one's own feelings, acts, and words—not blaming another but accepting behaviors and feelings as belonging to oneself. This means a sense of power in that only oneself has the power to cause feelings and only oneself "makes" one do something. This responsibility for oneself is a free choice. "I choose to respond or not, to feel or not, to speak or not—therefore I am responsible." "You made me do it" is not, nor ever can be, part of the growing, maturing, caring relationship. "You make me mad, you make me sad, you make me anxious" are alien to responsibility for oneself. "I make me mad, sad, anxious, joyful, glad" are symptoms of the growing maturing relationship.

Responsibility means not violating trust,

infringing on rights, encroaching on space, intruding into other relationships, interfering in plans, decisions, or activities, or trespassing where forbidden or uninvited. In other words, responsibility is for one's own activities that affect the relationship or the one cared about. This is not to be construed as being responsible for what another does with the behavior or words but only the doing or saying of it. Being considerate, thoughtful, and reasonable is being responsible in caring.

Caring is a process of increasing vulnerability because of the regard, trust, sharing, self-revelation, and intimacy of all caring relationships. The task of responsibility, in addition to the foregoing, means that one is aware of the vulnerability of the one cared for and is *care*ful of it.

Another area of which responsibility is a component is communication. Individuals in caring relationships attempt to make communications explicit and clear so that no one feels it necessary to make assumptions or mind read. Mind reading occurs when one wants to meet another's needs and, lacking input or contracts around needs, the responses become irrational or based on history rather than current expressions. Being rationally consistent in meeting another's needs and having one's own needs met is part of responsibility. Irrational meeting of needs becomes ritualistic—in other words, meeting another's needs because someone feels that it is expected. This may lead to boredom or guilt, and according to Perls,[39] when guilt is experienced, there is resentment behind it. Expectations or demands perceived as unfair or as a constraint on behavior, growth, or freedom lead to resentment, a killer of caring. Men and women often fall into communication and expectation traps. Traditional male-female roles are conducive to situations where communications about expectations are not clear, and social role expectations and assumptions based on role conditioning serve in lieu of contracts. Responsibility rests with caring people to establish clear behavioral contracts

or expectations so that this destructive chain of events is avoided.

TASK 7—CONFIDENCE. Confidence is acknowledging to oneself and to others in the caring relationship a certainty in one's own ability to recognize and meet one's own needs. It is a belief in one's own competence that provides the individual with freedom essential to the voluntary nature of the relationship. If confidence is lacking, a series of events can occur that "hook" the caring partners into games, manipulations, and irresponsible need meeting. Symbiosis, which is feeding on each other and/or unhealthy dependence, can result from the absence of confidence. Confidence means that each person believes in his own ability to look after his own interests, to say when he needs help, to ask for assistance, and to acknowledge strengths. Confidence also means that one has trust that the other person can also speak for himself, act in his own behalf, and ask for help or assistance when needed. Without respect, confidence is empty; however, confidence goes further than respect. It is knowing that oneself and others have strengths and limitations, that each recognizes for himself, and that each can and will act on that knowledge. When this occurs, people meet only those needs which have been specifically expressed—they avoid the rescuer role which leads to the persecution-rescuer-victim triangle.[40] They avoid getting hooked into relationships where the other person "needs" them so much that they believe the other person will disintegrate, fail, or be helpless without them. Many relationships stick at this level and progress no further. Dependent relationships, those in which confidence does not exist, stagnate at this point and progress no further.

TASK 8—COURAGE. Courage, the last task in Stage II, provides the temerity to venture into the unknown of the third stage, intimacy. Courage is luck; it is doing what one wants or needs to do despite fear, vulnerability, cost, or repercussions, but only after those contingencies have been assessed and the goal has been deemed worthy of the price. Courage is required to proceed into intimacy, deeper levels of self-revelation, increased vulnerability, greater trust, and expanded relationships with more people.

Another aspect of courage is being what one is, being oneself, and being true to oneself, one's feelings, hopes, and dreams. It means not yielding to fantasies that real aspects of oneself will "make" the cared one care less. Courage provides the ability to be, to venture, to grow, and to pursue mutual self-actualization.

STAGE III—INTIMACY. Intimacy is the stage of caring in which the caring parties move into a level of closeness in which they share each other's innermost being and come to understand and know the other's essential nature. It is marked by close physical, mental, and/or social association and unreserved, easy confidential expression of self. In this stage there is a deep commitment to the relationship, and the relationship takes on feelings of permanence. Even if the caring relationship does not successfully attain all the tasks of this stage, each friend makes an indelible imprint and is never forgotten.

The stage of intimacy is marked by five tasks—probity, self-revelation (step 3), perspicacity, sexuality, and inclusiveness.

TASK 1—PROBITY. The three characteristics of probity are integrity, trust, and nonexploitiveness. In Stage III there is an integrity to the relationship, a wholeness and unity, and a total integration. There develops a consistency among the elements of the persons involved. Each becomes part of the other's experiences, past, present and future, and the relationship develops a sense of even flow.

Trust of a very high level develops in Stage III. It is the development of this trust that enables the sharing of intimate information (task 2). Trusting includes being willing to be vulnerable about oneself and knowing the other person will accept and not judge actions, feelings, and thoughts. It also means that the individual knows, beyond doubt, that the knowledge, infor-

mation, or experiences will not be divulged or used except for the benefit of the individual or that of the relationship. No promises about confidentiality need to be exacted. The intimacy will be shared with the sure knowledge that it will not be misused.

Nonexploitiveness, the last characteristic of task 1, means that no one gets "ripped off." Everyone involved has his needs met, gives and receives equally, and is not used. It means that everything about the relationship is treated by both parties fairly, justly, and honestly. Each is responsibly careful of the other and, when necessary, looks after the other's interests in a way perceived as being acceptable to the other.

TASK 2—SELF-REVELATION (STEP 3). This step in self-revelation includes items that make the parties feel extremely vulnerable. They are free to share knowledge about themselves of socially nonsanctioned experiences or behaviors. For example, illegal acts such as crimes, drug use, past love affairs, living with someone of the opposite sex, or homosexual feelings or experiences fit into this category. The individuals are also willing to share self-doubts or experiences in which they feel they disappointed themselves or someone they cared about. This is probably the most difficult of all areas to share, for example, the sharing of times when a person has perceived himself as being weak, inexperienced, naive, malicious, hurtful, out of control, or any other way that may violate the individual's value system or damage his self-esteem. When self-revelation includes this material, it has achieved the degree of honesty and depth that marks the stage of intimacy in caring.

TASK 3—PERSPICACITY. Perspicacity is a simple yet important task; it means having rapid and accurate insights into the other. The caring parties are quick to discern, find meaning in and understanding of the other's words, behaviors, and feelings. Perspicacity may occur without talking. It is the ability to look across a room and know, beyond doubt, that you have communicated with each other accurately. It is not mind reading but behavior reading, eye reading, and of course, meaning-behind-the-meaning reading. It does not lead to mind reading but to validation. It is not used in lieu of explicit communications; rather it is an adjunct to explicit communications.

TASK 4—SEXUALITY. Sexual feelings toward the one cared about are a normal part of intimacy. Society has placed heavy injunctions on sexuality. The "don't" messages cover people of like sex, family, married people of the same and opposite sex, and children. With cultural injunctions so prevalent, most people believe that sexual feelings in other than courting and marriage are "bad" (abnormal or depraved), and they may not allow themselves to feel sexual feelings, may translate them into other feelings, or may deny them. In caring, intimacy includes sexual intimacy in feelings, thoughts, and fantasy and sometimes in actual fact. Some caring people are afraid of their feelings because they think that the feelings may be translated into behaviors. Once one knows that feelings do not have to be acted on and that one may have the feeling and choose to act or not act, there is enough safety to allow the sexual feelings to occur.

On the other hand, as is well known, sexual feelings do not necessarily imply caring. Engaging in a sexual act can mean any number of things that may or may not involve caring at any level or stage. Sexuality may be a part of caring beginning in Stage I and may exist completely independently of the other stages. However, if sexual feelings have not emerged prior to Stage III, intimacy, they will emerge here. Many relationships stagnate or reverse when sexual feelings arise, especially if the one cared about is a person to whom social injunctions against sexuality apply. Men who are in a caring relationship with another man, or a woman with a woman, may become scared at this stage and begin to decelerate the relationship. Sexual feelings, whether or not they are allowed to surface into awareness, may be manifested in socially approved ways. For instance, in the United States arm wrestling, back pounding, and shoulder slapping are socially approved for men, hugging and kissing for women. Backrubs, foot massages, and visual caresses are socially approved ways of expressing sexuality.

The sexually aware person will explore his feelings with the one cared about and reach some mutually satisfactory way of dealing with them. As a general principle, the more explicitly and honestly the sexual feelings are dealt with the less will be the threat to the caring relationship; and conversely, the less straightforward the handling of sexual feelings aroused by intimacy the less likely the relationship will continue to grow and ultimately ripen into Stage IV.

Self-doubts about one's sexual orientation ("Am I a homosexual?"), one's sexual deviance ("Am I incestuous?"), or one's monogamy ("Am I a philanderer?") may plague the person who does not confront and work through the normal feelings of sexuality arising in this stage. This is a result of social injunctions and not because sexual feelings in caring are unusual.

TASK 5—INCLUSIVENESS. In Stage III the time comes when the caring persons can move out into other relationships without feeling that the time spent would be better spent together without others. Two things happen: First, the intensity of the assiduity period has decreased and intimacy has developed to the stage of feeling comfortable and secure so that the two enjoy the inclusion of others. Second, the caring parties realize and accept that no one individual can meet all their needs and that, in order not to strain the caring relationship, diversity must occur. In relationships one gets different things from different people because individuals are composites of various needs and each person has so many variables that no one friend or person can respond to all the needs. Caring relationships, privileges, and responsibilities are simultaneously maintained with several persons. Each relationship may be in a different stage of development, since each is separate and apart from the others. However, in this stage of caring no relationship detracts from the others. Each is synergistic with all others and potentiates other caring relationships.

STAGE IV—CONFIRMATION. Qualities and feelings developed through successful caring relationships provide one with the ability and desire to share the richness and positive feelings of those relationships. Successful attainment of the third stage enables one to feel sufficiently comfortable and safe to expand caring on a wider basis. Attaining Stage IV in a caring relationship also has positive benefits for maturing the individuals concerned. One seems to feel secure, willing to be vulnerable, to grow, expand, and be the best possible self.

The stage of confirmation is that in which one verifies oneself, one's own sense of being good, worthwhile, able, strong, capable, and unafraid of intimacy in relationships. The behaviors of caring are deeply ingrained and are consistently practiced. Confirmation means to validate, assure, strengthen, and authenticate. In caring this is a confirmation of oneself and of the relationship with others about whom one cares. Because of the personal validation that takes place in the fourth level, relationships with others are sustained and expanded. There are four tasks in this stage—personal validation, augmentation, sustainment, and expansiveness.

TASK 1—PERSONAL VALIDATION. In personal validation there is a sense of assurance, strength, and well-being. The positive experience of being loved and loving in an egalitarian relationship provides a firmly established sense of power over one's own life and behavior. A growth potential is tapped, and the individual becomes more mature. This maturity is reflected in the person's sense of his own value, strengths, and limitations and in a growth in wisdom, judgment, and insight. The individual is more self-aware, resourceful, self-assured, less aggressive and more assertive, more articulate, responsive to others, and perceptive of the subtle undercurrents in relationships and conversations. These attributes, although perhaps always present and somewhat available in the individual, simply become more fully developed and frequently used because of the affirming nature of caring and being cared about to the degree expressed by Stage III. In this task there is a similarity to Maslow's self-actualizing person.

TASK 2—AUGMENTATION. Augmentation is a task in which the caring relationship itself becomes enlarged, strengthened, and more at ease. There is a consolidation of the friendship, a knowledge of each other, a comfort in being with each other, and a feeling of settling down after the rapid pace of building the relationship. The caring relationship continues to grow, but there is no longer an urgency about it. The energy formerly spent in extending, deepening, and expanding the relationship is now freed for other tasks. A time interval is necessary for augmentation to take place. As in wine, time provides the aging that mellows the relationship and increases its worth. Any remaining doubts about the caring persons are dispelled, and a high degree of trust evolves. Behaviors toward each other are predictable in principle if not in detail. Each person knows that the other's behaviors are supportive, nurturing, and positive; each has a clear sense of the direction in which the other is growing and has a feel for the focus of the other's life.

TASK 3—SUSTAINMENT. Sustainment is the ability to maintain the relationship through difficulty, loss, grief, interruption, or separation. It means the relationship is durable and can be maintained at the same or increased strength without reinforcement by the other person. In the absence of outside reinforcement the relationship continues at the same intensity. Sustainment is the self-reinforcing aspect of caring. The feelings of caring about the relationship and about the person continue in the absence of contact. Memories and the conditioning of past experiences together and the self-fulfilling joy of loving provide the mechanisms for self-reinforcement with no return expression from the other person. This self-reinforcing mechanism is based on a realistic perception of the caring relationship and its meaning to the individual, not on distortion because of time or rose-colored memory.

Sustaining behaviors are those which perpetuate caring. One feels good about oneself and "strokes" oneself for having entered into, developed, maintained, and confirmed the self-revelation, intimacy, and nurturing necessary to such a rewarding relationship. Self-reinforcing and maintaining the feelings of caring in the absence of feedback are never used as a positive device against developing other relationships or as a comparison for all other relationships. Quite the contrary, the sustaining task is one in which the good feelings that foster self-reinforcement are also used to foster expansion, the last stage of the caring relationship.

TASK 4—EXPANSIVENESS. Expansiveness is the ability to care on a widening basis. It is extended caring—extended in the amount of caring, the number of people, and the scope of things one can care about. The word alone provides insight into this task. "Expansive" means to spread out, unfold, amplify, enlarge; it is an outgoing and outpouring of caring. Caring becomes multiplex, that is, is caring for more people, more readily, with greater ease and less expenditure of energy. Expansiveness is not just more people one at a time but more people in groups. It is different from inclusiveness; it is actually entering into a phase of willingness to take risk and to be open, vulnerable, trusting, nurturing, and helpful on a wider scale. It means that one moves through the phases of caring more rapidly with others and with groups, but not without judgment. There is a great deal of judgment involved, based on assessment of the risk, energy, time, and consequences of entering into caring relationships. A person does not take foolish risks or expose all his feelings all

the time. He simply is available for more caring relationships. Attainment of this task is marked with a feeling of warmth and "good vibes" that flow from the person. The caring person is a living, breathing, recycling force for caring.

Creative outcome. Creativity, the third aspect of a process, is manifested in caring by the many unique ways in which caring is experienced. Each caring relationship is unique. Although the components are the same, the individual's context, variables, experiences, and circumstances are different for each caring relationship. The caring pattern affects only the common denominator of feelings and behaviors, their sequence and form. The experience remains uniquely one's own.

Summary. There is in humans a tendency to be concerned for other humans, even strangers. Except when fear or other conditioning eradicates or prohibits the feelings, caring (for example, concern for others) is a common human experience. The feelings of caring need not be acted on. However, when they are, they lead to events such as strangers stopping to help change a tire or passersby rescuing children from burning buildings at their own peril. The generalized caring about others is not the type and kind of caring discussed here. Personal caring, caring about a specific person or group, is the subject for this discussion. The proposition is offered that those who enter into personal caring relationships with others and who reach the fourth stage more readily expand their caring to the impersonal generalized caring about people.

Knowledge about the caring process, its purpose, organization, and outcome, enables nurses to understand and interact with clients more wisely and with greater caring because they make choices based on knowledge. For instance, clients, when moving into Stage II, want time with "their nurse" alone, without sharing with others, and only during that time will they be interested in self-revelation. Nurses who readily accept patient self-revelation can know, by understanding the caring process, that the same degree of self-revelation is desired of them but that it is not essential to the client at that time. If the nurse expects to carry the caring process into Stage III or further, the nurse must reciprocate in every activity of every phase or the caring relationship will not mature.

Process of management/changing. The process of management/changing subsumes the processes of leadership, organizational structure, and management. It includes some aspects of the processes of adaptation and problem solving, maturation, and communication. By definition, planned change is planned adaptation to a shift in the environment. The word "planned" indicates collaboration and cooperative endeavor; the phrase "shift in environment" means an increase in the number of variables as opposed to the stability of environmental factors. (Stable factors require no new adjustments, whereas variables require new considerations, new coping mechanisms.) In the process of changing, the interdependent and mutually inclusive nature of all the processes meaningful to nursing is obvious. Planned change is change with a purpose, devised to solve problems of society through the use of the behavioral sciences. Planned change is a type of human engineering where theories of human behavior are applied so that intelligent choices and actions are the result. Thus the process of changing deals with change by choice and deliberation and is distinctly different from change by indoctrination, coercion, growth (natural), and accident. Skinner's *Walden Two*[41] is an example of the use of stimulus-response association as the mechanism for social engineeering. Skinner fantasizes a utopia where by mutual consent people create a community that successfully applies stimulus-response associationism theories of learning to all facets of human life. Planned-change theorists propose a utopia not too different from *Walden Two* in the respect that appropriately employed, behavioral scientists can enable changes that are the result of collective and collaborative choice to take place in all facets of organized society.

For nursing process to realize its goal, nurses must respond, through participation and collaboration, to the vast number of variables in the health needs system with constructive, deliberate changes in methods of coping with health problems. The use of theories of change in all three nursing care systems, intrapersonal, interpersonal, and community, is necessary to the creative element of nursing process.

One of the most difficult problems facing change agents is the lack of a conclusive theory of how to implement changes. Many studies have been done on the mechanics and the dynamics of change. But according to Bennis,[42] there is no theory of changing. However, Bennis' propositions about the use of laboratory training in effecting social change can be altered and used as guides for change.

Change theorists commonly refer to the components of the change process as follows:

Agent—Person, social scientist, nurse (trained in the science of change)

Rate—Speed at which change takes place (evolutionary, slow, revolutionary, galloping)

Arena—Organization, institution (the place in which the change occurs, the environment of change)

Person—Target of change (client of change, the client system; may be individual or group)

To systematize the change process, one needs at least some hypotheses of changing, some theories about what will promote or inhibit change taking place. There seems to be agreement among change scientists about the elements of the process of change but no agreement about an organized system for effecting change. In lieu of definitive theory several propositions about implementing changes are offered. Since change is a process, the discussion of change is organized around the components of process: purpose, organization, and creativity.

Planned change (changing)

1. *Purpose:* To anticipate and solve the problems of society and its subunits with maximum efficiency and effectiveness and minimum disruptions.
2. *System*
   a. Change occurs when needs arise with which standard procedures and organization cannot cope.
   b. The breakdown of effectiveness of standard procedures and organization causes an increase in anxiety of the individuals within the group.
   c. Anxiety provides a need to change or adapt that is accompanied by an increase in individual and collective energy.
   d. Need to change or adapt stimulates fantasies of solutions or the anticipation of the achievement of objectives.
   e. Free exchange of ideas about goals helps to establish specific legitimate goals.
   f. Free exchange of ideas about goals and subgoals enables collaboration of purposeful effort.
   g. Group commitment to the change process itself instead of specific changes enables continuing investigation, growth, and improvement.
   h. Certain conditions and ground rules provide the framework necessary for planned change to occur.
   i. Once goals are established, an explicit and definitive task analysis provides the client system with an overall view of the subgoals and tasks that must be accomplished to attain goals.
   j. The establishment of target dates around timing realities enables change participants to pace their work realistically.
   k. Organization of change participants around components of task analysis decreases "power" focus and in-

creases goal orientation of work groups.
   l. Formation and assignment of task groups according to the task, timing, and capabilities of the participants enables each member of the client system to contribute optimally.
3. *Creativity:* Creativity in change is the act of change itself—the evolution of a new system that, in the long process of change, will give rise to yet another new system.

UTILIZATION OF A THEORY OF NURSING

The elaboration of a theory of nursing and its components has been recorded to illustrate its use in curriculum building. Nursing as a process can be actualized or enacted: The enactment of a process is the practice of that process. Nursing practice, nursing action, or nursing intervention is what nursing theory is all about. One of the values of a theory is to provide an educated guess about what is occurring so that reality can be reproduced more efficiently and effectively in the future. Theorizing is a speculation about the past; that is, it arises from practice, but its only value lies in the future, in its use for reproducing desired practice. Dickoff, James, and Wiedenbach state: "Nursing theory may be deemed a good one if, by following it, activity can be brought about persistently, consistently, and extensively to create the kind of reality conceptually specified by the theory as desirable."[43]

The theory of nursing suggested here is an attempt to articulate a nursing theory as a curriculum base. According to Dickoff, James, and Wiedenbach, there may be more than one good nursing theory.[43] A quick perusal of the literature indicates that there most probably are many valid, reliable, and usable theories of nursing, although few have been explicitly so labeled. The one suggested here is only a beginning attempt to provide a workable theory that will enable the reproduction of reality, "persistently, consistently, and extensively."

It is interesting to note that Dickoff, James, and Wiedenbach[44] state that many nonnurses can be agents of nursing activities. In other words, the activity being carried out may be a specific nursing activity designed to achieve high-level wellness but enacted, practiced, or carried out by a person other than a nurse. So often nurses seek a theory of nursing that delineates nursing activities as those which can be performed only by nurses. This uniqueness of nursing practice is neither desirable nor possible and clouds the real issue—that of the unique way that theories deemed by the theorist as relevant are utilized.[45] Thus it is not in any specific act that nursing is a unique discipline nor in the components of nursing theory; nursing's uniqueness can be found only in the whole, the blending and melding of theories from other disciplines with nursing care and the practice or activities that arise from that theory pool.

A curriculum is "a plan for learning."[46] A theory of nursing process is a speculation about how to produce the situation in which optimum health can be facilitated; therefore a nursing curriculum is a plan for learning how to produce the situation or environment whereby people can facilitate individual or collective optimal health.

Example of the use of the nursing theory in one health-threatening situation. A brief topical recapitulation of the nursing theory used in this book is presented here as a reference point for the illustration.

Purpose	Target system (organization)	Creative components (relative contributing theories)
Optimal health	Intrapersonal	Stress response
	Interpersonal	Decision making
	Community	Communication
	Behaviors	Learning
	Protective	Human development
	Nurtrative	Change
	Generative	

Optimal health is the goal of all nursing activities; however, more specific goals arise when anything threatens health. For instance, a specific goal would be to negate the health hazard of measles.

Some *protective* behaviors within the target system of the *intrapersonal system* would be to immunize susceptible individuals, that is, infants, school children, pregnant women, and so forth. To achieve this, nurses would need to use theories of *learning* to teach about the necessity of immunization; theories of *communication* to communicate with the individuals involved; theories of *growth and development* to know how to communicate effectively with individuals of that age group and which age groups were most susceptible to measles; theories of *stress response* to know about the antigen-antibody response and whether or not immunization is necessary in individuals who have already had rubella. An example of *nurtrative behaviors* that are in the *interpersonal target system* would be seen in helping a family cope with a family member who has measles or in *caring* about a pregnant member exposed to measles. Theories from all seven specified subprocess or content areas would be used in the simple nursing activities involved in helping a family care for a member who is sick with a communicable disease.

Curriculum content implication

The curriculum content implications of devising a nursing theory are that through designing or identifying and utilizing nursing theories, constructs, and concepts, content becomes clearly organized to meet educational and nursing service goals. Theories are used as an integral part of every nursing course and every nursing class. All facets of nursing theories and concepts that are deemed important to the curriculum builders are utilized to provide integrity to the content. The subject or knowledge area of the conceptual framework pervades every course, every class, as the content selection and organized strategy. The setting and student sections of the conceptual framework are also utilized in this manner. It is the articulated concepts arising from setting and student needs as well as professional concepts and theories that are visible throughout the curriculum. If category systems that are organismic and not dualistic are taught, holism is achieved and nursing concepts are no longer artificially fragmented by either the (1) phase of illness (prevention-acute-chronic-rehabilitation), (2) arena of practice (industrial nursing, school nursing, community nursing, acute-hospital nursing), (3) medical specialty area (obstetrical, psychiatric, public health, pediatric, and so on), or (4) type of relevant theory (decision making in nursing, leadership in nursing, nurse as change agent, and so on).

Output

Nursing behaviors, nursing care, and nursing caring are the output of the nursing system, the creative element of nursing process. This is the reason why outcome criteria in the guise of terminal behaviors are so important to nursing curriculum building, since without criteria there is no way to determine if the output of the system is responsive to the system input and geared to the target and clients of care.

The first type of behaviors listed comprise *protective nursing behaviors*, which are those roles and functions which protect the vulnerable, promote attaining and maintaining one's goals with the least expenditure of energy, and facilitate client systems in achieving self-protection. Protective nursing behaviors correspond with Leavell and Clark's "primary prevention."[47] Activities that conform to the concept of primary prevention are (1) the provision of the conditions of health, that is, adequate housing, food, clothing, and environment conducive to attainment of the tasks of development central to the growth phases of life; (2) protection from disease through immunization, communi-

cable disease control, removal of noxious stimuli, and the institution of safety controls; and (3) shielding from threats to health, such as fish contaminated with mercury or insecticides or improperly or misleadingly labeled food or drugs, that may jeopardize the user. For example, some baby foods labeled "Meat and Vegetables" contain only minute amounts of meat, and parents who know the percentage of meat to vegetables in such combination jars would probably choose to feed their babies from two different jars, one meat and one vegetable, rather than depend on a combination jar for adequate nourishment for their youngsters. This kind of information given to parents by nurses is an act of protection and enables parents to prevent malnourishment in their children. Protective behaviors constitute one classification of nursing functions that helps to meet the purpose of nursing—high-level wellness.

The second type of behaviors listed comprise *nurtrative behaviors*, which are those roles and functions which provide for the care, comfort, and cure of client systems. It is the provision of supporting, sustaining, and succoring activities. It is the facilitation of clients to nurture themselves and to enter into nurturing relationships with others. These nursing activities are behaviors that are involved in the direct care of people, whether it be to increase their comfort, to help them get well, or to nourish them. Nurtrative activities are activities such as hygienic care and nursing procedures, both comforting and curative. Nurtrative nursing behaviors are involved in supporting, sustaining, and helping; this may be accomplished by relieving pain, positioning in bed, encouraging and motivating patients, modifying behaviors, socializing people with antisocial behavior, giving dialysis, or helping a family learn to cope with the trauma of an absent member. Some of the components of the nurtrative aspect of nursing behaviors correspond to Leavell and Clark's "secondary prevention."[48] However, to draw a complete parallel would be in error. The American Nurses' Association's position paper describes the care aspect of nursing as "caring for and caring about as well as taking care of."[49] This paper further states: "It is providing comfort and support in times of anxiety, loneliness, and helplessness. It is listening, evaluating, and intervening appropriately."[49] Nurtrative behaviors constitute one classification of nursing functions that helps to meet the purpose of nursing—high-level wellness.

The third type of behaviors listed comprise *generative behaviors,* which are those roles and functions which are creative, productive, reproductive, and rehabilitative. It is helping client systems and their significant others to be optimally productive with the least expenditure of energy and minimal disruption of their ecological system. It is helping client systems find meaning in health-illness experiences and life gains and losses. It is helping clients to feel good about themselves, to grow, to be productive and fulfilled. The behaviors are labeled "generative" because they bring together many elements to form one innovative expression of potential fulfillment. A simple example of this is the man who has had an arm amputated. No nurse can replace the arm and the arm will never grow back. But a nurse can help the man marshal his assets, stimulate his motivation, reinforce his attempts to compensate, help him learn to use his other arm, innovate alternative ways of doing things, and teach the use of a prosthesis so that he becomes adept without his arm. Other facets of the generative aspect of nursing are productive and reproductive behaviors. For instance, the manipulation of factors to produce a desired outcome is productive behavior. A nurse may work with a group of health workers in such a way that attitudes are changed, cooperation is increased, and consequently patients receive better care or a job is more efficiently done. That is productive behavior. An example of the reproductive aspect of generative nursing behaviors is the duplication or

replication of something that is effective in optimizing health. For instance, the "each one teach one" concept is reproductive behavior.[50] Teaching people to teach each other and to be accountable for teaching others ensures the spread of an idea about health. Replication of a successful formula, duplication and use of an idea, and innovation of ideas and activities are all generative forms of nursing behaviors. Generative behaviors are building, devising, formulating, and constructing ideas, plans, theories, solutions, devices, machines, and relationships. Generative behaviors are one classification of nursing functions that help to meet the purpose of nursing—high-level wellness.

Organization of nursing process. The three types of nursing behaviors discussed in the previous pages are carried out in three basic arenas or target systems, which comprise (1) individuals, designated as intrapersonal or self-systems, (2) groups, designated as interpersonal systems, and (3) communities, designated as community systems. These systems are not mutually exclusive categories. The target arena of the nurse, at any one time, is a matter of emphasis. For instance, all nursing activities—even those devised for promoting intrapersonal adaptation—are interpersonal by virtue of the interaction that must occur during the administration of nursing care. However, the emphasis or primary objective of the nursing activity is the strengthening of the intrapersonal system. The target arena of concern, then, refers to the purpose of the nursing activity, not to the mode of activity selected, since all modes of activity use interpersonal behaviors to some degree. A brief description of these three components follows.

Intrapersonal system. The human being as a single unit is the focal point of all nursing activities that are designed specifically for the intrapersonal system. Chapter 1 described the nursing tasks of the intrapersonal system as those activities which through "protective, nurtrative, and/or generative nursing behaviors . . .

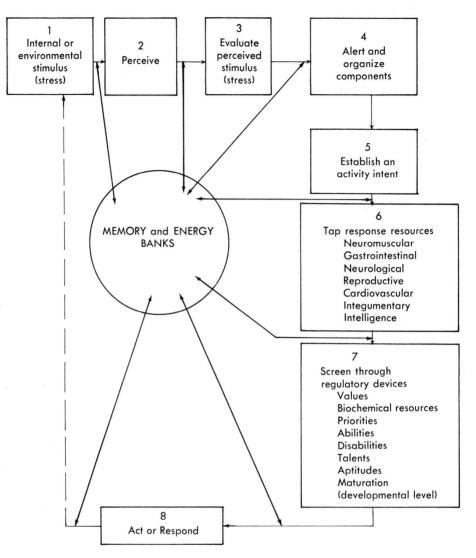

Fig. 5-7. Intrapersonal systems model.

promote the optimal functioning of all internal, biochemical, and physiological life processes, all biological growth processes, and individual personality formation and expression." The intrapersonal system could be described as an individual's internal communication system—open to and interconnected with his environment. The intrapersonal system is the human being's ability to receive stimuli or stressors, alert appropriate members (subsystems), and respond in an adaptive way.

The intrapersonal system has many components that enable this responsiveness to occur. It has memory and energy banks, levels of awareness and unawareness, perception apparatus, evaluation apparatus, selection-shuttling and communicating devices, and interconnections with the environment. Sending-receiving, action-reaction, evaluation, storage, or memory may occur in a chemical, cognitive, or electrical level and may occur with or without awareness. The nurse works to enhance the individual's ability to function optimally. For instance, providing proper nutrients is a supportive activity for the intrapersonal system, as are immunization and activities that promote attainment of the appropriate central task of development. Fig. 5-7 is a model of the intrapersonal system and its interconnection with the environment.

The intrapersonal system model can be explained as follows:

1. An *internal or environmental stimulus,* such as an infective organism, a drug, a pollutant, a death of a loved one, occurs.
2. *Perception* follows, which is the receiving and interpretation of the stimulus. Perception need not be cognitive or aware; it can be on an entirely organic level. Thus the response can also be limited to the organic level, for example, histamine released from damaged cellular walls.
3. *Evaluation* is determining what has been perceived—whether or not it is harmful, how harmful or to what extent, and what parts of the body will be most concerned.
4. *Alert components* is the notification, marshaling, and/or organizing of the many parts of the individual that will need to respond. This may be completely on a level requiring no awareness or it may be within the level of awareness.
5. *Activity intent* is planning the responses deemed appropriate by the system as a result of evaluation. These plans may or may not require awareness.

Memory and energy banks are available to each of the phases. Memory is used here to mean all previously established *patterns* of behavior from antigen-antibody formation to cognitive problem solving.

"Memory bank" is the label for a mechanism that enables reliance on preestablished patterns of behavior. Memory banks are available on both aware and nonaware levels. Many responses or patterns of behavior, such as the release of adrenocortical

hormones, are based on preestablished patterns of behavior and thus rely on the memory bank.

"Energy banks" are the nutrients, enzymes, muscle power, and so forth that can be tapped to promote the process at any state.

6. All activity must be implemented through some available *response resource,* that is, neuromuscular, gastrointestinal, neurological, cardiovascular, or integumentary system, native intelligence, hormonal maturity and integration.
7. All activity response has *regulatory devices,* such as the value system (priorities), abilities and disabilities, talents and aptitudes, developmental state, and biochemical materials. These regulatory devices may or may not be available from the memory and energy banks; they may be inherent in the nature of the person.
8. The final outcome is the *act or response* itself. This is the carrying out of the activity intent utilizing the response resources and memory and energy banks. This act or response is controlled by the regulatory devices and the memory and energy banks' potential. Notice that the memory and energy banks interact with and are an integral part of every stage of activity.

EXAMPLE OF INTRAPERSONAL MODEL IN USE. An infective organism, such as measles, threatens the intrapersonal system. The organism is the *environmental stimulus.* (1). The body *perceives* (2) exposure and entrance or presence of measles virus and *evaluates* (3) the nature of the threat, whether or not the virus is potentially harmful, and if it is, in what way and what forces of the body will be most effective in responding to the measles virus. As a result of evaluation, the body's mechanism for resistance to and combating measles is *alerted and organized* (4). For instance, antigen-antibody formation systems would be on notice that their services will be required, supply depots of raw material would be put in a state of readiness, and so on.

The *memory and energy banks* serve as the computer center, and all operations are programmed in, checked out, routed back, and stored for future use. *Memory banks* are concerned only in part with recall of experiences of awareness; memory banks store all patterns of response (even genetically built-in responses, such as the production of erythrocytes by bone marrow or antigen-antibody reactions). The *energy bank* is the source of energy for all system activities. The memory bank knows where all the available or potential energy is and how it can best be tapped; energy banks are all the body's storehouses, reserves, and resources.

Once the appropriate units of the body are on the alert and organized, a plan of response is formulated. This plan of response is *activity intent* (5). To combat the threat of measles, one can envision the plan as follows: (a) energy storehouses will make raw materials available; (b) transport facilities will pick up the raw materials and deliver to (c) antibody factories; (d) all other activities are reduced so that concerned units can carry out plans.

The *response resources* (6) are then tapped. In almost all responses many units combine together for each one response, and isolating and observing one component's response gives not only a partial picture but a completely false one. The response to measles' threat necessitates the tapping of such units or resources as neuromuscular, gastrointestinal, cardiovascular, fluid and electrolyte, antigen, antibody, and autonomic nervous systems.

The *regulatory devices* (7) are called into play to screen, modify, and regulate the planned responses. For instance, if the exposure to measles occurs while the person has hepatitis, the body's regulatory devices establish priorities about where energy and materials are to be spent—thus some of the potential plans are not carried out at all, whereas others are carried out minimally—sometimes the planned re-

sponse has so low a priority that the response is ineffective or out of balance. If it is ineffective, the person probably does indeed get measles and further perception-evaluation-alerting and organizing-planning-tapping resources and regulating will have to occur. If the response is out of balance, perhaps the response has more dire consequences than the measles would have had.

The *act or response* (8) itself occurs. After passing through all the previous phases, there is a response, many responses, or a series of responses to the stimulus of invasion of measles virus.

Activities within the level of awareness follow the same pattern. For instance, if the person were aware of his exposure to measles, he would:

Perceive the exposure (2)

Evaluate it (3)—"I'm run down; I could catch that disease"

Alert and organize components (4)—"I wonder if I shouldn't try to ward it off"

Demonstrate activity intent (5)—"I think I will take some vitamins and get more sleep for the next three days"

Tap response resources (6)—"I guess to do that I'd better get home early and watch TV or read a while so I can get my mind off things and relax, or I'll never get to sleep"

Use the *regulatory devices* (7)—"I really should get my class assignment done or my papers graded, but if I get sick I'd be out a week—I guess it is to bed for me tonight"

Act or respond (8)—go to bed and to sleep

Interpersonal system. The second system involved in nursing process is the interpersonal system, which is the interaction of two or more people. Chapter 1 described the interpersonal system as those nursing activities which through "protective, nurtrative, and/or generative nursing behaviors . . . promote the optimal functioning of two or more people. This includes the nurse and client, the nurse and other health persons, the nurse and other professionals, the client-family and nurse, and surrogate families . . . and nurse. . . ."

The interpersonal system is a social system; it is not just communications among people in groups of two or more, or families. The interpersonal system is the total effect people have on one another. The effect may be in terms of atmosphere, environment, or "vibes." The atmosphere or environment with one group of people may be happy, positive, and constructive, whereas another group are sad, negative, and destructive. Many components produce the total interactions of people. Things such as facial expression, general activity, posture, and head and hand movements or position all contribute to the total picture of atmosphere. However, interactions constitute more than communications between people; interpersonal systems are also the interaction of families or individuals and their environment. This interaction is responsive to social pressures of all kinds, such as the amount of leisure time available and the recreational facilities for using that leisure time. Some other factors are the values of the group as expressed in family social ambition, attitudes toward neighbors, police, material possessions, education, health, and civic responsibilities.

The interrelationship of the interpersonal and community system is expressed in the responsiveness of the family to such community conditions as crowding, pollution, high social pathology indices, and so on.

Two or more people interacting with each other constitute a social system. In any social system there are two primary categories of activities: activities (1) centered around making progress toward an identified goal and activities and (2) maintaining the internal equilibrium of the system.[51] These two activities must be conducted regardless of the size or function of the system. The interpersonal system is a social system; it may consist of the nurse-client, nurse-doctor-client, nurse-nurse, nurse-doctor, nurse-group, group-group, client-client, family-nurse, or any of innumerable other combinations.

There are certain assumptions that can be made about any social system as follows:

1. There is a purpose to its existence.
2. An individual belongs to a given social system as long as there is a purpose to be served (or it fulfills a need).
3. There are roles (functions) for the members of the system. Roles may shift, blur, or remain stable, but at any one moment in time roles exist in a definable way. The role may be primarily involved in goal identification or in movement toward the goal, or the role may be primarily involved with the maintenance of group equilibrium or integrity.
4. There are relationship controls.[52] In a family these relationships are exhibited by kinship structure and in other groups, by friendship structure or communication pathways. Sometimes these relationships are vertical, such as the hierarchy exhibited in authoritarian structured groups, or horizontal (peer), as exhibited in collegia-structured groups.[53]
5. There are communication pathways, which comprise both output and feedback pathways. They exist between elements of the social system regardless of the role or relationship that each member has to the other.

All interactions among people are governed by the processes of self-awareness, sensitivity and responsiveness, communications, group dynamics, and family dynamics. This section will not survey the relevant theories of these processes but will use the definition and description of a family as the focal point for the interpersonal system. Whether or not the nurse is relating to one person or a group of persons, the individuals are members of a family of some type. Furthermore, family, family structure, and family dynamics have parallels in all interpersonal systems. The interested reader is urged to explore theories about the interaction of people or theories about communication, group dynamics, family dynamics and sensitivity, self-awareness and responsiveness. Other helpful theories for exploration are psychological theories such as transactional analysis, Freudian analysis, gestalt-field theory, behaviorist theory, etc., which provide a more comprehensive knowledge about the interpersonal or "social" subsystem.

A *family*[54] is a group of persons who have kinship that is consanguinal (blood relative), affinal (marital), or fictive (invented) and are mutually concerned with each other's affairs and ambitions. A family may be a convenient assumption so that individuals' subsistence, nurturance, counseling, and dependency needs may be met. Members may or may not cohabit, but each member does participate through assuming one or more of the roles that mark family membership:

1. **Sustainer**—provides subsistence and livelihood by breadwinning, provision of basic material essentials
2. **Nurturer**—looks after health and welfare, training of children, feeding, clothing, and daily running of maintenance activities
3. **Counselor**—advises, sets limits, influences decisions about family member activities
4. **Dependent**—accepts shelter and protection, such as children who are being enculturated or the infirm or senile

Roles are independent of kinship. For instance, it is not uncommon to find a relatively young child fulfilling the role of nurturer and/or counselor while being financed, sustained, sheltered, and enculturated.

Kinship denotes relationships that are one or more of the following:

1. **Consanguinal**—blood relationships derived from the same genetic pool.
2. **Affinal**—marital ties; marriage designates the socially recognized and sometimes legally enforced relationships between a couple who wish to establish a nuclear family. Affinal ties are the way people relate to each other through marriage.
3. **Fictive**—invented relatives—people like godparents or adopted children. These are highly influential others who have feelings of

responsibility, identity, or belonging to the family. Some surrogate families are "invented families," thus fictive, e.g., some communes, holy orders, etc. Fictive kinships are tied by responsibilities, rites, or laws.

The family is a microcosm of society. Family coping for any one family varies from time to time and from condition to condition. Family coping, like community coping, depends on the total picture of several factors: (1) the communication skills and pathways; (2) the individual contributions of members to the welfare of the group; (3) the intrafamily congruence of values and behaviors; (4) the ability of the members to identify problems, articulate alternative solutions, negotiate and compromise, and make and implement decisions; (5) intermember care, respect, trust, or love; and (6) the family's response patterns to social stresses (poverty, members who vary from the family norm, sickness, drug addiction or alcoholism, crime, affluence, and so forth).

The family is one of the milieus in which nurses function. Nurses need to be able to recognize families and extended families, define their relationships, and identify family member roles.

To influence family health, the nurse must "get to" the key people in the family. An analysis of family structure delineates roles (by the functions members serve). Thus the family members can be approached by the nurse in the context of the role or roles they play and can influence the family's health more effectively.

Individual family members are influenced by other family members. For a nurse to be effective in health teaching, anticipatory guidance, modifying behavior, or in any way to augment adequate family coping mechanisms, the appropriate family members must be included regardless of their working hours, kinship, or role.

Family roles depend on ethnicity, timing, and expediency. Therefore families differ in their roles from family to family and from time to time in the same family. Constant review of family structure and role enables the nurse to work directly with appropriate family members to promote family coping mechanisms.

TYPICAL KINDS OF FAMILIES. Some examples of models typical of a variety of types of family configuration are presented. Roles and relationships are indicated, but communication and decision-making pathways are omitted. These models are presented simply to give examples of ways that nurses can translate actual families into small models to identify family relationships, roles, and so forth.

A *nuclear family* is traditionally composed of a mother, father, and their children. However, one or more of the members of a nuclear family may be absent (nonfunctioning), and the nuclear family may be one person.

An *extended family* is composed of the

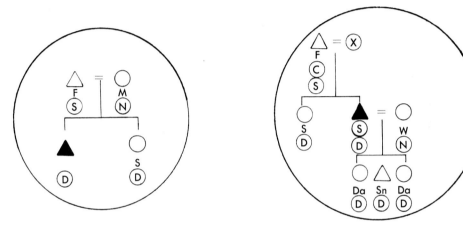

Model 1. Nuclear family.

Model 2. Extended family.

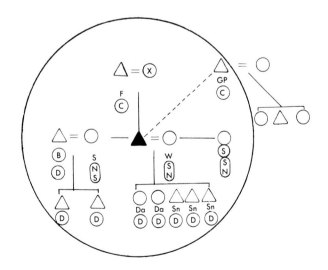

Model 3. Extended family model, relationships complex. In Models 2 and 3, Ego is a member of two nuclear families in which he plays different but important roles. Both families receive Ego's loyalty and support. Extended family is circled.

nuclear family plus meaningful other family members. Extended family members may or may not cohabit but must enter into the family structure in one of the preceding roles and participate regularly in family affairs. Extended families are cooperative individuals or groups that serve the general functions of the nuclear family. They may be two or more nuclear families that are linked by consanguinal ties or in some other meaningful, purposeful way.

Kinship group is not the same as extended family. Kinship group means all those related by consanguinal or affinal kinship ties; extended family refers to families that may or may not be united by these ties but are related by family roles, responsibilities, and fictive ties.

Another type of family tie classified as extended family is the tie of intimate friendship. Close friends often make the emotional commitment of family members to each other. Sometimes this commitment is articulated; sometimes it is not. But acts of intimacy, willingness to take risks, caring, concern, and love enable them to fulfill roles of support, dependence, nurturance, and mutual interdependence often fulfilled by other formal or legal relatives.

Perhaps one of the most important concepts about families is that the strength and usefulness to the client of the family tie is independent of the kind of tie involved. The client is the best source of information about who fulfills family roles and functions for him, and legal, moral, or religious ties can neither supplement nor replace choices of the heart and mind and practices of closeness and caring.

Communal families differ widely in composition, roles of members, and relationships among members. Some communal families are very loosely knit groups with members joining and withdrawing for short periods of time. Other communal families are very tightly knit groups, extremely selective in their family membership, and committed to the family group for long periods of time—in some cases for life. Model 4 represents one type of communal family.

The following key was used for Models 1 to 4.

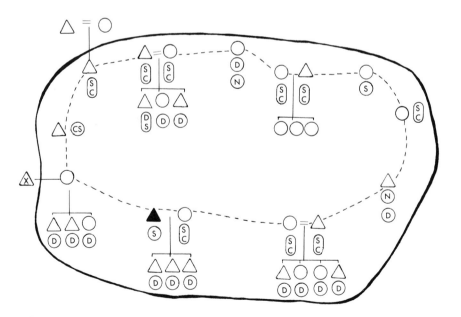

Model 4. One kind of commune. Communes exist in many forms, and roles of its members vary from group to group.

Code

△	Male
○	Female
=	Marriage
−	Kinship, consanguinal
.....	Kinship fictive
△⊗	Deceased, absent: nonfunctioning member
▲	Ego: or the person from whose point of view the labels are attached.

Role (function) code	Relationship code
S Sustainer	F = Father
	M = Mother
N Nurturer	B = Brother
	S = Sister
C Counselor	Sn = Son
	Da = Daughter
D Dependent	W = Wife
	H = Husband
	GP = Godparent
	Combinations of the above
	FF = Father's father
	FM = Father's mother
	FB = Father's brother
	BSn = Brother's son

Community system. The third organizing element in nursing process is the community system. The nurse has a substantial role to play in any community system. As a member of various health, education, welfare, and regulatory agencies and of civic organizations, the nurse functions as (1) an advocate for the health services client, (2) a concerned and active community member, (3) an expert in health affairs, and (4) a consumer of community services. The nurse who is at home with communities, their organizational structure, their composition, and their resources can operate within communities more effectively for the furtherance of health. Community surveys, assessments, demographic studies, epidemiological studies, and other means for assessing, evaluating, or appraising community-coping mechanisms are tools for the nurse's trade aimed specifically at the community system of nursing process.

A *community* is a group of people organized to achieve goals that are mutually important.[55] Communities are the actualization of the philosophy that supports the division of labor within a group for the mutual benefit of the group members. Communities arise in response to a basic human need or trait—gregariousness or

socialization. People band together for reasons such as protection, socialization, enculturation, and mutual welfare—such as the trading of goods and labor.

Communities may be conceptualized as having geographical boundaries (city limits, county lines, state lines) or natural borders (rivers, mountains). Communities can also be conceptualized as being problem centered and thus having boundaries of "solution."[56] Fig. 5-8 is a model of communities of solution. Such communities are temporal and exist only until problems are solved. They are communities of common interest, drawn around people, problems, and resources, for example, a community of scholars or a community of citizens concerned about pollution. Communities of solution may exist as a small part of a larger geographical county or across county and state lines. The community boundaries for any one person shift and change as the individual's movements, needs for services, and concerns change. The mobility of Americans is changing the popular concept of communities as localized geographical places to areas and regions primarily because geographical and political boundaries, even of regional, state, and national size, fail to consider relevance to specific problems of mutual concern over which local government and local communities may have little control.[57]

Even within communities that are primarily geographical or political in nature, community organization is devised around community problems of vital concern to individual citizen welfare and need. Almost all community organizations, both proprietary and official, are concerned with the mobilization of resources for responding to human needs and problems.

A community is a system, and all systems need to maintain themselves and fulfill their purposes. Communities have many of the same needs as individuals and families: mobility, health, maintenance and general welfare, protection, learning (including socialization and enculturation), recreation, economic sufficiency,

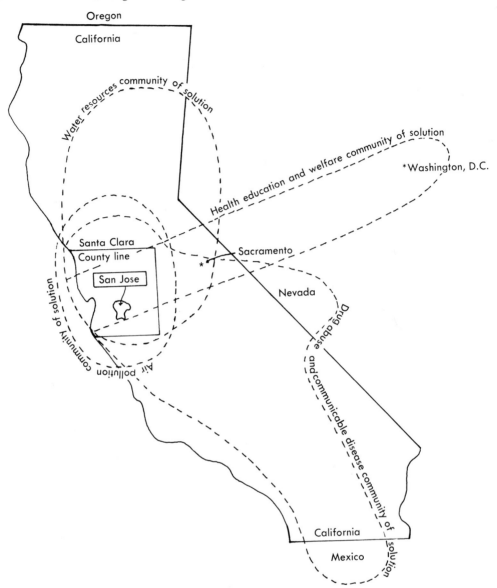

Fig. 5-8. Solid lines represent geographical and/or political boundaries of communities of solutions. (Modified from National Commission on Community Health Services: Health is a community affair, Cambridge, Mass., 1966., Harvard University Press.)

religious expression, and communication. In addition, communities have a need for leadership or organizing strategies for the support, coordination, and mobilization of resources to meet these needs. Any business, agency, group, club, or facility in a community can be classified or grouped under one or more of the preceding headings—in other words, grouped by the need it was designed to meet.

Social pathology is the failure of a community to respond to the needs of its citizenry. There are several reasons why communities fail in their responses. Communities are organized around the citizenry at any given time. Populations shift and change; conditions shift and change. Populations are characterized by ethnicity, educational level, age composition, economic characteristics, and values. There is a lag between community organization (response to needs) and the need arousal. In five years a city can have a significant population characteristic shift in ethnicity education, economic, health, and so forth. The response of community organizations tends to lag behind needs by months or even years. Social pathology is a signal of a lack of congruence between the population's needs and the community's mobilization in responding to those needs.

Nurses play a significant role in community affairs and influence the direction, speed, and comprehensiveness of community responsiveness to needs. Thus the more nurses know about the composition, organization, and characteristics of communities and the more able nurses are to operate within the community's political arena for response to citizen's needs, the better able nurses will be to facilitate community coping mechanisms that promote health.

Innovation component of the nursing process. Creativity, the third component of process is the output of the nursing system. It is the creation of "one" from the "many." It is the alchemy involved in the production from many ancestors in a long procession of "begats" of a new and unique individual; it is a unique act born from many contributing actions. Creativity is the inherent driving force of the universe that makes uniqueness the rule and sameness the exception. For instance, uniqueness is defined as "out of the ordinary," or being unlike other things. In truth, almost everything is unique; it is the identical that is unusual. Identical twins are relatively unusual, identical quadruplets are rare, but each person varies so much from other persons that fingerprints, voice patterns, and ear configurations can be used to distinguish one human from another. No two rocks are the same, no two trees are the same, few animals are identical—all because of the creative impetus of nature, the rendering of a "unique entity" from the amalgamation of "many."

Nursing is a unique process spawned from many processes, which makes it virtually impossible for nursing activities and functions not to be creative. All the processes that, when synthesized, form the nursing process have their own purpose, system, and creativity. For nursing to move toward the fulfillment of its creative potential, nurses must learn the basic or parent processes *and* their configuration in the unique holistic pattern of nursing. Nursing is a process and the elements comprising that process are many. These "many" unite in a unique and innovative way to bring into being a new "one": *Nursing*— holistic and dynamic.

No one element of the nursing process is more important than the others; no one element occurs in nursing activity more frequently than the others; each gives the necessary ingredients at any one time to unite to form a unique nursing activity, or behavioral outcome. One cannot deemphasize the psychological component and emphasize the pathophysiological component, or vice versa, since these divisions fracture nursing and deny its holism. Nursing is a new process—a unique process, born of many processes and combining with other processes to give rise to descendant processes.

HEURISTIC

The development of conceptual constructs, a theory of nursing, or an operational definition of nursing on which the curriculum can be built, becomes one of the major tasks for participants. It looms large at this particular stage of nursing history because so few schools of nursing actually attempt to develop a hypothesis for nursing. A few grounded theories are developing, but these are usually specific to an area of nursing action. A comprehensive general theory of nursing is yet to be developed and tested. A school of nursing may not wish to attempt to devise an operational theory; however, the outcome is well worth the effort, since it provides a model for all curriculum-building endeavors and a subsequent framework for learning about nursing. A nursing theory is an evolving concept. Initial attempts will become more and more useful as they are used and revised. The device suggested here is one way the group can begin to identify the components of nursing process and put it together as a working nursing hypothesis.

The purpose of this activity is to survey the literature, the faculty, and the present curriculum to determine common elements around which a definition or theory may be fashioned.

Heuristic: *Identifying the common elements of nursing and forging these elements into a working conjecture about the process of nursing*

Activity. This activity involves a survey of the literature, a survey of the current course outlines in the curriculum, a survey of the behaviors and content previously acquired (Chapter 4, Heuristic 1), and a survey of the opinions of the faculty. A frequency scale is then established for the results of the survey. Data are then evaluated by frequency of occurrence, sorted into areas of common groupings, and developed into a hypothesis or theory. The theory is then used to determine if it can be a model for (1) making nursing action diagnosis, (2) content organization, and (3) nursing intervention strategies.

Example 1. Opinionnaire distributed to faculty

To: Faculty

List below (using *any* or *no* sources, as you wish) the concepts/content/ideas/etc. that you think are central and common to all of nursing, regardless of clinical specialty or setting. Please return by _____ (date). Work in groups of three.

Example 2. Frequency scale of responses to opinionnaire and data from course outlines (a partial sample)

	Betty	Janet	Ken	Julia	Joyce	Susan	Steve	June	Mary	Sr. outlines	Jr. outlines	Soph. outlines
Homeostasis-equilibrium-disequilibrium			x		x	x				x		x
Hospital												x
Treatment											x	
Intervention		x								x	x	
Technical skills	x											
Protection											x	
Rehabilitation		x					x		x	x	x	x
Health												x
Health education	x									x	x	
Prevention	x	x					x			x	x	
Asepsis		x								x		
Acute and chronic disease pathology, morbidity										x		
Community	x			x						x	x	x
Environment	x						x			x	x	
Culture											x	

Example 2. Frequency scale of responses to opinionnaire and data from course outlines (a partial sample)—cont'd

	Betty	Janet	Ken	Julia	Joyce	Susan	Steve	June	Mary	Sr. outlines	Jr. outlines	Soph. outlines
Social stress							x					
Changing society needs	x											
Social systems	x											
Legality										x	x	
Problem solving			x			x			x	x	x	x
Assessment				x					x			
Evaluation											x	
Decision making												x
Family		x		x					x	x	x	
Home	x								x			
Security									x			
Leadership, change agent	x	x	x	x			x		x			
Delegation, authority									x			
Interviewing									x			
Group process		x	x						x			x
Behavior patterns									x	x	x	
Anxiety		x				x			x			x
Grief												x
Pharmacology		x							x		x	x
Fluid and electrolyte											x	x
Mental retardation									x			
High-level wellness		x	x	x		x	x		x			
Teaching-learning	x	x	x	x		x					x	
Communication (interpersonal)	x	x	x	x		x	x		x	x		x
Conflict						x						
Stress	x	x				x	x		x	x	x	x
Crisis		x							x			
Comfort						x						
Pain		x							x		x	x
Birth						x						
Death, mortality		x				x			x		x	x
Change, planned											x	x
Restorative		x										
Growth and development		x		x		x	x		x		x	x
Nutrition		x							x		x	

Materials
1. Concept list acquired from a wide variety of nursing literature
2. Course outlines from all current courses
3. Faculty opinionnaires
4. A task group for ascertaining frequency
5. A task group for sorting and categorizing
6. Three task groups for developing alternate nursing definitions or theories
7. Discussion time
8. Task groups using the theory to work simulated nursing problems or to develop a unity of specified content using the theory as an organizing strategy
9. A task group or individual to revise the theory as work proceeds

Procedure
1. Establish three task groups to comb the literature and collect concepts central to all of nursing.
2. Pass out open-ended opinionnaire.
3. Collect data from two above sources.

Example 3. Data sorted into categories (a partial sample)

Communication
Group dynamics
Writing
Self-awareness—sensitivity and responsiveness
Interpersonal relations
Interview
Use of feedback

Change
Leadership
Delegation of authority
Evaluating situation specific
Accountability

Learning
Learning theories
Teaching role
Prevention aspect
Facilitation
Conference
Reports
Teaching strategies
Learning modes

Nursing settings
Hospitals
Homes
Streets
County agencies
Clinics
Day care centers
Shelters
Jails
Schools

Nursing behaviors/roles
Care
Prevention
Rehabilitation
Therapy, treatment
Teaching
Technical skills
Comfort
Cure

Decision making
Problem solving
Judgment
Innovation
Generating alternatives
Setting priorities
Evaluation
Dependence-independence collaboration
Self-evaluation

Stress-stress response
Pathophysiology
Adaptive and maladaptive states:
    Individual
    Families
    Groups
    Communities
Anxiety states
Coping mechanisms
Pain

Human development
Assessment
Regression
Individual needs
Normal maturation
Levels of ability

Targets of nursing care
Individual
Families
Groups
Communities
Nations
Health care agencies

Example 4. Nursing theory stated as a definition and a hypothesis

Nursing is a process. Its purpose is to promote optimum health through protective, nurtrative, and generative activities. These activities are carried out within the intrapersonal system, the interpersonal system, and the community system. Nursing's protective, nurtrative, and generative activities are a unique synthesis of theories eclectically combined into nursing hypotheses that are validated or refuted in practice.

The following is the above definition of nursing stated as a hypothesis:

The unique synthesis of life process theories enables the enactment of protective, nurtrative, and generative nursing behaviors, which when carried out in intrapersonal, interpersonal, and community target systems, promote and maintain optimal health.

Example 5. Sample of symptom of edema and its correlative factors using stress response model from Fig. 5-2

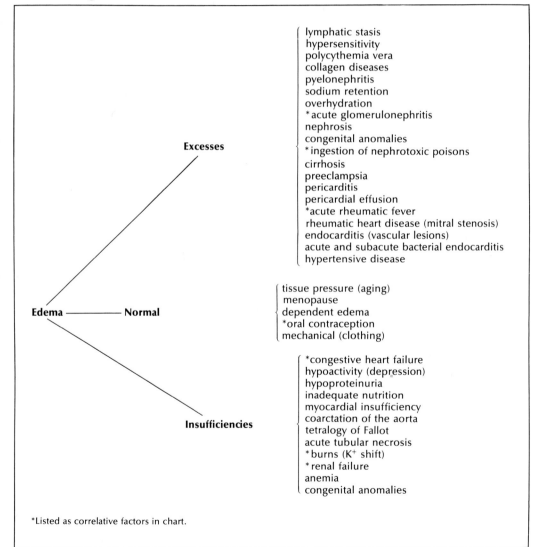

Edema ——————— Normal

Excesses
lymphatic stasis
hypersensitivity
polycythemia vera
collagen diseases
pyelonephritis
sodium retention
overhydration
*acute glomerulonephritis
nephrosis
congenital anomalies
*ingestion of nephrotoxic poisons
cirrhosis
preeclampsia
pericarditis
pericardial effusion
*acute rheumatic fever
rheumatic heart disease (mitral stenosis)
endocarditis (vascular lesions)
acute and subacute bacterial endocarditis
hypertensive disease

tissue pressure (aging)
menopause
dependent edema
*oral contraception
mechanical (clothing)

Insufficiencies
*congestive heart failure
hypoactivity (depression)
hypoproteinuria
inadequate nutrition
myocardial insufficiency
coarctation of the aorta
tetralogy of Fallot
acute tubular necrosis
*burns (K^+ shift)
*renal failure
anemia
congenital anomalies

*Listed as correlative factors in chart.

Example 6

Correlative factors	Manifestations (common)	Interventions (common)
	Intrapersonal system Interpersonal system Community system	Intrapersonal Protective Nurtrative Generative Interpersonal Protective Nurtrative Generative Community Protective Nurtrative Generative

Correlative factors	Manifestations (distinctive)	Interventions (distinctive)
	Intrapersonal system Interpersonal system Community system	Intrapersonal Protective Nurtrative Generative Interpersonal Protective Nurtrative Generative Community Protective Nurtrative Generative

Correlative factors	→	Common manifestations	→	Common nursing interventions
Correlative factors	→	Distinctive manifestations	→	Distinctive nursing interventions

4. Make a frequency scale of common concepts.
5. Assign a task group to establish some trial categories for sorting data.
6. Sort data.
7. Produce a list of categories and data that fit under each category.
8. Assign two or three task groups to generate a nursing hypothesis or operational definition that is suggested by the data.
9. Present all the lists, categorizations, and suggested definitions and theories to the faculty.
10. Discuss the strength and weakness of the theories.
11. Revise the theories using faculty feedback.
12. Ask task groups to test the definition/theory
    a. Using a simulated problem to make a nursing diagnosis and possible intervention within the framework of the theory.
    b. Choosing some area of content to use the theory as an organizing strategy.
13. Revise theory/definition based on feedback from trial groups.
14. Write theory as operational definition and as hypothesis.

Puissance
1. Facilitates whole faculty participation in theory development.
2. Is of instructional value to the faculty.
3. Provides a strong sense of unity in search for provisional nursing process model.
4. Generates a working organizing strategy that is *nursing* oriented and not "lifted" directly from another discipline, i.e., synthesizes theory.
5. Begins to provide focal point for change in faculty identity system from nursing specialty area to holistic framework.
6. Provides informational input and focus for content development.

Contingencies
1. May receive so much investment that it becomes "permanent" instead of "provisional."
2. Can be allowed to bog the faculty and prevent progress.
3. May generate anxiety over evolving holistic framework and threatened loss of specialty area "uniqueness."

The above examples are illustrative of progressive stages of group theory building activities.

Example 7. Use of the nursing theory as a content organization strategy

Correlative factors	Common manifestations	Common interventions
Congestive heart failure Renal failure Burns, severe thermal Oral contraception Ingestion of poisons (nephrotoxic)	Intrapersonal system Lowered resistance Arrhythmias Nausea Apprehension and depression Hypotension Hypertension Pain Edema Fatigue, weakness Fluid shift External dyspnea Anorexia Hypoxia Confusion Tissue damage Anemia Change in urinary output Restlessness	Nurtrative 1. Observe and report location of edema. 2. Give medication when appropriate. 3. Keep an intake and output record. 4. Check laboratory slips for electrolyte and hematocrit state of patient. 5. Observe patient for skin color, energy output, mood swings, changes in orientation and affect; report significant findings. 6. Give small frequent feedings. 7. Determine patient's food preferences that would not violate therapeutic diet. 8. Encourage patient to eat and reinforce his efforts. 9. Reposition patient for comfort, protection of skin, and promotion of venous return. Protective 1. Take vital signs, record, report significant findings (temperature; rate, character, quality of pulse; respirations; check blood pressure for deviation). 2. Protect from exposure to infection. 3. Provide or encourage scrupulous hygienic care. 4. Decrease external stimuli. Generative 1. Identify noxious environmental factors that increase nausea, pain, and anorexia and remove if possible or manipulate environment.
Congestive heart failure Renal failure Burns, severe thermal Oral contraception Ingestion of poisons (nephrotoxic)	Interpersonal system Changes in roles Economic changes Changes in activity Changes in communication Changes in personality or self-image Family anxiety for patient Need for coordinated care for patient Need for family to be involved in planning care of patient	Nurtrative 1. Help family accept changes in patient and his relationships. 2. Help family members identify family roles that need adjusting while patient is malfunctioning. 3. Offer approval and encouragement of progress. Protective 1. Promote and facilitate constructive communication. 2. If indicated, help family and patient to adjust to irreversible or fatal processes. 3. Encourage routine yearly physical examinations. Generative 1. Help family members adjust to new roles while patient is malfunctioning. 2. Provide and reinforce information; refer to appropriate agencies for provision of follow-up or home care. 3. Refer to appropriate community agencies if necessary for financial support and rehabilitation.

Continued.

Example 7. Use of the nursing theory as a content organization strategy—cont'd

Correlative factors	Common manifestations	Common interventions

Congestive heart failure
Renal failure
Burns, severe thermal
Oral contraception
Ingestion of poisons
  (nephrotoxic)
	Community system
	  Increased need for financial support
	  Changes in employment picture
	  Increased number of nonproductive members of community
	  Increased number of nonfunctional families
	  Changes in patterns of health care
		Nurtrative
		1. Provide vocational and family counseling centers.
		2. Refer to available agencies.
		
		Protective
		1. Provide educational programs dealing with prevention and detection.
		
		Generative
		1. Collect funds for establishing and maintaining communication to meet health need:
		    Public Health Department
		    Visiting Nurses Association
		    Mental health agency
		2. Form social action groups (political).

Correlative factors	Distinctive manifestations	Distinctive interventions

Congestive heart failure	Intrapersonal system
	  Paroxysmal nocturnal dyspnea
	  Dyspnea at rest
	  Orthopnea
	  Cough (productive, nonproductive)
	  Hemoptysis
	  Rhonchi
	  Rales
	  Cyanosis
	  Stupor
	  Cheyne-Stokes respirations
	  Hepatomegaly
	  Ankle edema
	  Dependent edema
	  Anxiety and/or fear
	  Restlessness
	  Behaves as "cardiac cripple"
	  Anasarca
	  Disturbed electrolyte imbalance
		Nurtrative
		1. Elevate head and chest while sleeping e.g., extra pillows, rent/buy hospital bed, sleep in chair.
		2. Give oxygen.
		3. Place patient in high Fowler's position, support small of back.
		4. Change bed linen top to bottom; "cardiac bed."
		5. Give digitalis to slow, strengthen heartbeat.
		6. Give diuretic as ordered.
		7. Apply rotating tourniquets.
		8. Keep open IVs.
		9. Apply leads; hook up monitor.
		
		Protective
		1. Special skin care to areas under monitor leads.
		2. Move leads as necessary.
		3. Explain use and purpose of cardiac monitor.
		4. Time alternating periods of apnea and dyspnea, record and report.
		5. Keep bedrails up for support and safety.
		6. Insert/maintain patency of drainage catheters.
		7. Do specific gravity test if urine becomes scanty.
		8. Check laboratory slips for results of gas studies.
		9. Take apical-radial pulse simultaneously to determine pulse deficit; record and report.
		10. Report any blood in sputum.
		11. Measure C.V.P. and report significant findings.

Example 7. Use of the nursing theory as a content organization strategy—cont'd

Correlative factors	Distinctive manifestations	Distinctive interventions
Congestive heart failure	Interpersonal system Family fear—implications of disease and technical equipment Family fear—patient's death due to heart involvement Family treatment of patient as a "cardiac cripple" Family fear of "hereditary" heart problems Family recognition of indication of symptoms Decrease or obliteration of sexual intercourse	Nurtrative 1. Demonstrate a warm, friendly manner. 2. Listen to family express their feelings. 3. Help family sort out reality from fantasy. Protective 1. Explain purpose and use of equipment, e.g., monitor C.V.P., IV. Generative 1. Provide information to family concerning activity status of the patient and help family identify ways in which they can help patient live within his cardiac reserve.
Congestive heart failure	Community system Increased number of nutritionists who teach about value of low-sodium diet for heart Emphasis on dissemination of information on heart disease to public Decreased number of physicians who smoke Increased number of people who diet to lose weight to protect heart; increased interest in low-cholesterol diets Legislation created Classes to teach heart patients to live within their cardiac reserve Increased number of people who exercise e.g., bicycling, jogging, using gyms	Protective 1. Disseminate information (radio, TV, pamphlets) concerning judicious exercises as opposed to danger of sudden or excessive exercising on heart. 2. Disseminate accurate information on low-sodium, low-cholesterol, reducing diets. Generative 1. Reinforce research findings on heart by modeling behavior that represents research. 2. Use examples of legislation to bring about other types of heart legislation, e.g., concerning diet pills, pollution, etc. 3. Work for legislation in truth in advertising.
Renal failure	Intrapersonal system High blood pressure Hypertension Calcium phosphorus imbalance Rales Rhonchi Hematuria Anuria Acidotic vertigo Convulsions High specific gravity Vision changes Subcutaneous hemorrhage Uremic frost Pruritus Thrombocytopenia Bad breath Twitching Hiccough High K^+ (intoxication) Severe headache	Nurtrative 1. Administer diuretics by IV. 2. Push IV fluids. 3. Limit fluids. 4. Give Amphojel as ordered (for mobilization of phosphates). 5. Decrease external stimuli. 6. Administer blood. 7. Observe and record for constipation (due to Amphojel). 8. Apply lotions to skin for pruritus. 9. Administer drugs to allay pruritus. Protective 1. Measure I&O. 2. Give frequent special mouth care. 3. Weigh patient same time each day, same amount of clothing, etc. 4. Keep side rails up and padded; padded tongue blade at bedside. 5. Maintain patent airway. 6. Note color, sediment, odor of urine. 7. Collect urine for kidney function tests. 8. Draw arterial blood for blood gases. 9. Administer electrolytes by IV as ordered by physician. 10. Draw venous blood for electrolyte studies.

Continued.

Example 7. Use of the nursing theory as a content organization strategy—cont'd

Correlative factors	Distinctive manifestations	Distinctive interventions
Renal failure	Interpersonal system 1. Possibility of family member becoming a kidney donor 2. Possible loss of family member 3. Cost and inconvenience of treatment usually beyond ability of average family to handle, as well as stressful 4. Highly emotional experience while waiting for kidney machine or transplant 5. Need for hospitalization Community system 1. Frequently need to leave home community for treatment 2. Community appeals for money for assistance for an *individual*	Nurtrative 1. Help family through grieving process (death or separation for treatment). Generative 1. Teach family how to use kidney machine. 2. Refer to social welfare department for financial aid. 3. Explore with family the possibility of surgery for donor kidney and its implications. Generative 1. Establish community kidney centers.
Glomerulonephritis (acute)	Intrapersonal system Fever (high) 101° to 104° F Pharyngitis Malaise Microscopic hematuria Puffiness of eyes Ankle edema Scanty urine (color of cola, weak coffee) Abdominal pain Headache, convulsion, high blood pressure Enlarged heart Elevated specific gravity Loin pain (colic like or steady) Albuminurea Azotemia Irritability Apathy Preceding infection by Group A beta-hemolytic streptococci (usually U.R.I. infection)	Nurtrative 1. Culture the throat. 2. Use tepid sponges. 3. Give salicylates by rectum. 4. Advise bed rest until proteinurea and microscopic hematuria is only symptom left after 6 to 8 weeks of bed rest. 5. Force fluids by mouth or IV (for fever). 6. NPO if vomiting; gradually introduce easily digested diet (while edema is present salt should be restricted). 7. Limit fluids (if edema is present). Protective 1. Decrease external stimuli. 2. Give antibiotics as ordered by physician.
Glomerulonephritis (acute)	Interpersonal system 1. Possible exposure of other family members to Group A beta-hemolytic streptococci; types 12, 4, 25, and redlike (nephrogenic) attack kidney more than other types of streptococci 2. Often difficult to keep child at rest 3. Affects family's social life 4. Need for long-term prophylactic drug regime 5. Taxes family's ingenuity in providing diversional and/or occupational therapy (goldfish, ant farms) 6. Possibility of shortened hospitalization if individual can receive adequate or knowledgeable home care	Protective 1. Teach parent to keep infected individual isolated from other family members. 2. Teach parent (or family member) to measure I & O and observe for gross change in color and report to physician. 3. Teach considerations necessary for correctly weighing sick individual (same time daily, same amount of clothing, etc.) Generative 1. Make suggestions to family members about ways to interest child in activities that promote required rest. 2. Work with family members so that responsibility for care of individual is shared. 3. Whenever possible, get physician to prescribe drug by generic name to save the family money.

Example 7. Use of the nursing theory as a content organization strategy—cont'd

Correlative factors	Distinctive manifestations	Distinctive interventions
Glomerulonephritis (acute)	Community system 1. Tendency for silent or undiagnosed cases to have recurrences that lead to renal failure 2. Need for school teachers to be able to recognize symptoms of glomerulonephritis 3. Indiscriminate use of antibiotics (penicillin, tetracycline) that produce sensitivity or resistant organisms	Generative 1. Use PTA to teach parents and teachers how to recognize symptoms and implications of U.R.I. leading to acute glomerulonephritis (rheumatic fever). 2. Have school nurse hold faculty meeting about signs and symptoms and predisposing factors associated with glomerulonephritis. 3. Warn friends, neighbors, community, groups about indiscriminate use of antibiotics. 4. Accept invitations to educate public against indiscriminate use of antibiotics. 5. Encourage schools, child-care centers to establish policies that will protect children from cross-contamination.

Example 8. Symptom: behavior changes—excesses, hyperactivity

Correlative factor	Common manifestations	Common interventions

Hyperthyroidism
Manic phase of manic-depressive psychosis-continuum
Amphetamine toxicity
Psychedelic drug toxicity
Alcohol toxicity
Delirium tremens
	Intrapersonal system
	Fatigue
	Hyperactivity
	Increased body heat
	Insomnia
	Dehydration
	Weight loss
	Decreased personal hygiene
	Purposeless movement
	Short attention span
	Poor judgment
	Incomplete activities
	Feelings of acute anxiety
	Feelings of depression-euphoria (depression-euphoria is a continuum)
	In thyrotoxicosis, depression generally present; in amphetamine poisoning, euphoria present in beginning of a "run" and depression follows
	Sensitivity to all types of sensory stimuli
	If the condition continues unchecked and/or becomes extreme, following are manifested:
	    Exhaustion
	    Hallucinations
	    Delusions
	    Paranoia
	    Altered self-image
	    Death
		Intrapersonal system
		Reduce stimuli: noise, light, odors, people, motion, commotion.
		Reduce intake of chemotherapeutic central nervous system stimulants.
		Push fluids; provide frequent small feedings of high-calorie, high-vitamin, high-protein diets.
		Establish a hygienic and bodily function regimen.
		Maintain calm, accepting atmosphere for behavior, set consistent and realistic limits. This provides security because patient has less self-control and needs someone to provide control.
		Redirect energy when possible.
		Reduce activity to prevent exhaustion.
		Administer physical or chemical sedatives.
		Observe for indicators of mounting tension and anxiety.
		Observe, record, and/or report manifestations.
		Refer or call in other health workers as needed.
		Listen, help sort thoughts, structure activities within capabilities (reduces anxiety).
		Provide something to do when possible.
		If condition is severe and exhaustion, hallucinations, delusions, or paranoia manifested, provide rest and/or sedation.
		Reinforce reality and do not get caught up in the hallucinatory or delusional system; i.e., tell them what you see, how you perceive the situation, what really is going on.
		Talk them down; i.e., reassure them that the hallucination, etc., will go away, that you will stay with them; provide loving, caring behaviors and physical contact when appropriate.

Continued.

Example 8. Symptom: behavior changes—excesses, hyperactivity—cont'd

Correlative factor	Common manifestations	Common interventions

Hyperthyroidism
Manic phase of manic-depressive psychosis-continuum
Amphetamine toxicity
Psychedelic drug toxicity
Alcohol toxicity
Delirium tremens
	Interpersonal system
	  Alienation of family members and friends
	  Contagious behavior (spreading of anxiety)
	  Incompletion of tasks makes them unable to fulfill family role
	  Dysfunction of family
	  Abusiveness of others
	  Irritability
	  Aggressiveness
	  Hostility
	  Wearing others out
	  Noncontinuity of family membership
	  Rapid speech that inhibits communications
		Interpersonal system
		  Help family members identify family role that may need supplementing while member is malfunctioning.
		  Refer to appropriate family agencies if necessary.
		  Help provide family therapy where needed.
		  Instruct how to deal with hostile, aggressive, or irritable family member.
		  Protect other family members from fatigue, e.g., such things as scheduling rest-responsibility cycles, cooperation for family maintenance chores.
		  Teach families how to promote normal and healthy growth and maturation in young children (prevention of drug abuse, alcoholism, manic-depressive syndrome, promotion of self-awareness).
		  Strengthen family communications.
		  Help family members understand what is going on.
		  Teach family members how to perceive and interpret behaviors.
		  Help family members learn how to intervene in anxiety and not become part of the anxiety system.

Hyperthyroidism
Manic phase of manic-depressive psychosis-continuum
Amphetamine toxicity
Psychedelic drug toxicity
Alcohol toxicity
Delirium tremens
	Community system
	  Disruptions in school
	  Disruptions in job
	  Dangerous drivers
	  Noncontributing community members
	  Increased production possible if symptoms not too severe
		Community system
		  Become involved in the following:
		    Health education for prevention and detection
		    Social action groups (nurse advocate and concerned citizen role)
		    Adequate community treatment and rehabilitative facilities and services
		    Education of interpretation with employers (management) about behavior manifestations, treatment, prognosis, and return to work
		    Child care centers, Head Start, etc., for family cohesion, promotion of normal growth and development
		    Community nursing services to promote adequate home prevention, detection, treatment, and rehabilitation

Example 8. Symptom: behavior changes—excesses, hyperactivity—cont'd

Correlative factor	Common manifestations	Common interventions

Seizures
Disorders
	Intrapersonal system
	   Tonic and clonic seizures
	      Petit mal
	      Psychomotor
	      Grand mal
	      Jacksonian
	   Abnormal EEG
	   Brevity and rapidity of attacks of
	      unconsciousness
	   Secrecy, hostility, guilt, shame
	   Fecal and urinary incontinence
	   Post-seizure sleep with head-
	      ache
		Intrapersonal system
		   Protect patient from injury (side rail pad-
		      ded, tongue blade).
		   Loosen clothing.
		   Observe patient for how and where seizure
		      begins.
		   Stay with patient.
		   Preserve patient's dignity by preserving
		      modesty.
		   Suction mouth and throat to maintain open
		      airway.
		   Medicate with anticonvulsants.
		   Provide skin care—wash and keep clean
		      and dry.
		   Educate for taking medication: conse-
		      quences and precautions.
		   Reduce stimuli (quiet, calm, no bright
		      lights).

	Interpersonal system
	   Frightening to people
	   Arousal of morbid curiosity
	   Stigma
		Interpersonal system
		   Provide privacy during seizure.
		   Teach members of family to care for person
		      during and after seizure.
		   Be calm and accepting in regard to seizure.
		   Educate to diminish stigma and fantasies
		      about insanity.

	Community system
	   Accidents due to seizures
	   Accidents and injuries due to
	      operating equipment while
	      taking medication (anticon-
	      vulsant medication causes
	      slowed reflexes and drowsi-
	      ness) at time of seizure
	   On-the-job injuries
	   Automobile accident and se-
	      quelae (legal hassle, etc.)
	   Myths about madness
	   Stigma
		Community system
		   Educate public to diminish stigma and
		      fantasies about insanity.
		   Educate employers, supervisors, teachers,
		      and .employees regarding safety pre-
		      cautions, likelihood of seizures and care
		      during seizures.

Manic phase of manic-
   depressive psychosis-
   continuum
Amphetamine toxicity
Alcoholism
Psychedelic drug toxic-
   ity
	Intrapersonal system
	   Decreased appetite
	   Undernutrition
	   Malnutrition
	   Dehydration
	   Self-destructive acts
		Intrapersonal system
		   Set and enforce firm limits.
		   Provide small, frequent feedings.
		   Tempt with favorite foods.
		   Encourage frequent drinks of water and
		      fruit juices.
		   Prohibit coffee, tea, cola, and other stimu-
		      lants.
		   Provide diet with increased vitamins, min-
		      erals, proteins, and calories.
		   Provide special constant observation and in-
		      tensive one-to-one relationship aimed at
		      helping client to "come down" and pro-
		      tecting him while he does.
		   Help patient learn to recognize periodicity
		      of illness and seek help at first sign of
		      recurrence.

Continued.

Example 8. Symptom: behavior changes—excesses, hyperactivity—cont'd

Correlative factor	Common manifestations	Common interventions
	Intrapersonal system Grandiosity expressed toward world, depleted family resource, big spending Pathological giving Playing "God," which makes for unequal interpersonal relationships; difficulty in approaching, understanding and getting through to "God" Hyperactivity, which wears others out and precipitates avoidance	Interpersonal system Help family members understand what is going on. Teach family members how to perceive and interpret behaviors. Help family members learn how to intervene in anxiety and not become part of the anxiety system. Help family members identify family role that may need supplementing while member is malfunctioning. Refer to appropriate family agencies if necessary. Help provide family therapy where needed. Instruct how to deal with hostile, aggressive, or irritable family member. Protect other family members from fatigue, e.g., such things as scheduling rest-responsibility cycles, cooperation for family maintenance chores. Teach families how to promote normal and healthy growth and maturation in young children (prevention of drug abuse, alcoholism, manic-depressive syndrome and promotion of self-awareness). Strengthen family communications. Help family set and enforce firm limits. Help family recognize periodicity of illness and get patient to help at first sign of recurrence.
Manic phase of manic-depressive psychosis-continuum Amphetamine toxicity Alcoholism Psychedelic drug toxicity	Community system Grandiosity and extravagance added to diminished judgment, leading to crime and legal and financial problems	Community system Obtain legal aid. Educate merchants and public to check credit closely, limit charge accounts and do not fall for big-talking expensive "Diamond Jim(s)—the last of the big spenders."
Amphetamine toxicity Alcoholism	Intrapersonal system Drug dependency initially Addiction Agitation, anxiety Posttoxicity depression Severe withdrawal Delirium tremens (alcoholism) or convulsions (amphetamine) Paranoia: fear of others harming him, delusions of persecution	Intrapersonal system Provide intensive nursing care during withdrawal, including the following: Restraints (chemical, interpersonal, mechanical) Fluids (IVs may be required) Decrease in stimuli (noise, lights, provide seclusion from IPR contact) Maintain one-to-one relationship with special constant observation Avoid personal touch or intimate contact; sudden movement or surprising events; threatening scenes; power struggles; authoritarian approaches. Reassure patient, remember he is hostile and aggressive because he is more frightened of you.

Example 8. Symptom: behavior changes—excesses, hyperactivity—cont'd

Correlative factor	Common manifestations	Common interventions
Amphetamine toxicity Alcoholism	Community system Disturbances in school or job performance Failure to succeed	Community system Take part in the following: Health education for prevention and detection Social action groups (nurse advocate and concerned citizen role) Adequate community treatment and rehabilitation facilities and services Education of interpretation with employers (management) about behavior manifestations, treatment, prognosis, and return to work Child care centers, Head Start, etc., for family cohesion, promotion of normal growth and development Community nursing services to promote adequate home prevention, detection, treatment and rehabilitation Suicide prevention centers Crisis clinics and telephone service; listen to despondent person; help sort out concerns; get person to an agency for help Community mental health centers
Hyperthyroidism	Intrapersonal system Increased metabolic rate Increased appetite: Protein bound iodine (PBI) Thyroxine (T_3) Radioactive iodine uptake Hyperplasia of thyroid gland Exophthalmia Fine tremor Increased pulse rate Interpersonal system Family anxiety about member's health: Treatment with radioactive materials or surgery Long-term exhaustion, debilitation and/or malnutrition Altered image of exophthalmic family member	Intrapersonal system Administer chemotherapeutic agents as ordered such as propylthiouracil, Lugol's solution, central nervous system depressants. Prepare for and assist with care for patient during reflex radioactive isotope therapy, radioactive iodine, x-ray therapy. Prepare patient for and assist with diagnostic tests. Provide preoperative, operative, and postoperative care. Teach importance of regularity in taking maintenance doses of thyroxine; reinforce taking medication. Interpersonal system Teach families the ease with which the disease can be treated. Involve family in continuing care of family member, i.e., taking medication, proper rest, nutrition, etc. Alert family to symptoms or recurrence.

Examples 5 to 8[58] illustrate how the nursing theory can be used to provide an organizing strategy for nursing content. Along with the accompanying diagrams, example 5 sets the pattern to be followed throughout the curriculum. The symptom tree is based on the model of stress response (strain). The unit introduces edema as the entree to a group of conditions that will demonstrate the normal excesses and insufficiencies predominantly manifested by the stress of an increase of fluid in the extravascular spaces. The correlative factors chosen for elaboration and discussion include important examples that illustrate the various underlying reasons for edema.

Example 6 demonstrates how the use of common and distinctive manifestations, and common and distinctive interventions within the three target systems, intrapersonal, interpersonal, and community, allows for specific identification of protective, nurtrative, and generative activities as outlined in the nursing process model. To use this format the system is entered initially at the manifestation phase where common symptoms and/or signs are identified to form a "clinical picture" of how the patient manifests his problem(s). One can then work backward to identify correlative factors and forward to identify possible common nursing interventions. The second step is to identify the distinctive manifestations of each correlative factor and the distinctive nursing interventions that are appropriate. Examples 7 and 8 illustrate this.

NOTES

1. Abdellah, Faye G., and Levine, Eugene: Better patient care through nursing research, New York, 1965, The Macmillan Co., p. 69.
2. Ibid., pp. 68-71.
3. Information about general systems theory is taken from the following sources:
   a. Groy, William, and Rizzo, Nicholas: History and development of general systems theory. In Groy, W. Dukes, and Rizzo, N., editors: General system theory and psychiatry, Boston, 1969, Little, Brown & Co., Inc.
   b. Von Bertalanffy, Ludwig: General systems theory: foundations, development, applications, New York, 1968, George Braziller, Inc.
4. An excellent discussion of high-level wellness can be found in Ford, Loretta C., Cobb, Marguerite, and Taylor, Margaret: Defining clinical content—graduate nursing programs: community health nursing, Boulder, Colo., Feb., 1967, Western Interstate Commission for Higher Education.
5. Rogers, Martha: An introduction to the theoretical basis of nursing, Philadelphia, 1970, F. A. Davis Co., p. 86.
6. American Nurses' Association: Educational preparation for nurse practitioners and assistants to nursing: a position paper, New York, 1965, The Association, p. 4.
7. Dunn, Halbert L.: High-level wellness, Arlington, Va., 1961, R. W. Beatty Co.
8. Maslow, Abraham H.: Toward a psychology of being, ed. 2, New York, 1968, Van Nostrand-Reinhold Co.
9. Dunn, Halbert L.: What high level wellness means, Canadian Journal of Public Health **50:**447-457, 1959.
10. Dubos, René: Mirage of health, New York, 1959, Harper & Row, Publishers, Inc.
11. Gove, Philip B., editor: Webster's third new international dictionary of the English language unabridged, Springfield, Mass., 1971, G. & C. Merriam Co., Publishers, p. 1043.
12. Abdellah, Faye G., et al.: Patient centered approaches to nursing, New York, 1960, The Macmillan Co.
13. Peplau, Hildegarde: Interpersonal relations in nursing, a conceptual frame of reference for psychodynamics in nursing, New York, 1952, G. P. Putnam's Sons.
14. This group of nonnurse theorists represents a wide variety of interactional theories, for example, Carl Rogers, self-development; Berne, transactional analysis; Perls, gestalt; and Skinner, behaviorism.
15. Travelbee, Joyce: Interpersonal aspects of nursing, Philadelphia, 1966, F. A. Davis Co.
16. Selye, Hans: The stress of life, New York, 1956, McGraw-Hill Book Co.
17. Riehl, Joan P., and Roy, Sister Callista: Conceptual models for nursing practice, New York, 1974, Appleton-Century-Crofts.
18. This arrangement is suggested by Verle Waters, of the Institute of Nursing Consultants.
19. Engel, George L.: Homeostasis, behavioral adjustment and the concept of health and disease. In Grinker, Roy R., editor: Mid-century psychiatry, Springfield, Ill., 1953, Charles C Thomas, Publisher, p. 51.
20. Erikson, Erik H.: Childhood and society, ed. 2, New York, 1963, W. W. Norton & Co., Inc., Publishers.
21. Gesell, Arnold, et al.: Infant and child in the culture of today, New York, 1943, Harper & Row, Publishers.
22. a. Newell, A., and Simon, H.: Computer stimulation of human thinking, Science **134:**2011-2016, 1961.
    b. Newell, Allen, Shaw, C., and Simon, Herbert A.: Elements of a theory of human problem solving, Psychological Review **45:**151-166, 1958.
23. McDonald, Frederick J.: Educational psychology, ed. 2, Belmont, Cal., 1967, Wadsworth Publishing Co., Inc., pp. 256-302.
24. Creativity is the process of actualizing a *new* solution from the many composite input data, that is, a choice of one alternative intervention which is an outgrowth of the whole process of problem solving.
25. McDonald, pp. 253-254.
26. Bower, Fay L.: The process of planning nursing care: a theoretical model, ed. 2, St. Louis, 1977, The C. V. Mosby Co.
27. Peplau, p. 85.
28. Ibid., p. 99.
29. McDonald, p. 49.
30. Interaction Associates, Inc.: Strategy notebook: tools for change, ed. 2, San Francisco, 1972, Interaction Associates, Inc.

31. McDonald, p. 293.
32. Torrance, E. Paul: Explorations in creative thinking, Education **81:**216, 1960.
33. Torrance, E. Paul, and Mason, Raigh: Instructor effort to influence creativity: an experimental evaluation of six approaches, Journal of Educational Psychology **49:**211-218, 1958.
34. Resources for this section primarily include the following:
    a. Ruesch, Jurgen: Therapeutic communication, New York, 1961, W. W. Norton & Co., Inc., Publishers.
    b. Ruesch, Jurgen: General theory of communication. In Arieti, Silvano, editor: American handbook of psychiatry, New York, 1959, Basic Books, Inc., Publishers.
    c. Ruesch, Jurgen, and Bateson, Gregory: Communication: the social matrix of psychiatry, New York, 1968, W. W. Norton & Co., Inc., Publishers.
    d. Ruesch, Jurgen, Shannon, C. A., and Weaver, Warren: The mathematical theory of communication, Urbana, 1949, University of Illinois Press.
35. The process holds consistent whether or not the communication is intrapersonal, interpersonal, or group (community). Thus the word "unit" will be used to indicate a section, organ, or part of the body in intrapersonal communication, an individual person in interpersonal communication, and a person or group of persons in group communication.
36. Murray, Joyce, and Bevis, Em O.: Caring: process and practice, 1977, unpublished manuscript.
37. Fromm, Erick: The art of love: an inquiry into the nature of love, New York, 1956, Harper & Row, Publishers, pp. 8-10.
38. Mayeroff, Milton: On caring, New York, 1971, Perennial Library, Harper & Row, Publishers, p. 2.
39. Perls, Frederick S.: Gestalt therapy verbatim. In Stevens, John O., Lafayette, Calif., 1969, Real People Press, pp. 48-49.
40. Karpman, Steven B.: Fairy tales and script drama analysis, Transactional Analysis Bulletin **7:**39-43, April, 1968.
41. Skinner, B. F.: Walden two, New York, 1962, The Macmillan Co.
42. Bennis, Warren G.: Changing organizations, New York, 1966, McGraw-Hill Book Co., pp. 81-94, 99-108.
43. Dickoff, James, James, Patricia, and Wiedenbach, Ernestine: Theory in a practice discipline, Nursing Research **17:**415-435, 1968.
44. Ibid., p. 426.
45. Ibid., p. 423.
46. Taba, Hilda: Curriculum development: theory and practice, New York, 1962, Harcourt, Brace & World, Inc., p. 293.
47. Leavell, H., and Clark, E. G.: Preventive medicine for the doctor in his community, ed. 3, New York, 1965, McGraw-Hill Book Co.
48. Ibid., pp. 24-26.
49. American Nurses' Association, pp. 1-9.
50. Laubach, Frank: Everyday reading and writing, Syracuse, N.Y., 1976, New Readers Press.
51. Johnson, Miriam M., and Martin, Harry W.: A sociological analysis of the nurse role, American Journal of Nursing **58:**373-377, March, 1958.
52. Lawrence, Mary R.: Relationship control. In Carlson, Carolyn E., coordinator: Behavioral concepts and nursing intervention, Philadelphia, 1970, J. B. Lippincott Co.
53. Bennis, pp. 200-207.
54. The material on families is basically derived from the following sources:
    a. Schusky, Ernest L.: Manual for kinship analysis, New York, 1966, Holt, Rinehart & Winston, Inc., pp. 5-8.
    b. Honigmann, John J.: The world of man, New York, 1959, Harper & Row, Publishers.
55. Hayes, Wayland J., and Gazaway, Rena: Human relations in nursing, Philadelphia, 1955, W. B. Saunders Co., p. 175.
56. National Commission on Community Health Services: Health is a community affair, Cambridge, Mass., 1966, Harvard University Press, p. 1.
57. Ibid., p. 2.
58. Nursing Faculty Publications Association: Theoretical foundations of nursing II, San Jose, Calif., 1973, The Association.

BIBLIOGRAPHY

Abdellah, Faye G., and Levine, Eugene: Better patient care through nursing research, New York, 1965, The Macmillan Co.

American Nurses' Association: Educational preparation for nurse practitioners and assistants to nursing: a position paper, New York, 1965, The Association.

Bailey, June T., and Claus, Karen E.: Decision making in nursing, tools for change, St. Louis, 1975, The C. V. Mosby Co.

Bennis, Warren G.: Changing organizations, New York, 1966, McGraw-Hill Book Co.

Bower, Fay L.: The process of planning nursing care—a theoretical model, ed. 2, St. Louis, 1977, The C. V. Mosby Co.

Byrne, Marjory L., and Thompson, Lida F.: Key concepts for the study and practice of nursing, St. Louis, 1972, The C. V. Mosby Co.

Dunn, Halbert L.: High-level wellness, Arlington, Va., 1961, R. W. Beatty Co.

Engel, George L.: Homeostasis, behavioral adjustment and the concept of health and disease. In Grinker, Roy R., editor: Mid-century psychiatry, Springfield, Ill., 1953, Charles C Thomas, Publisher.

Erikson, Erik H.: Childhood and society, ed. 2, New York, 1963, W. W. Norton & Co., Inc., Publishers.

Ford, Loretta C., Cobb, Marguerite, and Taylor, Margaret: Defining clinical content—graduate nursing programs: community health nursing, Boulder, Colo., Feb., 1967, Western Interstate Commission for Higher Education.

Gesell, Arnold, et al.: Infant and child in the culture of today, New York, 1943, Harper & Row, Publishers.

Honigmann, John J.: The world of man, New York, 1959, Harper & Row, Publishers.

Interaction Associates, Inc.: Participatory decision-making, San Francisco, 1972, Interaction Associates, Inc.

Interaction Associates, Inc.: Strategy notebook: tools for change, ed. 2, San Francisco, 1972, Interaction Associates, Inc.

Johnson, Miriam M., and Martin, Harry W.: A sociological analysis of the nurses' role, American Journal of Nursing **58:**373-377, March, 1958.

Lawrence, Mary R.: Relationship control. In Carlson, Carolyn E., coordinator: Behavioral concepts and nursing intervention, Philadelphia, 1970, J. B. Lippincott Co.

Leavell, H., and Clark, E. G.: Preventive medicine for the doctor in his community, ed. 3, New York, 1965, McGraw-Hill Book Co.

Lidz, Theodore: The person: his development throughout the life cycle, New York, 1968, Basic Books, Inc., Publishers.

Maslow, Abraham H.: Toward a psychology of being, ed. 2, New York, 1968, Van Nostrand-Reinhold Co.

Mayeroff, Milton: On caring, New York, 1971, Perennial Library, Harper & Row, Publishers.

McDonald, Frederick J.: Educational psychology, ed. 2, Belmont, Calif., 1967, Wadsworth Publishing Co., Inc.

McGinnis, Thomas C., and Finnegan, Dana G.: Open family and marriage, a guide to personal growth, St. Louis, 1976, The C. V. Mosby Co.

National Commission on Community Health Services: Health is a community affair, Cambridge, Mass., 1966, Harvard University Press.

Newell, Allen, and Simon, Herbert A.: Computer stimulation of human thinking, Science **134:**2011-2016, 1961.

Newell, Allen, Shaw, C., and Simon, Herbert A.: Elements of a theory of human problem solving, Psychological Review **45:**151-166, 1958.

Nursing Faculty Publications Association: Theoretical foundations of nursing II, San Jose, Calif., 1973, The Association.

Peplau, Hildegard E.: Interpersonal relations in nursing, New York, 1952, G. P. Putnam's Sons.

Reinhardt, Adina M., and Quinn, Mildred D.: Family centered community nursing, a sociocultural framework, St. Louis, 1973, The C. V. Mosby Co.

Ruesch, Jurgen: Therapeutic communication, New York, 1961, W. W. Norton & Co., Inc., Publishers.

Ruesch, Jurgen: General theory of communication. In Arieti, Silvano, editor: American handbook of psychiatry, New York, 1959, Basic Books, Inc., Publishers.

Ruesch, Jurgen, and Bateson, Gregory: Communication: the social matrix of psychiatry, New York, 1968, W. W. Norton & Co., Inc., Publishers.

Ruesch, Jurgen, Shannon, C. A., and Weaver, Warren: The mathematical theory of communication, Urbana, 1949, University of Illinois Press.

Rogers, Martha: An introduction to the theoretical basis of nursing, Philadelphia, 1970, F. A. Davis Co.

Schusky, Ernest L.: Manual for kinship analysis, New York, 1966, Holt, Rinehart & Winston, Inc.

Skinner, B. F.: Walden two, New York, 1962, The Macmillan Co.

Sobol, Evelyn G., and Robischon, Paulette: Family nursing, a study guide, ed. 2, St. Louis, 1975, The C. V. Mosby Co.

Spradley, Barbara W.: Contemporary community nursing, Boston, 1975, Little, Brown & Co., Inc.

Thomas, Rhys W.: Introduction to socialization, human culture transmitted, St. Louis, 1972, The C. V. Mosby Co.

Thompson, Lida F., Miller, Michael H., and Bigler, Helen F.: Sociology, nurses and their patients in a modern society, St. Louis, 1975, The C. V. Mosby Co.

Torrance, E. Paul: Explorations in creative thinking, Education **81:**216, 1960.

Torrance, E. Paul, and Mason, Raigh: Instructor effort to influence creativity: an experimental evaluation of six approaches, Journal of Educational Psychology **49:**211-218, 1958.

Wallach, Michael A.: The intelligence/creativity distinction, New York, 1971, General Learning Press.

Wayland, J. Hayes, and Gazaway, Rena: Human relations in nursing, Philadelphia, 1955, W. B. Saunders Co.

Whaley, Lucille, Dunbar, Jacqueline, and Horton, Cleora: A human development survey, 1971, unpublished manuscript.

6

CURRICULUM VIVIFICATION

Vivification means to bring to life. Life is the inner reality or substance of process. From a study of biological life, Jan Smuts first drew the concept of holism; from observations of life, Alfred North Whitehead proposed process as life's reality. Curriculum vivification means to bring to life the individual courses of the curriculum—to take the "many" elements of curriculum and combine them into one living, growing, changing group of learning activities that are relevant to the health needs of society and appropriate to the students and the school. Curriculum vivification is the creative element of the process of curriculum building. It is the creation of one holistic new curriculum from the many parts; it is the translation of the substance of the framework into functional forms. Thus curriculum vivification is the beginning of a dynamic curriculum—a growing, changing, becoming curriculum that is always assimilating new elements, utilizing feedback, adapting, and innovating.

Curriculum structure, pattern, or design refers to the arrangement of courses within given time periods. Curriculum design is, to a great extent, the choices made by faculty based on the following:

1. The conceptual framework
2. The structure of the educational setting
3. The preferences of faculty and students

An infinite variety of curriculum patterns can arise from a single conceptual framework. A conceptual framework dictates the content, the sequencing of the content, and some of the factors about the curriculum structure for the content. Within general guidelines there is much variety for patterning the courses.

Some of the factors that influence curriculum design are structural. These are the givens in any situation over which the faculty has little influence:

1. The time pattern of the sponsoring agency, for example, semester, trimester, quarter, etc.
2. The time patterns of institutions offering support courses
3. The accepted average number of credits per course recommended by the curriculum committee of the sponsoring agency
4. The clock hours, credit, or unit ratio policy of the agency
5. The support courses, prerequisite courses, and cognate field courses available from educational institutions

Some factors are choices made by the faculty based on their preferences, their philosophy, and/or the conceptual framework:

1. The preference of a faculty about courses that include or exclude laboratory and classroom work within the same course
2. The degree of correlation between classroom work and practicum work
3. The degree of correlation among courses themselves, for example, which courses are prerequisite to which other courses and which courses must be taken concurrently with other courses

Many of the choices faculty make depend directly on statements in the conceptual framework that provide guidelines for decision making about curriculum patterns. For instance, if the conceptual framework states that students have choices, the curriculum pattern must include courses for electives that are choices in nursing and non-nursing subjects for students. If the conceptual framework states that the curriculum is responsive to individual student needs, to a great extent self-pacing and choices about subject matter must be provided for students. If the conceptual framework states that the curriculum will be responsive to individual student needs, structure must be provided so that modules, units, or courses may be omitted if students can substantiate that they have acquired the knowledge. In other words, curriculum patterns must accommodate to the conceptual framework as well as to the structure of a sponsoring institution and the preferences of faculty and students.

CRITERIA FOR A DESIRABLE CURRICULUM

The problems of curriculum change become the criteria for determining the desirability of a curriculum. A list of the problems of curriculum development, recapped and stated as criteria, follows.

The curriculum, that is, the pattern of courses and the selected learning activities, must do the following:

1. Be consistent with the conceptual framework and implement the conceptual framework commitments
2. Derive and test its concepts and theories in the practice of nursing in a real community of health need
3. Respond to the health needs of society and the immediate concerns of students
4. Cope with the knowledge explosion and the short "half-life" of scientific knowledge
5. Use the logical, precise, effective, and efficient educational technology that is currently available

6. Use teaching personnel in the most economical and efficient way (time, energy, and money)
7. Enable utilization of simulated nursing practice of cognitive nursing input
8. Provide for student testing of learned behaviors in reality situations
9. Produce a graduate capable of delivering creative nursing care for the next fifteen to twenty years
10. Spend a *reasonable* length of time accomplishing the goals of the curriculum

A "good" or desirable course pattern and implementation strategy will meet the foregoing criteria and will utilize all data generated in the previous stages of curriculum development. There are many ways the curriculum commitments can be implemented that will meet the foregoing criteria and therefore be a "desirable" curriculum. All the effective patterns have one common element—the capacity to continue to change and grow without the necessity of rebuilding the entire structure. Curriculum vivification is not the final step in curriculum building; there is no final step. Curriculum vivification is only a beginning or trial validation of ideas. From the first day of the first class of the implementation of the "new" or "revised" curriculum, feedback about implementation begins to enable plans to be made for continuing changes. Courses must change, grow, and improve; teachers must develop new teaching skills, learn new teaching strategies and tactics; and students must acquire new patterns of learning. All this is a continuing process—a process of trial, feedback, alteration—trial into infinity. The curriculum is like the limerick of the lady and the tiger:

> There was a young lady from Niger
> Who smiled as she rode on a tiger.
>   They returned from the ride
>   With the lady inside
> And the smile on the face of the tiger.

The curriculum "tiger" consumes the "lady" or those who ride him, since the processes of change, when built into the curriculum, continue to operate through the graduation of class after class of students and the attrition of faculty member after faculty member. This tiger with a smile on his face, is the antithesis of another curriculum tiger, the "saber-toothed curriculum."[1] The saber-toothed curriculum was allowed to continue to decimate the brain power, initiative, and creativity of students and faculty long after it was extinct because somehow it had become sacred, ritualistic, and frozen into a time and space that no longer existed. The tiger with a smile on his face is an ever-changing beast who is never to become extinct because he adapts to his ever-changing environment.

DEVISING COURSE PATTERNS AND DEVELOPING EACH COURSE

There are many ways to develop course patterns from the mass of data that the curriculum groups have created to date. The conceptual framework, program purposes, objectives, and the behaviors and content based on the future are like the bits and pieces of brightly colored glass in a kaleidoscope; they can be twisted and turned into many shapes and forms, all beautiful, all with symmetry, and all with a sense of unity and purpose. The task for the curriculum development group centers around developing, kaleidoscopically, alternative course patterns from the same component materials developed to date that are workable for the group. The methodology suggested here is just one of many ways that alternatives for courses and course sequences can be devised. It is suggested because it is simple and pragmatic and enables the faculty to collaborate in generating two or more alternative plans from which to choose or synthesize a plan suitable to their needs and wishes.

The suggested heuristic device for involving all faculty in course vivification is at the end of this chapter. The following is a discussion of the order and sequence of tasks for devising the pattern of courses

and developing each course. This discussion presumes use of the suggested heuristic.

I. Develop aims, purposes, and/or objectives consistent with the conceptual framework.
II. Devise alternative organization and course configuration patterns.
III. Develop each individual course in detail:
Objectives
Content packaging (units, modules, learning activities)
Evaluation and measurement of learner progress devices

The following is a list of activities necessary in designing the actual pattern of courses in the curriculum:

I. Aims, purposes, and/or objectives
  1. Develop aims and purposes of the program that are consistent with the sponsoring institution and expressive of the intent of the conceptual framework.
  2. Formulate program objectives from the accumulated data (conceptual framework, desired behaviors, and content).
II. Devising alternative organization and course configuration patterns
  1. Ask all faculty to build the curriculum of their dreams using all curriculum materials accrued to date.
  2. Identify the commonalities and differences among dream curricula and give written feedback to the faculty about commonalities of the dream curricula.
  3. List the possible organization patterns suggested by the faculty that are consistent with the theory of nursing and the conceptual framework commitments.
  4. Make models of the curriculum structure suggested by the organizing strategies that the faculty finds consistent with the nursing theory and other conceptual framework components.
  5. Create, for further development, not more than four nor less than two curriculum-organization models that are reflective of many of the commonalities in the dream curricula.
  6. Assign task groups to design the courses based on the models.
  7. Provide copies of the dream curricula to all task groups.
  8. Elaborate specific objectives for each course that will contribute to meeting the program objectives.
  9. Suggest possible learning activities and teaching strategies that will facilitate meeting the objectives.
  10. List the types of prerequisite knowledge

necessary to the students' ability to be successful in the tentative course.

11. Present all plans to the faculty. Ask the task groups to explain plans and answer questions.
12. Provide time to study, think, and discuss (one to two weeks).
13. Brainstorm ways to pull the best components from all plans.
14. Assign task groups to evaluate and choose ideas and to synthesize the plans as directed by the faculty.
15. Obtain consensus from the faculty to "try" one plan.

III. Devising each individual course in detail
1. Assign faculty in task groups for each course to do the following:
   a. Describe the intent of the course.
   b. Formulate the behavioral objectives.
   c. List content (processes and information) of each course that is necessary to promote learning of the desired behaviors.
   d. Suggest teaching strategies and learning activities.
   e. Propose a course "outline" or content to be covered.
   f. Decide on "unit" learning activity or "modular" structure or a combination of both.
   g. Suggest evaluation methods.
   h. Suggest grading techniques.
2. Ensure continuity, progression, and realization of program objectives by the following:
   a. Look at all behavioral objectives in a sequence to provide for progression between levels of learning.
   b. Check for content continuity by looking for the elaboration of essential processes throughout the courses and in each level of courses.
   c. Evaluate suggested learning activities and teaching strategies for consistency with the conceptual framework commitments about learning theories.
   d. Prognosticate the efficiency of proposed learning strategies.

Each of these major topic areas will be discussed to provide some data about each phase of curriculum vivification.

Aims, purposes, and objectives

Nursing is a practice discipline, and curricula for teaching practice disciplines are different from curricula for teaching cognitive disciplines. These differences are reflected in the purposes and objectives. In a practice discipline the objectives do not reflect so much what the graduate will know as what the graduate will be able to *do,* since what the graduate will be able to do is the ultimate test of any practice-oriented curriculum. Almost every statement of purpose that one can read in the catalog of any school of nursing speaks of critical thinking, the educated mind, or the liberally educated person. These are legitimate goals and are consistent with the conceptual frameworks of most curricula. What is seldom clear is what is meant by the educated mind. What are the behaviors of the person who thinks critically?

Borton[2] suggests that the education of the mind involves the processes of gathering, evaluating, and acting on information. The processes necessary to "think" creatively are the methods, skills, and purposive behaviors of processing information. He further states that these skills cut across subject matter disciplines and are of fundamental applicability in all areas of student life, not just the major subject area. His proposition is that no one subject area lends itself to process education more than another; nursing, social studies, physics, history, and philosophy all lend themselves to the element of education most often left to chance—the process of using a logical system of cognitive processes. For nursing, a process curriculum can realize the goal of critical thinking and/or an educated mind through identifying the explicit process goals necessary to function in the discipline and designing learning activities necessary to achieve those goals. Traditionally, nursing has been taught in the same way in which cognitive disciplines have been taught, that is, identifying the *knowledges* one needs to have to practice. The "application of theory to practice" has been left to the student to devise in the real situation in a place called the "clinical area." If the student had difficulty in applying theory to practice, something was obviously wrong with the student—perhaps not enough study. In a process curriculum *the theory is the practice,* and the classroom is one place it occurs. The classroom is a safe place where no patients can be hurt, no families disrupted, no students scared out of their careers, no physicians offended, and no graduate nurses made anxious.

The knowledge explosion puts educators in an uncomfortable position. One half of what is being taught in the science areas will be obsolete in two and a half years, and each year there is at least one tenth more information than there was the previous year. Add to this phenomenon the fact that 75% of what is memorized will be forgotten in two years and one is confronted with a startling fact: Most of the effort geared to pouring information into nursing students' heads is wasted effort. If nursing curricula do no more than sensitize students to the jargon of health work, orient them to some of the sources of information about health problems, provide them with a framework for nursing functions, guide them in the processing of data toward the solving of nursing problems and in responding effectively to each other and to clients, and help them know how best to use the energy generated by caring, it has done a magnificent job, since it will have provided the students with behaviors that are timeless.

The problem in specifying purposes and objectives becomes one of identifying those behaviors that the faculty thinks necessary to the functions of nursing as defined in the conceptual framework. There are many sources for this task. Several are listed in the bibliography of this chapter. The primary task involved in specifying the objectives is one of teasing the desired behaviors out of the conceptual framework materials and out of the "predicted nurse behaviors and content" outlines produced by the faculty (p. 61).

Behavioral objectives. Since the emphasis of nursing curricula is on *practice* and practice "doing," it behooves nurse educators to spell out objectives behaviorally on all levels. Program aims, goals, or purposes tell *where* one is going; program objectives tell *what* one can do when one has arrived.

Program objectives are, in effect, end-product criteria. Course, unit, module, and/or learning activity objectives are stepping-stones along the way. They are the building blocks whose cumulative effect is the end product criteria spelled out as program objectives. Program objectives are derived from the conceptual framework. Course, unit, module, and/or learning activity objectives cannot be developed until a curriculum organization has been devised that will enable the meeting of the program objectives. The program objectives must be spelled out prior to any other step in curriculum vivification.

The process of writing objectives in behavioral terms is well programmed. There are many excellent and adequate sources for this activity, and it will not be elaborated here. The bibliography contains several basic references about construction and use of behavioral objectives. Some general guidelines are offered on p. 168.

Alternative organizing strategies and course configuration patterns

There are as many ways to organize the content of a curriculum as there are philosophical views of nursing. There are no "bad" ways; there are just some that are better than others for given situations. Some organizing strategies include the following:

1. Organize by teaching strategy to be used:
   a. Lecture courses for information
   b. Process courses for utilization of information
   c. Simulation courses for practice
   d. Reality validating courses for application and testing
2. Organize by sequence of content:
   a. Simple to complex using Gagné's stages of learning
   b. Chronological order or growth and development phases
   c. Life crisis periods
   d. Practice implications—or clinical setting situation
   e. Specialty area or medical model
   f. Physiological systems
   g. Stress—stress response phase
3. Organize by process or nursing function to be emphasized:
   a. Courses in teaching-learning role of the nurse

b. Courses in communicative role of the nurse
c. Courses in the decision-making role of the nurse
d. Courses in change and changing
e. Manipulative or motor nursing skills
4. Organize by target system problems:
   a. Self-system—intrapersonal problems
   b. Group-system problems
   c. Family-system problems
   d. Health care delivery systems problems
   e. Community-system problems
   f. National-system problems
   g. World-system problems

Almost all patterns devised as effective educational systems are syntheses of more than one approach or organizing stratagem.

Devising and organizing courses into a curriculum pattern is neither the most difficult nor the most important part of curriculum development but seems to hold a key place in the minds of the participants of curriculum building. Perhaps the reason is that it is actually the *real* implementation of the conceptual framework, behaviors and content selection, and philosophical commitment. In the imagination of the builders it is the acid test. In actual fact the acid test comes later in the planning and implementing of the content of the courses. Course patterns can facilitate or inhibit the flow of content because of the structure of material, but only slightly; *the key factor is how the format is used*. There are as many ways to organize courses as one wishes to consider. The problem is not only to think up ways but also to choose ones that have greatest potential for fulfilling the conceptual framework commitments.

The faculty will have more commonalities than differences in expectations and desires about a curriculum format, and an effective strategy for generating alternatives will capitalize on most of those commonalities. This will leave defined areas of differences to be negotiated.

One of the activities that will enable the faculty to bring the common work of the whole group to bear on course patterning and planning will be a recapitulation of what has gone before. Periodically, facul-

ties lose perspective because they are so preoccupied with the job of today that the achievements of the past, such as identifying and formulating conceptual framework, philosophy, and objectives become blurred. The major task of this phase of curriculum building is to facilitate the participation of every faculty member in the actual planning and choosing of a curriculum organization plan. The pinion gear of this operation is a summary of all work. Even though each person has had finished copies of all materials distributed at the completion of each task, the work should be collated and redistributed as a packet of provisional accomplishment. This packet should contain at a minimum the conceptual framework (both structural and cognitive), including the theory of nursing and the theory of learning that has been tentatively accepted, the philosophy, and the program objectives. Using this summary, the faculty is in a position to envision how best to create a curriculum pattern that will fulfill the expectations inherent in the work to date. A heuristic device for facilitating the process is suggested at the end of the chapter.

The use of models for envisioning the curriculum enables people to communicate whole ideas or complete pictures with few words or short phrases. It illustrates abstractions in concrete ways, reduces detail and emphasizes the major or important aspects of the curriculum components, and shows the dynamics of flow of people and/or ideas, for example, content.

Curriculum patterns: some format options and their underlying assumptions. Curriculum patterns are as numerous as there are schools of nursing. There is an almost limitless number of ways one can group classroom and clinical experiences to potentiate learning. The following are some short discussions and graphic models of six selected curriculum patterns or formats.

Pattern 1: Progressive block (Fig. 6-1). The progressive block pattern is one in which groups of students in certain num-

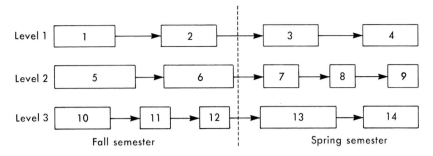

Fig. 6-1. Progressive block (classroom and practician).

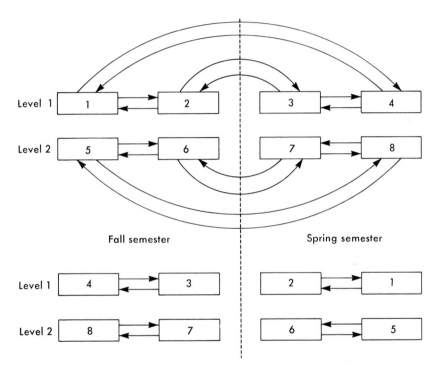

Fig. 6-2. Swap block (classroom and practician).

bers are "rotated" through specified classes and closely correlated practice. Usually the number of students in these classes is regulated by the number of students who can be accommodated by that clinical rotation. This method (Fig. 6-1) presupposes the following:

1. Clinical practice and classroom information must be closely correlated, and retroactive integration is minimal.

2. Each student must have essentially the same amount of time in each clinical practice area.

3. Each student who is provided with this practice is receiving a similar education.

Pattern 2: Swap block (Fig. 6-2). The swap block is a pattern in which the students are divided into two or more groups. Each group takes a specific course and its correlated clinical practice, then on signal

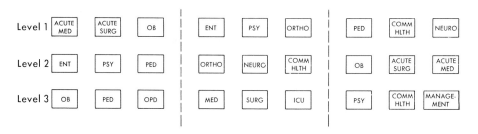

Level 1	ACUTE MED	ACUTE SURG	OB		ENT	PSY	ORTHO		PED	COMM HLTH	NEURO
Level 2	ENT	PSY	PED		ORTHO	NEURO	COMM HLTH		OB	ACUTE SURG	ACUTE MED
Level 3	OB	PED	OPD		MED	SURG	ICU		PSY	COMM HLTH	MANAGE-MENT

Fig. 6-3. Peat and repeat.

everyone swaps chairs, teachers, and clinical areas and takes the same course that the other group was taking. The presumptions on which this method is based are as follows:

1. Clinical practice and classroom information must be closely correlated, and retroactive integration is minimal.
2. Students must be at the same level in each new subject area and cannot start at a higher theory level because the content is new.
3. Each student must have essentially the same amount of time in each clinical practice area.
4. Each student is receiving a similar education.

Pattern 3: Peat and repeat (Fig. 6-3). The peat and repeat pattern is one in which each student and each teacher is provided with time together at each level of the curriculum so that two or more "mini" courses in each "specialty" area are taught. A modification of this pattern is to repeat each week or each day so that students on Monday go to public health, on Tuesday to acute hospitals, on Wednesday to psychiatric centers, and on Thursday to general clinics. This pattern has among its assumptions the following items:

1. As students mature, they are capable of attaining more depth in a specialty area.
2. Students are more capable of concentrating on the specialty after having some basics in all clinical areas.
3. Integration will take place by exposure to a variety of clinical areas.

4. The time interval between exposures to the subject matter provides more effective learning.
5. Learning materials in small doses provide a better inoculation than one large dose.
6. Those clinical areas to which students are exposed in their last year are more likely to attract the students' interest than those to which they are exposed in the first year.
7. Each student must have the same amount of time in each clinical area.
8. Each student provided with this type of practice is receiving a similar education.

Pattern 4: Concept clock (Fig. 6-4). The concept clock is the pattern in which courses proceed along a preconceived progression of conceptual constructs that are inclusive enough to provide clinical parallels regardless of the arena of clinical practice for the student. Emphasis is on the selected concepts and not on the clinical specialty. If electrolyte balance is the conceptual area emphasized, students are working with clients who have electrolyte problems in every clinical area. Rotation to various clinical areas is provided simply for exposure to varying diagnoses and the concomitant nursing care problems. Nursing care is emphasized as the organizing factor, and nursing care problems are tied to what is happening to the client and not to his diagnosis. Concepts are the unifying factor and not medical specialty areas. Some of the underlying assumptions for this structure are as follows:

1. Nursing care concepts are fairly uni-

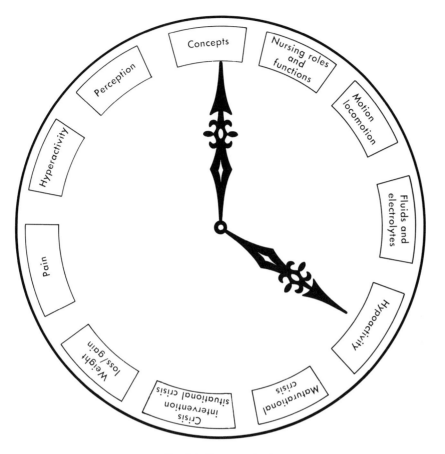

Fig. 6-4. Concept clock.

versal phenomena that we found in all types of clients in all settings.

2. Near replication of student learning experiences is not possible or necessarily desirable.
3. Nursing problems are more important than medical diagnoses.
4. Generalization, not specialization, is the legitimate business of generic programs.
5. Retroactive integration is an operational learning phenomenon, and therefore it is not necessary to teach all information concomitantly with practice, since students will retroactively assimilate and integrate learnings.

Pattern 5: Holistic hop-along (Fig. 6-5). The holistic hop-along is a further devel-

opment of the concept clock and not as "far out" as the smorgasbord. The holistic hop-along provides a series of classroom experiences or courses that has as its clinical component a series of required and/or optional learning activities that are highly structured and progress with the content of the class. These learning activities may be accomplished in specified clinical settings, in homes, on street corners, in health departments, with kid brothers and sisters, and elsewhere. The learning activities specify the type of clients to be used and where the clients may be found. If the subject is maturation, the learning activity may be assessing a child of specified age with the Denver Developmental Screening Test, and any child, regardless of place found (home, church, health department,

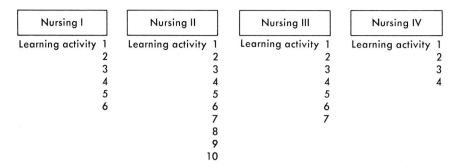

Fig. 6-5. Holistic hop-along.

or neighborhood) will do. On the other hand, the learning activity may be total support of the unresponsive client, and nursing homes and intensive care units may be the only places that students may select to care for these clients and complete the learning activity. The learning activity may have to be completed by contract within specified times to enable the correct number of students to be accommodated by the correct number of teachers supervising the activity. This pattern has the following assumptions:

1. Within specified constraints, all learners are capable of selecting the time and place most appropriate for them to accomplish learning activities.
2. Learning experiences are different for each student, and commonality can be found in the generalizations derived from experiences and not in the specifics.
3. Many nursing problems are found in a wide number of clients with a variety of health problems and medical diagnoses. Nursing focuses primarily on what happens to the client who has health problems and secondarily on the diagnosis.
4. The most valuable nursing-oriented learning activities focus on common manifestations of health problems and common nursing care interventions.
5. There are learning objectives that all students must attain, and the

way and pace at which the objectives are attained can be individualized by each learner.
6. Retroactive integration is an operational learning phenomenon and enables students retroactively to assimilate and integrate learning.
7. "Specialty area" nursing can be minimized or eliminated in given programs because most general nursing care is applicable in all specialty areas of practice.
8. Time needed for each student to complete a learning activity is different for each student and can, within broad limits, be provided.
9. Students who are provided with the same "time," kind of clients, and similar experiences will still learn different things.
10. Structured learning activities facilitate greater homogeneity of student learning than simple exposure to arena, type of clients, and time on specific units.

Pattern 6: Smorgasbord (Fig. 6-6). The smorgasbord pattern offers learning experiences that are arranged in discrete episodes that can be selected to compile an individualized curriculum. The selection can be done by the learner, by the teacher, or by learners and teachers collaboratively selecting desired or appropriate experiences. The episodes can be informational, simulated, or reality practice or any combination of these ingredients. Smorgasbord patterns enable individuals to select learn-

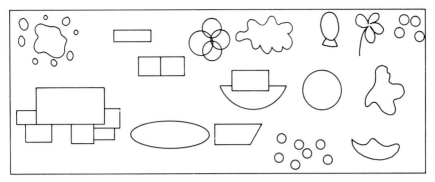

NOTE: MODULES ARE WEIGHTED
    5 mini modules = 1 module = 1/5 unit of credit
    5 modules = 1 maxie module = 1 unit of credit
    5 maxie modules = 5 units of credit = 1 course
    Normal load = 3 courses = 15 units of credit per quarter

Fig. 6-6. Smorgasbord.

ing experiences that build directly on past experiences and build toward individualized goals.

The smorgasbord is based on some of the following assumptions:

1. Students have unique life experiences that make their learning needs different.
2. It is legitimate to have student learning experiences different for each student.
3. Student homogeneity in a program is achieved through terminal criteria (behavioral objectives), consistency with the conceptual framework, and internal structure of the learning activity, not through identical requirements for each learner.
4. Faculty and students are committed to individualized learning and are appropriately organized for it.
5. Retroactive integration is an operational learning phenomenon, and progression through a curriculum follows a "natural" sequence that may differ from student to student.

Each of the described patterns has many more assumptions than those listed here. Each reader can list the assumptions for possible patterns for his curriculum in the light of his own faculty, philosophy, and conceptual framework. Patterns vary in degree and kind from those listed. However, these are the most common ones, and most schools use a variation of one of the foregoing patterns or a combination of several of them.

Selecting a format. Selecting a curriculum pattern, format, or plan is a task that follows exploring the possible patterns potentially useful to the faculty, consistent with the conceptual framework, and appealing to the preferences of the faculty. To select a pattern that will provide optimal usefulness, consistency, and appropriateness, faculties take two or more plans and weigh the advantages and disadvantages. One maxim in this stage of curriculum development is never to offer the faculty only one choice of a plan. The more choices offered the better able the faculty will be to synthesize the best features of the alternatives and to generate a plan pleasing to most faculty members. Task groups working independently to devise alternative plans usually produce two or more different plans. If the faculty wishes more plans, more task groups will be utilized. The following discussion depicts some of the considerations a faculty might give to alternative plans.

The examples in Fig. 6-7 depict two dif-

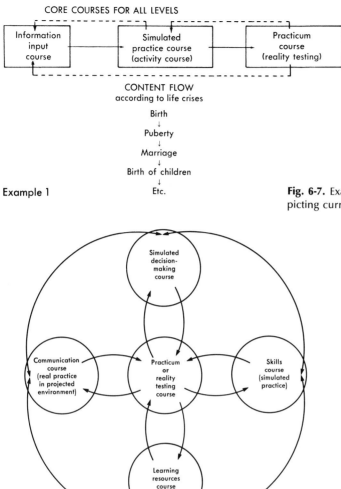

CORE COURSES FOR ALL LEVELS

Information input course → Simulated practice course (activity course) → Practicum course (reality testing)

CONTENT FLOW
according to life crises

Birth
↓
Puberty
↓
Marriage
↓
Birth of children
↓
Etc.

Example 1

Fig. 6-7. Examples of the use of models for depicting curriculum structure.

Example 2

ferent types of approaches to curriculum, and each type represents different problems in planning for course content. Example 1 in Fig. 6-7 is a curriculum that is "prefabricated," that is, built to specifications around a fixed sequence of procession of materials. This plan has the advantage of a certain amount of stability of structure so that both students and teachers can know the exact content areas to be covered at any given period of time. Whether or not the content is organized around life crises, growth and development periods, target-system problems, major health concepts, primary nursing functions, or any other organizing idea,

the course is fixed and predictable. Some of the advantages of such a plan follow:

1. Topical outlines on a "fixed time" schedule are available to faculty and students.
2. The curriculum for each student is similar within the same level.
3. All students in a level are able to take the same examinations.
4. All students in a level can do similar learning activities at a common time.

The disadvantages are as follows:

1. It is sometimes difficult to find enough practicum experiences to enable the simultaneous application of the selected concepts.

2. Conflict often arises between the practicum specialty area objectives and the curriculum objectives during a specified practicum experience time.
3. Individual learning needs of students (interest, style, tempo) are often sacrificed for the learning needs of the group.

Example 2 in Fig. 6-7 represents the independent modular form of curriculum. Structure is in small, compact learning packages so that teacher and student can pick and choose those modules most appropriate at a given time to fulfill specific needs. In this kind of curriculum, student progression from level to level must be measured in performance criteria, not in normative criteria. Another progression measuring rod can be the proportion of total materials to be learned by a given date. Each module must be complete and have its behavioral objectives, its basic information, and its learning activities. The information delivery system can be packaged for any format available to the school: super-8 single-concept movies, slides, television, filmstrips, audio cassettes, written programs, and books. Lectures (live) must necessarily be extremely limited. Simulation learning activities can be drawn from practicum experiences and planned for achieving specified objectives and thus form the stable backbone of the curriculum. Following are some of the advantages of such a plan:

1. It allows very close correlation of practicum experiences and classroom experiences.
2. It makes some provision for progression within students' learning tempo and style.
3. It makes information available to students around "need" or problems.
4. It enables selection of materials from a wide variety of sources and packaging of faculty information in an efficient and effective format.

Following are some of the disadvantages of such a plan:

1. It requires a real change in teaching style.
2. It requires most students to change learning style from accepting teacher-set structure and pace to assuming more responsibility for their own learning needs.
3. It requires a lot of time to prepare the modules and to continue to improve them.
4. It causes a disruption in the use of "quarter" or "semester" time spans as learning intervals.

The group can devise many plans, and each plan deserves consideration for feasibility, congruence with conceptual framework commitments, efficiency in learning, cost in time, materials, energy, and money, and legality (state board standards and requirements). Each plan can be evaluated by listing the strengths and limitations or liabilities as perceived by the group. An acceptable plan will probably be one that synthesizes the advantages and minimizes the liabilities of several plans.

When plans are formulated, they tend to be vague and slightly unreal to even those who have participated in their development. Major problems of curriculum will have been worked out by this stage, but there will be many unknown factors, which will be a source of anxiety. If the faculty can agree together that at this stage of development there are details for which it is impossible to know the answer, that there are "how to's" which will take a lot of work to develop, and that initial trials will only form the foundation for further evolution, then a mutual agreement to risk something different from previous patterns can be reached. Curricula do not jump full blown onto paper; they begin with a skeleton structure, like a house, and gradually over the months the details of the roof, walls, interior, paint, and household goods provide the fulfillment of the architectural plans that began it. If a curriculum group can reach a consensus about the form and shape of a plan and "trial" implementation, ongoing feedback or natural maturation will continually add more and more functional details.

Devising each course in detail

The first task in devising the details of courses within the curriculum pattern is to develop a thorough description of the intent of the course. Definitive course objectives are unnecessary at this stage, but general objectives are inherent in the course description. The specific objectives are easier to devise once thorough course descriptions are articulated. The wording or flow of the paragraphs needed to do this is not important, in that they are not for publication and distribution. This task is necessary to provide the curriculum group with a sense of the components of the pattern that has been adopted. To agree on a pattern at all, some thought and discussion have been given to the courses; perhaps even brief descriptions have been written. For the work on course development to progress, more definitive and explicit descriptions need to be recorded. Following is an example of such a description:

Course name: **Clinical Practicum in Nursing I**
Catalogue No.: N95
Units: 3. Type course: Laboratory. Total hours per week: 9 (2 days, 4½ hours per day).

Course description. This is the first course in a series of four practicum nursing courses and is the course in which students may reality-validate the nursing content acquired in all the informational and simulated practice courses that precede or are concurrent with this course. Competence can be learned in the classroom under simulated conditions, but confidence comes only from reality testing. Expertise is not an expected outcome but a beginning confidence from reality practice, and testing of learned behaviors is expected. All or any nursing environments may be used, and all settings will be viewed as community efforts to meet the health needs of its citizens. Learning activities in this course will be designed to facilitate a holistic view of nursing and will be completed by each student in every setting.

Learning activities will stress protective, nurtrative, and generative behaviors with the focus on protective and nurtrative behaviors. Intrapersonal, interpersonal, and community target systems will be used regardless of the student's clinical setting assignment. Practicum course requirements in the form of learning activities will facilitate the students' working with each of the target systems.

Learning activities will be designed to facilitate the students' identification of community demography, community health needs and problems, and community agencies that are a response to those problems. The study of family roles and structure will be begun, and each student will study a client and his family in depth. Assessment of the developmental levels and nutritional patterns of clients will be started. Cognitive, communicative, and motor skills learned in the multimedia laboratory will be practiced and tested. Overall course objectives and required projects, activities, and/or modules will take precedence over specialty area or setting objectives.

Special skills, techniques, or information that is dictated by the setting to which the student is assigned must be defined and programmed using one or more of the available media. A feedback group will monitor these programs or modules so that they are consistent with the conceptual framework, the level of the student, and the objectives of the course and are feasible for concurrent student load.

Use of course description. As the course details are completed, the description will be altered to conform to the evolving concept of the course. The course description simply preserves the intent of each course in the pattern while courses are being developed one at a time. It will also orient the task group to the original intent of the course. If the original intent of the course alters because of other contingencies (for example, concurrent course changes that encroach on content originally intended for a different course), corresponding changes in the course under consideration can be made. These descriptions are not a law about what must be included in a course; they are options and statements of intent, which like real estate options can be a matter of exercising choice at one's discretion.

All courses cannot be developed in detail at once. Faculties usually develop courses in detail that will be offered to students first in the curriculum; then as the earlier courses are developed, later courses are commenced. In this way curriculum vivification proceeds in the same manner in which students proceed through a curriculum. Most often faculty implement the early courses of a curriculum at the same time that they are developing subsequent levels of courses. This has the happy effect of allowing development based on the testing of ideas in early level courses. It has the unhappy side effect of being extremely stress producing and contributing to faculty overload.

Formulating course objectives. Once a course description has been agreed on, a task group can begin to consider what the desired behavioral outcomes of the course will be. There are six basic sources that the task group must use when devising the behavioral expectations of each individual course:

1. A conceptual framework so that all objectives are congruent with the setting, student, and subject components
2. Curriculum commitments so that they are fulfilled by the various objectives
3. The behaviors necessary to function in the predicted environment and the content necessary to facilitate the development of those behaviors
4. The program objectives so that level and course objectives contribute in definable and explicit ways to the achievement of program objectives
5. The level objectives so that course objectives are consistent with and contribute to the achievement of level objectives
6. The course description or intent so that the objectives fulfill the intent of the course as it fits into the curriculum plan

Legitimate course objectives must reflect the level of theory attained through previous educational experiences (pp. 168 and 169) and the changing trends in education. The accompanying McBeath Model depicting change illustrates the stages of development of society and the appropriate educational outcomes for the age in which we live. Stage III of the model provides a quick overview of the developments in technology, the accompanying developments in science, and the concurrent developments in education. McBeath has categorized principles, practices, and outcomes so that with a quick overview one can see the trends in educational development and the areas for objectives to emphasize.

Ideally, the model flows from Stage I to Stage III. If Stage III is to be realized, nursing education must adopt the objectives and instructional system appropriate to those objectives.

Waters[4] has provided two approaches useful for devising behavioral objectives or for checking those already devised to ensure that they are behaviorally stated. These "Verle's Pearls" are provided here as a brief survey for objectives. For further information, see the Bibliography.

McBEATH MODEL[3]
A model depicting change as sequential, emergent, and transformational

Stage I (Agrarian society)	Stage II (Industrial society)	Stage III (Technological society)
Developments in technology		
Wheel	Motor	Jet propulsion
Manpower	Machine power	Electronic controls
Cottage industry	Mechanization	Automation
Structures and functions	Functions in structures	Structures for functions
Units	Networks	Constellations
Explore	Exploit	Conserve
Developments in science		
Certainties	Confusion	Probabilities
Absolutes	Relative absolutes	Relatives
Metaphor	Toward models	Functional models
Linear sets	Rationalized structures	Emerging patterns
Closed system	Open system	Organic systems
Static	Dynamic (in-flux)	Dynamic (evolving)

Developments in education
Principles

Active mind	Reactive mind	Transactive mind
Unity (dualism)	Unity (monism)	Plural
Autocratic	Laissez-faire	Democratic

Practices

Teacher dominated	Permissive	Inquiry centered
Do things to	Do things for	Do things with
Subject emphasis	Method emphasis	Interdisciplinary emphasis
Product oriented	Process oriented	Performance oriented
Extrinsic manipulation	Random reinforcement	Meaningful involvement
Standards grouping	Age grouping	Readiness grouping
Class teaching	Group teaching	Independent study
Fixed stimulus	Multiple stimuli	Organized stimuli
Limited access	Random access	Systematic access
Limited resources	Multiple resources	Instructional systems
Teaching aids	Audiovisual techniques	Instructional technology

Outcomes

Fixed response	Varied response	Response mastery
Convergent thinking and rote memory	Convergent thinking plus free expression	Convergent and divergent thinking
Competitive	Cooperative	Adventure
Inner directed	Other directed	Self-actualizing

VERLE'S PEARLS[4]
Recipe for writing behavioral objectives

Five basic steps in writing an objective:
1. State the objective from the learner's point of view.
2. Make the type of learning explicit: cognitive, psychomotor, affective.
3. State the terminal behavior.
4. Specify conditions under which behavior will be performed.
5. State the degree of proficiency you expect.

Put another way, every objective should answer these five questions:
1. Who is to perform?
2. What category of learning is involved?
3. What is the terminal behavior?
4. Under what conditions will it be demonstrated?
5. What degree or level of proficiency is to be met in order to succeed?

Seven secrets: Keys to objectives that will work for you:
1. Be clear and concise. (Avoid global phrases—appreciate the dignity and worth of each individual point, etc.)
2. Be realistic and appropriate to the level of your learner (vocabulary).
3. Be attainable by instruction (e.g., character and personality).
4. Be significant (e.g., nursing's preoccupation with forms of dress and grooming).
5. Be developed cooperatively between teacher and learner.
6. Be stated so that each objective is separate.
7. Be measurable.

Probably the most difficult part of composing behavioral objectives for either courses or learning activities is finding behavioral words that are descriptive of the task to be performed and the level expected of the performance. The taxonomy below lists some verbs or phrases that are helpful in expressing behaviors in the four levels of theory suggested by Dickoff, James, and Wiedenbach.[5]

TAXONOMY OF THEORY-BUILDING LEVELS

Theory-building level[5]	Taxonomy of appropriate activities for mastery of level[6]
Level I: Factor-isolating theories	Perceive Name Label Name parts Classify (simple) List Identify Recognize Inspect Record Recall Repeat Restate Tell Report Examine Copy
Level II: Factor-relating theories	Depict Describe Relate factors Draw, sketch Schedule Discuss Express Translate Inventory Diagram Compare factors Analyze factors Distinguish Differentiate Categorize Sort Define Chart

TAXONOMY OF THEORY-BUILDING LEVELS

Theory-building level[5]	Taxonomy of appropriate activities for mastery of level[6]
Level III: Situation-relating theories a. Predictive theories b. Promoting or inhibitory theories	Interpret Demonstrate Explain Assemble Order Hypothesize Theorize Measure Predict Estimate Compare situations Rate Value Apprise Assess Relate situations Analyze situation Synthesize Question Critique Employ Combine Guess Systematize Randomize
Level IV: Situation-producing theories a. Prescriptive theories b. Creative theories	Use Set up Manage Plan Design Arrange Organize Prepare Create Formulate Compose Propose Choose Select Index Evaluate Test Experiment Solve Utilize Practice Apply Substitute Adapt Build Change Vary Commit Implement Devise Generate Generalize Transform

Beginning level courses usually focus on Level I and II objectives. Naturally, there are some Level III and a few Level IV objectives, but the Level I and II predominate. As courses move up the continuum of difficulty, increasing numbers of Level III and IV objectives appear. The last courses of baccalaureate curricula and graduate courses have few Level I and II objectives (although usually some do appear) and a predominance of Level IV objectives.

Complexity in courses is a function of (1) the number of variables with which the student must deal at one time; (2) the degree or amount of structure imposed by the setting (environment), the teacher, and the course (curriculum), which affects how difficult or easy it is to monitor the variables; and (3) the level of theory with which the content deals. Course objectives must, when formulated, address themselves to all three of these elements to enable students to progress along the difficulty continuum.

Each level of taxonomy presumes mastery (inclusive) of previous levels. There are some unclear categorizations between levels.

Course target behaviors give rise to unit, learning activity, or learning module objectives. Courses are constructed around the content deemed necessary to produce the desired target behaviors. The structure of a specific course in the curriculum can be organized in units, in learning modules or learning activities, or in any combination of these components. Units are convenient ways to group areas of content. Units can be organized around broad concepts, common denominators, a process, a phase of a process, or any functional division of content. Units are not necessary to the organization of a course; units of study are merely a format of traditional course organization. Learning activities are ways in which objectives are accomplished. Learning activities are the heuristic devices of education. They are things the learner is to do that will promote the desired changes

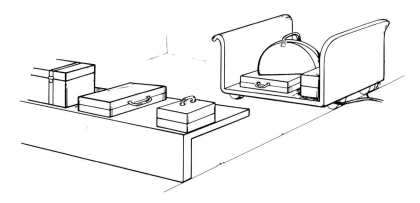

Fig. 6-8. A module is like a luggage gondola: a device for transporting learning activities going to the same objective.

in behaviors. They may be passive, cognitive activities such as reading; cognitive interactive processes with a machine such as programmed instruction; a manipulation of a skill such as bedmaking; or any kind of activity that requires the learner to *do* something.

Learning modules

A learning module is a package containing the whole of the instructional materials necessary for the learning of an entity. Modules are like the gondolas used to transport luggage by airlines (Fig. 6-8). These gondolas have unity, can be transported as a package, and contain luggage that is going to only one place. Inside the gondola are many or a few pieces of luggage (depending on how much luggage needs to be transported to a given location). Each piece of luggage inside the gondola can belong to a different passenger, can have a different appearance, can be manufactured by different companies, and can be of a wide variety of sizes. They all have in common one thing: they are headed for the same destination. Modules are the same way. Modules contain learning activities that are devised to accomplish a given, defined behavioral objective or group of behavioral objectives. Learning modules contain the following items:

1. The behavioral objective or objectives for the module

2. The module pretest
3. Content resource material or resource reference (software)
4. Evaluative checkpoints
5. Passive or active learning activities and the equipment necessary to the tasks (syringes, paper and pen, models, dolls, etc.)
6. A list of the hardware or audiovisual equipment necessary to the use of the software and directions about where it can be found or obtained
7. Posttest

Constructing learning modules is made simple by following the design for constructing units depicted in the Kemp model.[7] Following are the basic activities for developing modules:

1. Analyze the concept or behavior topic of the module.
2. Describe the intent of the module. List the course objectives for which the module is expected to facilitate attainment. Show its relationship and congruency with the conceptual framework program objective, expected graduate behaviors, and level objectives.
3. List the target behaviors or the behavioral outcomes expected when the module is completed by the learner.
4. Hypothesize the content necessary to promote the described changes

of behavior by (a) listing the information necessary to the attainment of the behavior(s) and (b) listing the processes inherent in the content.

5. Generate some possible activities that would enable the learner to self-appropriate the information and the behaviors.

6. Delete information, processes, and behaviors learned in previous courses, in other modules, or in earlier states of maturation. Derive from this a list of prerequisite knowledge and behavior.

7. Choose a series of activities that (a) will promote or facilitate the attainment of the behavior, (b) will provide a variety of levels of concreteness and abstractness (to accommodate different learning styles), and (c) are simple components of the "whole" module intent.

8. Select the media that will best deliver the content of each learning activity in the module.

9. Select one or more performance activities for each content area of the module. (Performance activities are things that the learner does which require that he use the information and thus self-appropriate the content.)

10. Devise pretests and/or posttests and/or checkpoints that allow evaluation of both affective and cognitive domains.

11. Package the objectives, information (software), learning activity directions and materials, affective and cognitive evaluation tools, test, and/or criteria in one container if possible.

A concept analysis is a methodology for defining the subconcepts within a concept or topic and establishing the perimeters and hierarchy, the preknowledges and postknowledges and behaviors, and the configuration or flow of knowledge and skill. A concept analysis is a way to break a concept or topic down into small enough

components to make learning episodes or activities that center on one or a few subconcepts. Begin with a concept and see what ideas come to mind. The ideas thus generated are then evaluated for true relevance to the topic and the appropriate ones selected. The selected subconcepts are then arranged in sequence. Those which are dependent on others are placed in descending order; those which are not dependent cluster around common objectives or spin off to stand alone. For instance, the concepts in the topic of behavior modification could be analyzed to provide the following pattern:

Behavior modification
Antecedent events
Target behavior
Consequence
Reinforcement (negative, positive, avertive)
Contingency management

These topics could be broken down further if necessary. In addition, they could be placed under larger concepts such as learning or therapeutic modes. A diagrammatic model patterned after Fig. 6-9 and combining the forms suggested there is helpful in visualizing what the series of modules on behavior modification will look like when completed. Such a diagram furnishes an overview for students and helps the learner attain insights into how the concepts fit into the overall learning schema for the course.

Modules have specific target behaviors, a test of learning readiness and/or accomplishment, definitive cognitive input, a selected operational activity, and a test of achievement—all in one compact, exportable package. They may be devised for independent learning or built for use with a teacher facilitator; they may be constructed for individuals or for groups. They can contain programmed instruction, filmstrips, audio cassettes, televised programs, study questions, games, field trips, interactive processes with peers or teacher, pretest, posttest, cognitive test, and/or performance test.

Pretests need to test not only prereq-

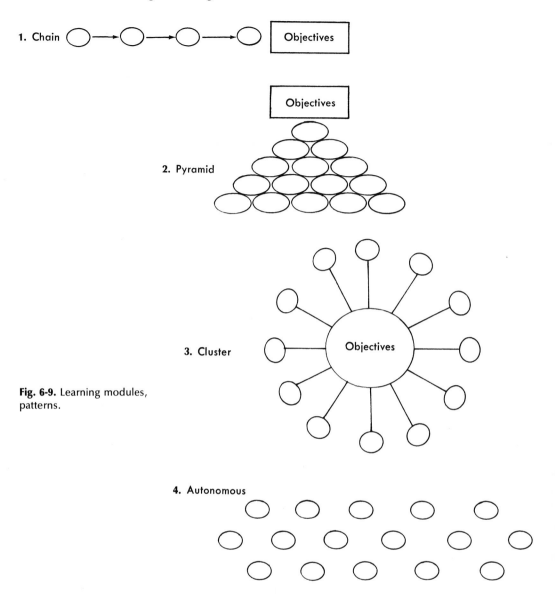

1. Chain

Objectives

Objectives

2. Pyramid

3. Cluster

Objectives

Fig. 6-9. Learning modules, patterns.

4. Autonomous

uisite knowledge for completing the module but also the knowledge that will be included in the module. Thus the pretest can achieve one or all of the following:

1. Determine if the learner has the knowledges deemed prerequisite to the content of the module
2. Determine if the learner already knows the content in the module and therefore can omit proceeding through the module

3. Focus the learner on the content of the module and guide his attention to the study areas particularly appropriate for his learning needs

Pretests need to be brief and easy to score by learner, peer, or teacher. Part or all of the posttest can be included in the pretest without jeopardizing the validity of the evaluation.

Checkpoints are formative evaluation activities that enable the learner to determine direction and rate of progress toward meeting the goals of the module. Checkpoints are interim tests within the module that can help the learner refocus, start anew, continue as is, and know how he is doing. Checkpoints are also reinforcing and motivating to learners.

The cognitive input of the learning module need follow no set pattern. The input can be an outcome of some process-oriented learning activity wherein the learner draws observations and concepts from the activity experience, or input can precede or follow some type of active learning experience. The content input needs to be an inherent, but explicit, part of the module. Explicitness is desirable because it crystallizes or surfaces concepts that are learned while engaged in the activity.

Learning activities can follow several patterns: (1) they can follow formats similar to programmed learning; (2) they can be active learning experiences that require the student to handle equipment, put puzzles together, and interact with friends, strangers, or teachers; (3) they can require the learner to perform an experiment, observe, and record; (4) they can be a paper that must be written and submitted for feedback; and (5) they can be passive learning activities such as looking at a film or a television program or listening to an audiotape.

All learning activities will be more effective if followed by a learner summary of what he has learned. This can be done by simple recall and listing, by reproducing what he did in the activity, by creating a similar activity or model, by generating another way that the concept would be used, or by taking a cognitive or performance test on the content.

Modules may be treated as independent entities within a course or grouped in clusters to form units of study. Fig. 6-9 depicts several ways in which modules can be used.

The chaining of learning modules is an effect created when one learning module is built on the presumption that the content of the previous module is prerequisite.

Each module in the chain is built on the one preceding. In such an arrangement posttests for previous modules become part of the pretest for the next module.

Modules pyramid when one wishes the learner to be able to gain depth in a subject. Modules 1 to 4 in Fig. 6-9 are considered the basic behaviors for the objectives. Some students may require or desire to know more about the subject. Learners who have a special interest in pursuing the subject may do modules 5 to 7 or complete all modules in the pyramid. Using the pyramid type of module format, modules 1 to 4 might be done in any order or they might be chained, but all four must be completed before the next tier is begun. The same pattern would then apply to the subsequent tiers.

Modules cluster when there is an objective or a group of objectives to be achieved. Many learning modules are designed to facilitate the achievement of the objective(s). The modules form clusters because each one contributes to meeting the objectives or part of the objectives. They may not all be necessary to the learning of one individual learner. Learners may select any module or group of modules in any order to achieve the objectives of the cluster.

Modules are autonomous when they stand completely alone. They can be taken smorgasbord fashion by the learner. The learner is completely free to arrange his own curriculum. Depth can be achieved through the selection of modules that add increasingly complex behaviors. The learner practices a self-selection process. Learners do retroactively integrate concepts effectively so that the smorgasbord approach can work whether or not modules are selected in set patterns.

Hardware and software

Hardware is the audiovisual equipment necessary to provide the means for using the software (programs). Hardware can be computers, projectors (overhead transparency, movie, slides, and so forth), record players, tape recorders and playback recorders, headsets, teaching machines, and a host of other types of equipment. There is a plethora of audiovisual hardware on the market, and each month new varieties and more sophisticated machines are produced. Software includes the programs for learning, either commercially prepared or homemade. They can be programmed learning books, single-concept movie films, super-8 movies with sound, slides, overhead transparencies, television programs, and so forth.

The most difficult thing about establishing a format for learning modules is that the software must match the hardware, and there is such a wide variety of formats available on the market that the expense

```
Content Subject Area_____

Name of Item_____

Published or Distributed by_____

FORMAT
—Filmstrip
—Audio cassette
—Film strip with attached cassette
—Slide with sound disc
—Slide
—Overhead transparancy
—Record, 45rpm, 33-1/3rpm
—Reel to Reel audio tape
—Television tape, 2", 1/2"
—Super 8 movie cassette
—Super 8 movie cassette with sound
—8mm movie
—16mm movie
—Autotutor
—Computer program
—Book or workbook
—Programmed handbook or pamphlet

Cost per unit_____

Description of material




Evaluation of material clarity, succinctness, accuracy,
congruence with our theoretical framework, depth, etc.



Recommendation:     Purchase           Rent
                    ____yes            ____yes

                    ____no             ____no

                    ____later          ____later

For use in which course?_____


Previewer_____Date_____
```

Fig. 6-10. Instructional materials record form.

of the equipment alone can be prohibitive. There are some general guidelines that will provide teachers who are reviewing materials and equipment with some ideas about how to make choices.

1. Review a large number of commercially prepared learning materials.
2. Keep careful notes on content (see Fig. 6-10 for sample record card).
3. Evaluate material for congruency with conceptual framework, depth and breadth, and efficiency in time, energy, and expense.
4. Keep a record of which programs are most likely to be ones that the faculty will wish to use.
5. Determine the kind of equipment available for use with software that will most probably be useful to the school of nursing.

Select hardware that fulfills the following criteria:

1. *Simple.* The more complex a machine the more difficult it is to keep in repair.
2. *Sturdy.* Many students and faculty will use the equipment and it will be moved about frequently; therefore it should not be delicate.
3. *Lightweight.* If the equipment is made available to student or faculty to check out and take home or to transport to classrooms, it should be light and compact.
4. *Inexpensive.* Expense is not always connected with quality—it is sometimes a function of sophistication. Playback machines cost a small fraction of the price of recorder-playbacks but are all that is needed for hearing tapes. Filmstrip viewers and playback recorders as a twosome cost about three fourths to one half the price of a single piece of equipment that will do both audio and filmstrip viewing.
5. *Flexible.* Some programs are created that are audio only, some that are visual (silent super-8 movies). Formats containing both slide and playback require that the whole large

piece of equipment be transported when only sound is required.
6. *Has variety.* Several alternative formats are desirable and can be put together rather inexpensively. A basically flexible laboratory that provides variety for learning has television, 16 mm movie, super-8 single-concept movie, audio cassette playback recorders, slide projectors, and filmstrip viewers. Other materials can be provided as money becomes available.

This chapter has been based on the premise that some independent learning and the use of modern instructional technology are essential in every nursing program regardless of the conceptual framework, the program objectives, the course pattern, the organizing strategy employed, or the course content organization and structure. Inherent in every curriculum and in every course in the curriculum is a consideration of the educational delivery systems to be used. It is impossible to consider educational delivery systems without investigating the use of learning modules; it is impossible to examine the use of learning modules without considering instructional technology. Once one begins to investigate instructional technology and educational delivery systems, one is already deeply in the realm of learning strategies. Thus it becomes difficult to determine when the subject of content has been left and the subject of learning strategies has been begun. It is sufficient to restate a valid educational maxim: Once you know what you wish to teach, you can proceed to discover a way to teach it.

HEURISTIC

Any curriculum coordinator can sit in splendid isolation and construct a curriculum that is theoretically sound, has a design that is congruent with the conceptual base, and is efficient and economical. However, the faculty will have no ownership of the curriculum, and in all probability it will be implemented poorly. The problem then becomes how to involve the total faculty in curriculum vivification and retain the quality desired. Curriculum builders tend to

Example

To: Faculty
From: Steering Committee

Directions for generating your "dream" curriculum:
- Pretend there are no constraints on you and you could implement any type of curriculum that you desire so long as it is consistent with our conceptual framework, philosophy, and objectives (attached).
- Work alone, with a friend, or in groups of not more than three (three is the limit so that we will get a broad view of everyone's vision).
- Present your responses in as much or little detail as you wish. Remember, the more detail that you provide the more likely the task groups will be able to visualize your ideas and use them in forming curriculum pattern alternatives. Do not write on the back of the paper. Use more paper if you need it.

(The following questions should be printed, providing enough space for detailed elaboration—perhaps one question per page.)

1. Is there a central theme, concept, process, or theory around which you would organize the courses? (It may or may not be explicit in the conceptual framework.) If so, describe it.

2. What kind of courses do you visualize in the curriculum? Name them. Draw a model or course flow chart.

3. If you designated an organizing strategy in item 1, illustrate how it influences item 2.

4. Describe the content or type of content you think might be appropriate to the courses named in 2.

5. What are some of the outcomes that you expect from each of the courses?

6. Do you have any special preference about the teaching strategies appropriate to each of the courses?

7. Are there special teacher development areas that you believe would be essential to the implementation of this curriculum?

have fantasies about some "hodgepodge" pattern of courses resulting from the participation of large numbers of faculty. Another popular misconception is that it takes more time for large numbers of people to participate. Both time factors and numbers of people participating are functions of the heuristic designed for use in this phase of development. Any heuristic device that will collect opinions about course patterns and organizing strategies, categorize and sort the data, use the data in making alternative plans, and involve the whole group in decision making will facilitate total faculty participation and get the job done efficiently and effectively. The device suggested here is just one of several that could be developed for this purpose.

Heuristic: *Generating alternative course patterns and selecting an organizing strategy*

Activity. A packet of materials containing the conceptual framework, the philosophy, and the program objectives will be distributed along with a form to be filled out by faculty individually or in groups of not more than three. These forms will be collected and given as raw data to three task groups. The task groups will use the data to generate a curriculum pattern. The three alternative patterns will be distributed to the faculty for discussion. Faculty recommendations will be used to return the three alternatives to one task group to revise as directed by faculty feedback. Faculty will then discuss, revise as necessary, and tentatively agree to implement.

Materials
1. A packet containing the conceptual framework, philosophy, and program objectives
2. A sheet of directions and a blank questionnaire
3. Three small task groups of three people each, and a set of definitive directions for their assignment
4. A set of criteria for desired curriculum

Procedure
1. Distribute the packet with the conceptual framework, philosophy, and program objectives criteria for desired curriculum, the sheet of directions, and the blank questionnaire.
2. Provide a written description of the process to all participants.
3. Ask faculty to follow the directions on the kit.
4. Collect the responses.
5. Make photoelectric copies of the responses for each task group.
6. Distribute the responses to the task groups with the directions about their task.
7. Set a 4- to 7-day time limit on the task.
8. Duplicate the task groups' plans (all) for distribution to all participants.
9. Set aside at least 3 hours for discussion.

Use basic feedback-type–discussion-session ground rules.
10. Allow 3 to 7 days to elapse.
11. Ask the faculty to reconvene and make recommendations for final pulling together of feedback.
12. Assign one task group to use the feedback of the faculty to revamp the plans, synthesize them, or whatever is necessary according to the directions from the faculty.
13. Resubmit the one plan to the faculty. Get feedback.
14. Use feedback.
15. Resubmit to the faculty. Get tentative consensus to try the plan.
16. Organize task groups for developing courses in detail.

Puissance
1. Identifies the commonalities and differences in actual course pattern preferences among the faculty.
2. Makes the commonalities very concrete and easy to identify.
3. Makes the differences in preference among the faculty explicit.
4. Gets preferences concretized and shared.
5. Allows faculty to participate to the limits of their own abilities and desires.
6. Allows each participant to have an equal "say" in developing pattern.

Contingencies
1. May draw lines of battle between power groups.
2. Could be misused as a premature "vote" about directions that course pattern will take.
3. Could cause degree of investment that would make curriculum outcome "permanent" rather than vested with the power of ongoing change.
4. May become time consuming if allowed to become "win-lose" instead of "win-win."

NOTES

1. Benjamin, Harold [Peddiwell, J. Abner]: The sabertooth curriculum, New York, 1939, McGraw-Hill Book Co.
2. Borton, Terry: What's left when school's forgotten? Saturday Review, pp. 69-80, April 18, 1970.
3. McBeath, R. J.: Is education becoming, Audio-Visual Communication Review **17:**36-40, Spring, 1969.
4. Waters, Verle: Verle's pearls—recipe for writing behavioral objectives. In Developing learning modules, Woodside, Calif., 1976, Institute of Nursing Consultants.
5. Dickoff, James, James, Patricia, and Wiedenbach, Ernestine: Theory in a practice discipline. I. Practice oriented theory, Nursing Research **17:**415-435, Sept.-Oct., 1968.
6. Bloom, Benjamin S., et al.: Taxonomy of educational objectives.

a. Handbook I. Cognitive domain, New York, 1956, David McKay Co., Inc.
b. Interaction Associates, Inc.: Tools for change, ed. 2, San Francisco, 1972, Interaction Associates, Inc., pp. 54-60.
7. Kemp, Jerrold E.: Instructional design, a plan for unit and course development, Belmont, Calif., 1971, Fearon Publishers.

BIBLIOGRAPHY

Banathy, Bela H.: Instructional systems, Belmont, Calif., 1968, Fearon Publishers.

Beauchamp, George A.: Curriculum theory, ed. 2, Wilmette, Ill., The Kagg Press.

Benjamin, Harold [Peddiwell, J. Abner]: The sabertooth curriculum, New York, 1939, McGraw-Hill Book Co.

Bloom, Benjamin S., et al.: Taxonomy of educational objectives. Handbook I. Cognitive domain, New York, 1956, David McKay Co., Inc.

Bruner, Jerome S.: The process of education, Cambridge, Mass., 1960, Harvard University Press.

Conley, Virginia C.: Curriculum and instruction in nursing, Boston, 1973, Little, Brown & Co., Inc.

DeTornyay, Rheba: Strategies for teaching nursing, New York, 1971, John Wiley & Sons, Inc.

Gronlund, Norman E.: Individualizing classroom instruction, New York, 1974, The Macmillan Co.

Gronlund, Norman E.: Stating behavioral objectives for classroom instruction, New York, 1970, The Macmillan Co.

Kemp, Jerrold E.: Instructional design, a plan for unit and course development, Belmont, Calif., 1971, Fearon Publishers.

Lenburg, Carrie B.: Open learning and career mobility in nursing, St. Louis, 1975, The C. V. Mosby Co.

Mager, Robert F.: Preparing instructional objectives, Belmont, Calif., 1962, Fearon Publishers.

Mager, Robert F., and Beach, Kenneth M., Jr.: Developing vocational instruction, Belmont, Calif., 1967, Fearon Publishers.

Mager, Robert F., and Pipe, Peter: Analyzing performance problems or "You really oughta wanna," Belmont, Calif., 1970, Fearon Publishers.

Notter, Lucille, and Robey, Marguerite, editors: Proceedings of Open Curriculum Conferences I, II, and III: a project of the NLN Study of the Open Curriculum in Nursing Education, New York, 1974, 1975, The National League for Nursing.

Parker, J. Cecil, and Rubin, Louis J.: Process as content: curriculum design and the application of knowledge, Chicago, 1966, Rand McNally & Co.

Postlethwait, S. N., Novak, J., and Murry, H.: The audio-tutorial approach to learning, Minneapolis, 1969, Burgess Publishing Co.

Russell, John D.: Modular instruction, a guide to the design, selection, utilization and evaluation of modular materials, Minneapolis, 1974, Burgess Publishing Co.

Taba, Hilda: Curriculum development, theory and practice, New York, 1962, Harcourt, Brace & World, Inc.

Tyler, Ralph W.: Basic principles of curriculum and instruction, Chicago, 1950, University of Chicago Press.

White, Dorothy T.: The scenic route: modes of student progression. In non-traditional developments in nursing education, Proceedings of the 24th and 25th Meetings of the Council on Collegiate Education for Nursing, Atlanta, 1976, Southern Regional Education Board.

7

LEARNING STRATEGIES AND MEASURING ACHIEVEMENT

Imagine yourself on an airplane thousands of feet over Denver. The communication system crackles and a voice says, "I am your head stewardess. Both the pilot and the copilot are ill and cannot fly the plane; however, I read a book on flying this kind of plane and heard a lecture on it once. I will try to get us safely landed." Or think of yourself visiting a friend in an office building. You are sitting in the back of an office on the sixteenth floor and a bomb is placed between you and the other occupants and the only exit. The bomb squad arrives and a nice-looking chap tells you, "Do not worry, I've had a lecture or two on dismantling this kind of bomb, and I know that they are very sensitive." Then, of course, there is the old cartoon that shows the patient on the operating table when the surgeon, gowned, gloved, and masked, comforts the patient with, "I understand how frightened you are; this is my first operation, too." Situations of this kind are only funny if you are *not* the victim. Practice disciplines require practice learning in noncritical, safe, simulated environments.

Nurses are usually given passive learning opportunities and placed immediately in live environments to "practice" with people. If any practice in simulated environments is provided, it is usually motor skill practice, for example, manipulation of equipment for the learning of procedures. This small segment of nursing functions receives the best efforts for simulation. The nonmotor skills of nursing need equal time

and effort so that simulated practice of desired behaviors can occur under safe conditions with peer and teacher support. This chapter primarily concerns process learning strategies and a brief discussion of measurement and grading.

In Chapter 3, learning was described as having three aspects: an *input* aspect, an *operational* aspect, and a *feedback* aspect. The development of skill in anything requires that all three aspects be completed more than once, since skill requires practice and practice is repetition using feedback for improvement. All teaching strategies that qualify as "process" teaching strategies have these three aspects. The model of a process learning episode presented in Fig. 7-1 separates the aspects of process learning into five categories. The input aspect has been divided into three categories: (1) the collection of information, (2) cognition about the information, and (3) articulation of synthesization and feedback data. The operational aspect has one category: (4) actualization (real or simulated). The output and feedback aspect has one category: (5) validation.

To have a complete process learning episode, all five categories must have been enacted. The more explicit the enactment of each category the more likely learning is to take place. A process teaching strategy is a learning episode wherein students engage in real or simulated activities that require the use of specified kinds of information, cognition about that information, validation of behavior, and articulation of

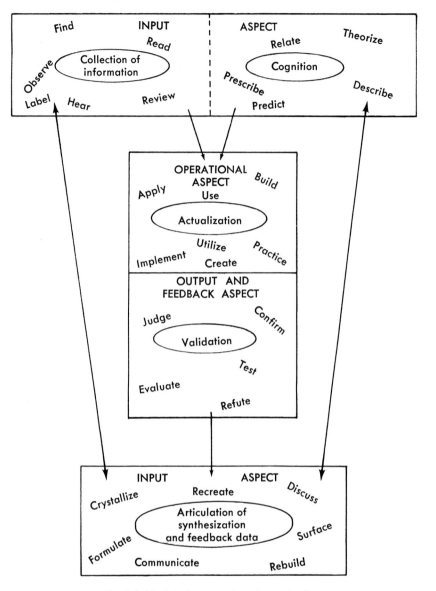

Fig. 7-1. Model of process learning episodes.

learnings. The aspects of the learning episode may come in any order, and all feed into each other. Actualization and validation are so closely aligned that it is impossible to separate the outcomes functionally. However, explicit emphasis on validation will help the feedback to become input so that the process can be improved. Most often process learning is conceived as being the experiential portion of learning only (whether that experience be real or simulated). The experiential portion (actualization) is only one aspect and *alone* probably will achieve minimal or no changes of behavior. However, almost all experiential learning has inherent feedback, and thus learning can take place.

SELECTING TEACHING STRATEGIES AND OPERATIONS

Teaching strategies and operations are those things the teacher does that facilitate learning. Technically, a strategy is an over-all plan of attack, or a conceptual plan. Operations are the actions through which strategies are implemented. For instance, brainstorming is a strategy that can be operationalized by listing, tape recording, or the making of index cards. Often a single strategy can be operationalized in several ways. Methods, on the other hand, are more complex and are the use of sever-al strategies to achieve an objective.

Strategies must be planned so that they meet the following criteria:

1. Be consistent with the conceptual framework of the school of nursing, especially the accepted learning theo-ries and the student model.
2. Provide for the level of concreteness or abstractness of the learner's think-ing processes (style).
3. Consider the learner's learning tempo (rate).
4. Be appropriate to the target behav-ior(s).

Passive and active learning

Passive learning occurs when the learner uses his senses to absorb information and makes some effort to remember that infor-mation. Teaching by way of lecture, films, tapes (television and audio), and reading are all strategies for passive learning. Pas-sive learning methods are, at present, the most frequently employed and are devised solely for the purpose of acquiring informa-tion. They are efficient neither for retention nor for the use of the information. The curriculum that relies primarily on passive learning is confronted with a dichotomy be-tween the input and operational aspect of learning. Under these conditions grading students is fraught with frustration, since students who test well on informational as-pects may or may not perform well in prac-tice. Passive learning utilizes the input phase of learning to the exclusion of any simulated situation or any learning activi-ties that require the higher levels of learn-ing such as building, devising, creating, prescribing, or utilizing. The operational

phase is minimal, and the feedback phase is restricted to examination or test of cog-nitive recall or left to the learner to "apply" without a transitional episode in a safe environment.

Active learning involves the learner through actual participation and invest-ment in all phases of the learning process. Active learning enables the learner to self-appropriate and self-experience learning. The teacher must simulate reality or par-ticipate with the student in the reality set-ting. In active learning the teacher is a resource person—providing information input when asked or needed, guiding or steering processes so that they are system-atized, and suggesting heuristic devices for widening experiences and testing pro-cesses. Active learning involves the student in operations and behaviors that require his participation in all three phases of learning, that is, input, operation, and feed-back. To be complete every active learning episode has information, cognition, actual-ization, synthesization, and validation. All phases need not occur during one time interval, but as a general rule the more closely the aspects are aligned in time and the more meaningful and related the as-pects of the episode the greater is the learn-ing. Explicitness is an important aspect of active learning. The learner needs to be aware of what he did that made the activity (trial) a success or failure, and the success must carry with it some reinforcement that will sustain or "fix" the experience so that it can be repeated when needed.

Nursing, as a practice discipline, re-quires active learning. A concert pianist never studies music theory and then offers a concert; he studies music theory and "practices," perfecting his skill until he offers his music to the public in concert. One never hears the remark, "I'm practic-ing my history lesson," but never blinks over "I'm practicing my piano lesson." Music theory is a complex science, but without the practice aspect—either in composition, analysis, or performance—it is a speculative science. History lessons can be practiced, but practice is not an essential ingredient. Nursing, like music, must be practiced because without the practice aspect it is *not* nursing. Therefore the postulate is offered that all practice-oriented disciplines must have, as essential ingredients, active learning modes for self-appropriation of the discipline.

Active learning requires teaching strategies that require learners to engage in processes (a purposive series of activities) that are deemed essential to the subject under study. Information (input) necessary to the activities is provided through any method that seems appropriate (reading, lecturing, consulting, attending seminars), but the information is always secondary to the process. The basic philosophy of process learning is that the person who is skilled in the essential processes of a discipline can identify the input which is needed and can find a source for that information. Thus information, activity, and feedback are equally used, but the activity provides the leverage through which the information and the feedback operate.

In any form of active learning the learner is *required* to participate in some way. If there are specific readings which the teacher thinks are necessary for learner preparation for a given class, commitment to active learning requires the teacher to make some assignment which necessitates that the student *do* something with the information—not just read it. Reading assignments can be used as a focal point for requiring students to formulate predictive theories from the data presented in a required bibliography. Formulating "promoting and inhibiting theories" from data collected through reading is a strategy that enables the student to *do* something with the material and takes the passivity out of learning from simple reading. Process teaching in the classroom is predicated on some prior preparation by the students so that classroom activities do not become a pooling of ignorance but rather a pooling of talent and information. Classroom preparation handled in some way which requires that the information be

used by the student promotes the greater accessibility of the information to the learners during participatory learning in class.

The case for process education in nursing

Processes teach what to do with knowledge. Processes are suggested to the nurse teacher as worthy of teaching specific content. As students learn content selected from the expanding and changing world of knowledge, they can become skilled in the basic processes for *using* data for accomplishing nursing goals. Nursing teachers have traditionally assumed that, given information about the pathophysiology of a health condition, students would "transfer" the knowledge to the clinical situation and "use" it in nursing care. Process teaching ensures this transfer by making it necessary to use the information as it is learned so that one learns the processes inherent in a planned, organized way *at the same time* that one learns the information.

Four factors mandate the use of teaching processes to nursing students: (1) it is a way of selecting only essential content from the masses of data being generated by the knowledge explosion; (2) it teaches a logical, precise, computer type of cognitive process that is easily applied to simulated nursing problems; (3) it responds to the immediate concerns of students for immediate relevance and usefulness (and thus provides motivation, interest, and reinforcement); and (4) it uses teaching personnel and classroom time in the most economical way.

Discovery learning. Discovery learning is a form of process learning. Discovery learning was described by Rogers as "self appropriated and self experienced." In its early form, Thorndyke, the famous stimulus-response associationist, called it "trial and error learning." It is more reasonably called learning by trial and accidental success. In actual practice, discovery learning is learning that places emphasis on guidance of the activity phase of learning rather than the input or information phase. For example, students are presented with a real or simulated problem, and the information to solve that problem is made available. The guidance or teaching role is one of helping the student learn to organize and process the information in a system that will promote synthesis of the information and alternative solutions to the problem rather than stereotyped answers. The teacher also provides some feedback so that information can be reprocessed. The teacher, however, is only one source of feedback. Most feedback in discovery learning is provided by the peer group and by the success or failure of the outcome of the process.

Modeling. Modeling is providing an example that can be imitated by the learner. Someone (a model) who has the behavior needed by the learner exhibits that needed behavior, and the learner copies the model's behavior as closely as possible. The model provides both the input and the mechanism for feedback so that the learner can compare his behavior to the model's behavior and make the appropriate adjustments to simulate the model's actions more closely. The model can be an illustrative movie, slides, a fellow student, a teacher, a nurse practitioner, or a diagrammatic illustration of the desired behavior. The use of modeling primarily emphasizes the activity phase of learning, and the input is so closely intertwined with the activity that separation is, for practical purposes, difficult. The use of modeling is, then, an active form of learning. Demonstration and return demonstration is a form of modeling, but the more common form is less formal and occurs constantly as people function together. Enculturation occurs because of modeling; language develops through modeling; nursing attitudes, habits, and group culture are learned through modeling. Modeling is a powerful influence on all learning—thus the cliché, "What you do speaks so loudly I cannot hear what you say." Modeling is self-experienced learning, with *observation being the major input phase mode* and *self-comparison the major feedback mode*. If the modeled behavior is reinforced by social approval, sat-

isfaction, lowered anxiety, or tangible reward, the modeled behavior tends to become habit.

Heuristics. Heuristics are employed in all forms of process learning. Heuristics are tests, tools, or devices for finding some way of achieving a goal or solving a problem. The heuristic is a mechanism to an end, not an end in itself. For instance, brainstorming is a heuristic device for generating a quantity of ideas about a given subject, without reference to the quality or practicality of those ideas. Each idea theoretically stimulates members of the brainstorming group to think of other ideas. But brainstorming is not the end, or objective— it is simply a device for thinking up alternatives. Groups involved in active learning situations need a storehouse of heuristic devices and need to learn to employ heuristics to prevent "locking" into a single-track line of thinking. Heuristics test an idea and provide alternative ideas. In other words, heuristics provide input, operational test, and feedback and play a part in all three phases of learning.

Learning style and tempo

Learning styles differ from person to person, as do learning rates. Both style and rate are related to the characteristics of the learner and to the teaching strategies employed in the learning episode. Learners grasp concepts on a wide variety of levels of abstractness to concreteness, and a curriculum devised to deliver instruction to learners who have a wide variety of learning styles employs several modalities for learning a single essential concept. Simulation—games and programmed learning that require the learner to participate through formulation of promoting and inhibiting theories, prescribing, and other high levels of creative activity—enables individual learners to participate and attain a given concept, utilizing a level of concreteness or abstraction suitable to themselves.

For example, if the conceptual framework of the school of nursing establishes a commitment to problem solving, decision making, creativity, and learning theories and propositions that include self-experiencing learning according to the learner's style and rate, then the learning activities would achieve those things through active participation of the learner. The following programmed activity about theory building illustrates this point. Theory building is a highly abstract concept. The following episode illustrates a way to concretize learning about theory building.

Games

The use of games as a learning strategy has been developing rapidly over the last half-century. Children have always learned through games and devised games that simulate real life situations. Little girls and boys devise games that model adult life roles such as "playing house" and "dressing up." Some highly sophisticated games have been devised for business and industry to teach administrative skills and decision making. Nursing has lately come to the conclusion that gaming and simulation strategies have great potential for learning nursing. "*A game is any contest played according to rules and decided by skill, strength, or apparent luck,*"[1] and is not "for real." All games have players (single persons, teams, or groups) and have a win-lose element, but they are not necessarily competitive with others.[2] For instance, solitaire and puzzle games sold in peg, block, or color combination format are games that force the player to play against the game itself. Motivation to win or "beat the system" is high in these games just as in competition against other people. With some cultural groups, where competition with other people is not sanctioned, competition against the system is acceptable and can be used as a strategy. Simulation and/or games are useful for teaching under the following conditions[3]:

1. There are specific complex skills to be learned.
2. The components of the task are complex and difficult to analyze.
3. Equipment necessary for the task is

costly or can be broken or destroyed easily.
4. The behavior to be learned is hazardous to life or potentially places people in unsafe, uncomfortable, or unhealthy situations.

Simulation and gaming will work under almost any conditions and for learning almost any skill or concept. The teacher and/or students may have to be highly creative in generating games structured for specific concepts, but that effort too can be exciting. There is an enthusiasm about learning through games that is stimulating both for teacher and learner. Only 2% to 7% of the population do not enjoy educational games. Some authors believe that this small percentage who do not like learning in this mode dislike the competitive element that characterizes games.[3] The competitive element does have some specific advantages, and unless the learning population has the definite characteristic of noncompetitiveness, games should not be eliminated as a strategy for this reason. Team or group games teach cooperation as part of the competitive format; for example, members of one team must plan, implement, and carry through cooperatively to win against the other team. Learning through gaming removes learning from the totally cognitive domain and turns it into a participatory skill requiring interaction so that one valuable side effect is that much is learned about human relationships.[3] Teachers often think that gaming takes control from their hands and believe that games as a teaching strategy are too unstructured. In reality, games are a highly structured way to learn because some learner action must result in a "payoff" or real reward. Both the action and the reward are prestructured into the game by the teacher; thus the structure of content is in the hands of the teacher.[4] Furthermore, the experience of the game itself is insufficient. Cognition, reflection, interpretation, discussion, and so on are necessary to crystallize the process experience of the game and "fix" the concepts and

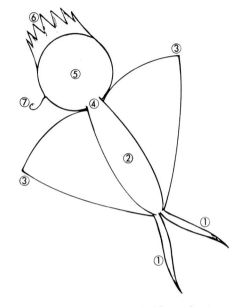

EXAMPLE OF CONCRETIZED, INDIVIDUALIZED ACTIVE LEARNING

Objective: At the end of this activity the learner will be able to create an imaginary theory and develop it through each of the four levels of theory designated by Dickoff, James, and Wiedenbach.

Directions to the learner: You will be shown a picture and asked to make up or imagine specific things about the picture. Relax and let your imagination run wild.

Directions:
Look at this picture (perceive it).
Make up a name for what you see (name it).

Number each part on the picture.
Name the parts of the item (isolate the factors).

Responses (as would be provided by student):
Fork-tongued batwinged Whourk
1. Fork tongued
2. Body
3. Batwinged appendages of body
4. Sluice gate
5. Food reservoir, also handle
6. Rake prongs
7. Hanging baffle hook

You have just completed Level 1 of theory building: *Factor-isolating theories.*

Directions:
Describe the item named in the first part and discuss briefly how each part relates to the whole.

Responses (as would be provided by student):
The fork-tongued, batwinged Whourk is an animal that is stiff like iron but is flexible. He has a forked tongue on one end and a rakelike appendage on the other. His body is shaped like a delta-winged airplane. Food flows through his mouth, into his body, and through the sluice gate creating energy at the rake prongs. The hanging baffle hook is affixed to the anterior caudal portion of the food reservoir and is left over from another nightmare.

You have just completed Level 2 of theory building: *Factor-relating theories.*

Directions:
Formulate two hypotheses about how the item works or what it does and under what circumstances it will so perform. In other words, predict how it works or performs.

State in cause-and-effect terms what would promote or inhibit the occurrence of your first prediction.

State in cause-and-effect terms what would promote or inhibit the occurrence of your second prediction.

Responses (as would be provided by student):
Under conditions of extreme cold, 8° F or below, the Whourk will break into small bits and pieces.

When grasped firmly around the food reservoir, just below the sluice gate, the Whourk will become stiff like iron.

Lowering the temperature to 8° F or below results in shattering the fork-tongued, batwinged Whourk.

Firmly grasping the Whourk by the food reservoir below the sluice gate produces ironlike stiffening of the Whourk.

You have just completed Level 3 of theory building: *Situation-relating theories: (a) predictive theories; (b) promoting or inhibiting theories.*
Continued.

EXAMPLE OF CONCRETIZED, INDIVIDUALIZED
ACTIVE LEARNING—cont'd

Directions:
Create a plan by which you could test one of the hypotheses above; put the plan in a sequential, step-by-step set of directions.

Responses (as would be provided by student):
1. Catch the Whourk sitting unaware daydreaming.
2. Put salt on his tail.
3. While he is under the "salt" spell, grasp him firmly around the food reservoir behind the sluice gate.
4. Take equal weight of iron forged in shape of Whourk.
5. Get stress reading from certified structural engineer.
6. Test Whourk for structural stress rating under same conditions or ask certified structural engineers to do so.
7. Do not remove grasp from Whourk while testing stress.
8. Compare findings.
9. If garden is weedy, use Whourk for hand weeder–rake combined while waiting for computer to compute findings.
10. Release Whourk (the species is protected by the SPCA).

You have just completed Level 4 of theory building: *Situation-producing theories: (a) prescriptive theories; (b) creative theories.*

The activity you have just completed is called working forward. You took an unknown and worked it into a fully matured theory.

Directions:
Now take a theory and work *backwards* by imagining it being taken by Pascal through each level: "Fluids and gases in a combined space exert pressure equally and undiminished in all directions."

Level 4:

Level 3:

Level 2:

Level 1:

Directions:
Take the following nursing action hypothesis and do the same thing, or formulate your own nursing action hypothesis for development. You may work in groups of up to four for this exercise. Turn your paper in within a week.

Suggested nursing action hypothesis: "Definitive structured plans when written or communicated to the client in concrete terms lower client anxiety when he is faced with unfamiliar diagnostic procedures and tests."

behaviors learned.[5] The efficiency of games as a learning strategy is evident in the retentive factor. Since gaming requires players to use themselves and their own tools for problem solving,[6] and the payoff or winning depends on the players' quickness and sophistication in abstracting, organizing, and using information from a variety of sources, gaming becomes experiential learning and retention is raised because retention is tied to reality.[7]

Games are particularly appropriate for the undermotivated learner, since while teaching skills and other content[5] they do so through providing goal orientation. Students must then seek the information necessary to achieve the goal and win the game. Thus games basically teach people to learn.[8] There are two fringe benefits of gaming: (1) tolerance for oneself and others and (2) a feeling of control and competence. Through participating in games as principal players or team members, learners must truly utilize selected principles. In gaming, students tend to grow much more tolerant and patient about how real-life situations are handled.[9] Through the experience of self-participation the learner believes that the practice has increased competence and feels better prepared to use the concepts in nursing situations out of the classroom.

Example games. A game called "Squirms," copyrighted and sold by the American Drama Association, provides a model for games for simulated active problem solving. The game has several problem situations from which players choose. An egg timer is then set and players have 3 minutes to interact and win the game. Nurses have added other rules, written more "squirm" situations, developed the predictive theories on which each situation solution is based, and scored players on the number of predictive theories that players employ in their nursing intervention strategies.

The following are two games currently being used in nursing classes. These two examples will only expose two types of games. The wide variety of types of games and subject matter for games makes it impossible to present a wide selection of example games here. Copyrighted and commercially prepared games provide good game models for the faculty who wish to embark on gaming as a teaching strategy. Enthusiasm for gaming will grow, and faculty will begin to build their own games for teaching particular content.

EXAMPLE GAME 1: HERE COMES THE JUDGE

Purpose: To facilitate participation in a group endeavor to solve simulated nursing problems.

Description: A game called "Here Comes the Judge" employs the team concept and intergroup cooperation to beat the other team. Each group solves a specific given problem about a topic selected by the teacher. The groups go through all phases of the problem-solving process; they carefully document each alternative that might be an acceptable intervention, select an intervention, and justify the intervention selection with sound documentation. One team presents the problem as they solved it going through each stage. The challengers must catch them out—find and prove the flaws. In cases of impasse a group of judges makes decisions about who wins the point.

Points accumulate, and the winning group is rewarded.

Objectives: This game is contrived so that to reach the established goal the participant will:
1. Gather, organize, document, and assimilate information collected by the participants.
2. Critically choose the information and predictive principles appropriate to specific problems.
3. Utilize data in the appropriate facets of problem solving.
4. Participate in a mutually accountable way in a group problem-solving endeavor.
5. Use other members of the group for information, validation, feedback, negotiation, and judgment.
6. Encourage communications, peer support, evaluation, and critiquing of the authoritative resources cited and question validity of resources by citing authoritative opposing views.
7. Utilize the problem-solving strengths of all members of the group by varying player roles and group composition.

Rules: The class is divided into three basic groups:
1. The group presenting (usually 3 to 5 students).
2. The group who have the first right of challenge (usually 3 to 5 students).
3. The group of judges who arbitrate challenges and rebuttals and award the decision to the group who best substantiate their statements. The awards are made in points, and the judges keep score. If the groups wish to award prizes, they may determine what these are to be—losers buy Cokes, and so forth.
4. If the class is larger than 15 to 18 students, the students not immediately involved in one of the three groups have the privilege of challenging any decision after it has been made and before the next phase of problem solving continues; however, their challenge must be substantiated as above. If in the opinion of the judges this group makes their challenge, they collect the point.

Procedure of play: The game may be used for the solving of a whole problem or for any selected part of problem solving, that is, problem identification phase, problem data phase, or decision phase. The game can be spread over several class periods or contained in one period. Several class periods permit additional research by enthusiastic players. Books and so forth are permitted in class.

1. Statements on transparencies or on butcher paper may be prepared ahead of time or as part of the class.
2. A member of the presenting group is chosen by that group to act as moderator for the group. However, it is the responsibility of all the presenting members to coach and strengthen the group's presentation, that is, to assume responsibility for making as valid and strong a case as possible for their portion of solving a problem.
3. The presenting group presents the whole problem briefly. This gives the players an overview and prevents challenging material that is covered later. During this overall presentation, challenge groups can take notes on incorrect, omitted, or extraneous material for use during the challenge part of the game.
4. Points are awarded by the judges as follows:
   a. The presenting group gets 1 point for correct and accepted presented material.
   b. The group citing data or material omitted by the presenting group collects 1 point for each concept area accepted by the judges as essential omitted material.
   c. Challenged material is arbitrated by the judges, and the group who are adjudged as correct win 1 point. If the presenting group are deemed correct, they are awarded 1 point for being incorrectly challenged; if the challenge group are deemed correct, they are awarded 1 point for being proper in their challenge.
   d. Material that is included by the presenting group that is challenged for being extraneous, inappropriate, tangential, or unnecessary to the solution of the problem can be awarded a point for the winning group in the same way.

EXAMPLE GAME 2: CLOTHESPIN GAME TO LEARN ABOUT LEARNING

Objectives: At the end of this activity you will be able to:

1. State the difference in discovery learning and modeling.
2. Compare the differences in time needed to learn a task among (a) those using exploration and discovery learning techniques, (b) those using modeling techniques, and (c) those who have the benefit of practice.
3. Identify the role of reinforcement in learning and name some of the forms that reinforcement takes.
4. List learning propositions that can be derived from this activity.

Directions:

1. Divide into groups of three players.
2. Designate one person as discovery learner, one person as modeling learner, and one person as timer-recorder.
3. Take six wooden pieces and three metal pieces from the clothespin box.
4. Give two wooden pieces and one metal piece to both the discovery learner and the modeling learner.
5. The discovery learner must put the clothespin together without prompting or guidance from the other members of the group.
6. The timer times, in seconds, how long it takes the discovery learner to complete the task.
7. The timer and the modeling learner smile, nod, encourage, clap, cheer, or do anything else they think will encourage and reinforce the discovery learner while he is doing his task as long as they think he is moving in the direction that will lead to success. They may not offer him any advice or directions.
8. The timer marks down the time used by the discovery learner in completing his task.
9. The modeling learner places the clothespin that is now back together in front of him. Using it as a model and having observed the discovery learner complete the task, the modeling learner proceeds to put the second clothespin together.
10. The timer again times the operation and records the time in seconds. The difference in the two times is calculated.
11. The discovery learner and the timer use the same reinforcing tactics listed in item 7 to encourage and reinforce the modeling learner.

12. The discovery learner takes the remaining two pieces of wood and one wire and puts the clothespin together. He can look at the clothespins that are put together, if he chooses. Reinforcing behaviors are again used by the other group members.
13. The timer again times the discovery learner and records the time as "practice number 2."
14. Someone collects the times, averages them, and puts the findings on the blackboard.
15. Each group uses assigned texts, class notes, any other available resources and experiences, feelings and observations made during the activity to list learning the propositions they saw enacted or experienced while participating.
16. The class may or may not wish to award a prize to the group identifying the most nearly complete and accurate list of learning propositions that they saw in actual operation during the activity.

Hints for teachers using experientially based learning

All process teaching requires particular behaviors from the teacher whether or not the process activity is simulation, games, discovery, modeling, or guided activities. The following paragraphs provide a list of hints or necessary activities for teachers to promote success in the use of process teaching strategies.

Definition of process teaching. Boiled down to one idea, one sentence—process is the continuing detection, selection, and use of feedback for change. Thus process teaching is the detection, selection, and use of feedback to facilitate changes in behaviors. Since the definition states "use of feedback," process teaching requires an *activity* mode for changing behaviors. For process learning to be deliberate learning and not learning by trial and accidental success, the experiential base for the process learning must be a prestructured, preplanned episode with reinforcements. Cognitive recognition of the input as an integral part of the teaching operation is a further adjunct to process learning and tends to strengthen retention and the ability to

generalize the learned behaviors. However, it is not an essential component of process learning. In other words, the use of feedback need not be on a rote level. Most nursing teachers are committed to cognition as a desirable aspect of learning even motor skills, and thus they include some activity that will surface or make explicit the content of the learning.

Teacher preparation. Teachers can prepare for their class in the following ways:
1. Formulate the student objectives (desired behavioral outcomes); make explicit the processes and information expected to be learned and the behaviors that will be outcomes.
2. Design (a) the teaching strategies, (b) possible teaching tactics, and (c) the evaluation tool.
3. Make preparatory assignment to students.
4. Require evidence of completion of assignment (optional).
5. Write a description of the learning activity for the class (if problem solving, write the problem situation).
6. Do the activity prior to requiring it of students.
7. Have a list of principles that pertain to the subject and are available for reference to ensure that appropriate content is used in the process as well as provide for comments on student activities.

Teacher's functions in experientially based learning episodes. The teacher's role is threefold. The first function is to devise the simulated experience or the game and provide the structure necessary to the successful playing of the game or the enactment of the simulated experience. The second function is to surface the learning so that it can be better retained. The third function is to provide for evaluation.

Devising the game or simulated experience and providing structure. The elements necessary to an effective and efficient game or simulated experience are the same elements necessary to any successful learning unit. The first activity is always a concept analysis followed by determining what kind of strategies and operations are most likely to be effective in teaching each subconcept.

Paradoxically, it is structure that enables freedom and independence. For instance, if the game or simulation experience is to be student devised, the structure needs to be inherent in the objectives, which are clear and specific, in the directions, in the limits and constraints, and in the expected product.

Providing no structure whatsoever is a teacher cop-out that reduces learning. Providing too much structure is overcontrol and places constraints on exploration and discovery, chokes independence, and reduces learning. The balance is as important as it is difficult to achieve.

Every experientially based learning activity must provide the amount of structure that enables students to have freedom to be independent. Whether explicit or implicit every experientially based learning activity must have these components:

1. Objectives.
2. Pretest (may be simple assessment of readiness or knowledge of the learner's previous behaviors, etc.).
3. Directions. These are explicit descriptions of the operations necessary to attain the goals. These may even be the options open to the learner.
4. Criteria of success (for example, recognizable behaviors). These can be, but do not have to be, in the form of posttest.
5. Grading mechanisms.

Elements of structuring educational games. Educational games have some additional elements. Below are elucidated the components of educational games that will provide guidelines for teachers who are building games:

1. State the object of the game or simulation. This is different from learning objectives. For instance, the object of chess (which was an ancient war game) is to win by capturing the king or placing him in check.
2. Give the educational purpose (if it is not a secret).
3. Give the directions for play. This includes such materials as how to get the game started, the materials needed, how the players are divided, and what the players do.
4. Give the rules for play. This is the legal aspect and concerns what is legitimate to do or not to do in the game.
5. Make explicit the winning payoff. In other words, the players must know how to recognize a win. It is a statement of the object of play and, if covered sufficiently there, need not be repeated. However, if prizes are awarded, this should be explicit. Prizes are not a recommended form of reinforcement, which should come in either the win itself or in the realization of the learning that has taken place. However, one does need to look at group values to determine an appealing winning payoff.

Surfacing the learning. This is one of the most important aspects of simulation, gaming, and other experientially based learning activities and is often neglected, thus almost negating the educational value of play. Surfacing the learning is an activity that can take place during or at the conclusion of play. The beauty of simulation and gaming is that one can freeze the action and stop for conceptualization. Learnings must be externalized or made explicit. This need not be done by the teacher, but must be provided for as an expected and regular part of the learning episode. It can be carried out through discussion, written assignment, and so forth. If the learning episode is an independent learning activity, crystallization of learned concepts or behaviors should be structured into the directions. Following are some hints for teacher activities to facilitate cognition of the learning experience:

1. Strategic decisions and their operations
   a. Find out if there are strategic mo-

ments. If so, when? What strategic decisions were made?

b. How were these decisions carried out (operations)?

c. What influenced the choices (time, constraints, panic, etc.)?

d. How were choices made? What problem-solving heuristics were used (trial and error, imagining the consequences, starting with desired results and working backwards, etc.)?[10]

2. Elicit all data that might contribute to concept generation. Eliciting comments from students can be aided by such statements as: "Describe what you were feeling when you discovered you were boxed in." "Help me to understand the sequence of events . . ." "Give me a clear picture of . . ." *Do not say,* "OK, what did you learn?"

3. Give feedback yourself and elicit from others in group. For example, "Joan, what did you think when you saw your partner do that?" "Bill, I wondered when I saw you do that, if you were aware of how beautifully you were using the principles of crisis intervention. You used every one of them that were appropriate to the crisis Mary was portraying."

4. Reenact play, if helpful. For example, one might say, "Let's freeze the play a moment and talk here." Then after play is over the discussion leader can say, "Now let's back up and reenact that sequence to see what effect the changes we made had" or "Let's go back now to such and such a point in play and try that again in the light of our present knowledge." It is a very important learning step to use learned behaviors quickly in a successful episode.

5. Summarize yourself, or elicit summary from the group. This is good closure and marks some perimeters for the group and gives a sense of completion on one plane that makes it easier to move on and to use what has been learned.

Features to be wary of while process teaching

1. Sidetracking or tangential activities
2. Being led into a student anxiety system
3. Spending huge amounts of time trying to untangle one or two students' thinking
4. Locking into *one* solution to a problem
5. Feeling as if you have to know everything or have all the answers
6. Solving the problem and/or helping win the game for the students
7. *Not* letting go of the group

Faculty development

All people learn through modeling behaviors of contacts within the role; thus the teaching role model of information-giver by way of lecture has been and is the primary strategy for teaching nursing. Most of the multimedia for teaching nursing have developed around the "information-giving" format. Filmstrips, tape cassettes, television, and movies are all information-transmitting devices when used without specially planned and constructed process-learning activities. Devising ways to help students in using information to build, construct, formulate, and utilize interventions takes teaching skills seldom taught in graduate schools or modeled in classrooms. Any faculty who are building a curriculum that evolves from a conceptual framework that has a commitment to active involvement of the learner in the learning process will need to work closely and determinedly on developing the teaching skills necessary to implement this commitment. Most faculty do not need lectures on process teaching, readings on process teaching, or any other cognitive input on process teaching strategies; there is generally an intellectual acceptance of process teaching as an efficient and effective learning mode. What is needed are actual experiences in simulation, games, and pro-

cess-learning activities and some structured sessions in generating process-learning activities. The experience of playing
several games and actually participating in
learning to use games and the experience
of selecting a concept, performing a concept analysis, and devising a game or an activity appropriate to that concept constitute
self-actualized, self-appropriated, self-rein-
forced learning for teachers. Teachers become frustrated and discouraged about
process teaching because they have more
desire to process teach than ability to do
so or guidance in doing so. Faculty development efforts in the direction of self-experience for teachers and active support
by consultants, colleagues, administration,
and students are necessary for faculty
growth in the ability to implement active
learning episodes for students.

There are within every faculty many resources available from the group itself.
There are a few basic procedures which
one can use to assess the faculty's own
strengths and to mobilize those strengths
so that faculty can train each other and
obtain outside help in areas where it is
necessary. Nursing faculty tend to be reluctant to accept each other as consultants,
teachers, and authorities. Validation by
outside authorities may be necessary to
increase the acceptance of group members
as able authorities, but the group needs to
establish habit patterns of utilizing the
resources within the group. The following
is a simple list of steps that will help in
planning and implementing faculty development activities to enable the faculty to
learn teacher behaviors that will facilitate
implementation of new teaching strategies:

1. Inventory skills of faculty.
2. Survey needed skills for new courses.
3. Match skills needed by all with those
   already possessed by some faculty
   members.
4. Bring in consultants for skills needed
   but not available within the faculty.
5. Form faculty support groups for sharing and helping each other while implementation proceeds.

NORMATIVE AND CRITERION REFERENCED EVALUATION FOR GRADING PURPOSES

Evaluation of student progress is done
for four basic purposes[11]:

1. To determine student attainment of
   the behaviors established as objectives.
2. To assess the success of the instructional delivery system and all its components.
3. To predict professional success, for
   example, with state boards and in
   the work world.
4. To determine grades. Grading is done
   to provide the learner and others with
   insights into his achievement either
   in relation to the course goals or in
   comparison with peers.

There are two basic kinds of evaluation
methods used to fulfill the purposes of evaluation just listed. They are designed to accomplish different purposes and are derived from two different philosophical van-
tage points. They are (1) criteria performance (or referenced) tests and (2) norm
performance (or referenced) tests.

Criteria performance methods of evaluation are those activities enacted by the
teacher, learner, peer, or group which enable the learner's behaviors to be compared
with the behavioral objectives that are the
educational target behaviors. Each student
then is measured in relation to his ability to
perform in the desired manner.[12]

Norm performance tests compare one
student with an established norm group or
groups. Norm referenced tests are activities
usually performed by the teacher that enable the teacher to rank and order one
learner's progress in relation to the other
learners in the class. The classical graphic
outcome is the bell-shaped curve; however,
all statistical manipulations of data that
use means, standard deviations, and other
intergroup or intragroup comparison methods are ways of comparing students with
each other or with groups.[13]

There are specific situations where each
frame of reference is more appropriate than

the other. The choice of which frame of reference to use entirely depends on the outcome desired. If the teacher is trying to determine whether or not the behaviors deemed necessary to the intent of the course have been achieved, the choice will be criteria performance methods. If, on the other hand, the teacher desires a point of reference for determining how a student is performing in relation to other students (either in the same class, in other sections of the class, or in other nursing programs), norm performance methods are indicated.

Criterion referenced evaluation is particularly well suited to a process curriculum or a curriculum where individualized instruction and active involvement of the learner in the learning process are stressed. Skinner[14] used criteria referencing when he devised programmed instruction. In any programmed instruction, when the learner has completed a portion of the program, he is asked a simple question designed to determine whether or not he learned the content of the program. If he answers correctly, he may proceed to the next section; if not, he must repeat the section until he successfully responds to the questions. The programmed instruction model utilizes the concept of mastery.

All programmed instruction uses criterion referenced testing because the only measurement relevant to the instruction is whether or not learners have mastered the content of the program. The concept of mastery learning has been around since the 1920s, when Washburne[15] developed the Winnetka Plan. With the work of Skinner,[14] Carroll,[16] and Bloom,[17] learning for mastery is becoming more acceptable. Probably one of the most difficult problems with which faculty must deal in using mastery learning and criterion referenced grading is that it is possible that every learner may achieve at an "A" or a "B" level. Opponents of this system of grading see this as an indictment of the system, and state that it is nondiscriminating. If discrimination among levels of learners is an objective (for example, to determine speed, cognitive

style, and "fitness for graduate school"), criteria must be established for measuring mastery of increasing levels of sophisticated or complex behaviors. Establishing levels of mastery can be quantitative or qualitative. Quantitative levels reflect the *amount of work* that must be done to master a specific level; qualitative levels reflect the *type of work* that must be done to attain specific levels of mastery. The mastery level need not be purely quantitative or qualitative, but most often it is a combination. If levels of mastery are designed, the learner should be able to choose or contract for the set of criteria he will master.

Contract grading is grading according to student attainment of a specified set of criteria that are deemed to be of "A," "B," or "C" level. A contract is then established between the learner and the teacher. This contract is a working agreement that can be negotiated and renegotiated as the learner becomes more realistic about his priorities, needs, motivation, and interest. Usually contracts may be renegotiated up as well as down the alphabet. Only the learner knows the amount of time, energy, and effort he wishes to commit to particular sets of learning objectives. Choice, being the most fundamental of freedoms, cannot be exercised by a teacher in behalf of a student—each learner must exercise his own choice based on his assessment of his own ability and motivation to attain.

Criteria performance techniques have the advantage of precise achievement in direct relation to the target behaviors. The student has a sense of his own merit in relation to specific, known expectations. Such techniques provide for implementation of learning for mastery of objectives. It is consistent with the concept that students may repeat a given learning activity or substitute other learning activities that will enable each student to find a learning style and tempo that promote his attainment of specific target behaviors. Criteria can be established for each level of achievement, for example, criteria for "A" performance, criteria for "B" performance, and so on, or numerical values may be placed on levels of criteria attainment. On the other hand, a system can be devised so that it *only* discriminates between mastery of specified objectives and nonmastery of those objectives. Individual learning goal attainments can be averaged as in any other evaluation system just as long as the items are considered to be of equal importance or weight. If not, some mathematical calculations will need to be done to provide for weighting. However, averaging all students' grades together violates the individuality of grading and immediately makes grading norm referenced. Criterion referenced evaluations decrease student competition with each other and facilitate cooperative learning and mutual support groups.[18] Students under this system can assume some responsibility for helping each other because the achievement of another does not influence his grade.

Norm referenced evaluation, on the other hand, enables the learners' achievement to be compared with (1) other students in the course, (2) other sections of the course, (3) populations from other schools, (4) standardized norm groups, (5) national norms, and (6) populations from other professions or occupations. National League for Nursing Achievement Tests are norm tests that allow the student to be compared with a national population. Most psychological tests have been standardized and are norm referenced tests. All teacher-made tests that put students from several sections or one section into a pool in which achievement is measured by deviations from a mean are norm tests and are especially suited for comparing one student's achievement with that of other students regardless of the number of sections in that specific course.

Grading and report systems are imposed programs of conformity, and to impose the system of assigning marks to process involvement is to court failure, since process is associated with human activities and by its nature is subject to the utilization of feedback and growth. Grading imposes a finality, and failure is death to the process. The two things are basically contradictory and impossible to reconcile.[19]

Most current grading systems are predicated on normative grading using a variation of the classic bell-shaped curve. The very use of this device communicates to learners two facts[20]:

1. I am in competition with my classmates for a place in relation to the class mean and therefore I do not help others learn because someone else might, through my help, make a better score in relation to that mean than I do.
2. Only about one third of us are going to get "A"s and "B"s, the rest of us are worth only "C"s or less.

In this way competition and a sense of poor performance is reinforced. Skinner, Carroll, and Bloom make a good case for reinforcing success by making it possible for students to *master* a criterion or set of criteria. All programmed learning is based on their work, and nursing content and experientially based learning is a natural vehicle for implementing this philosophy.

Most nursing problems propose, as part of their conceptual framework and part of their objectives, the concept of nursing response to social needs. Social responsibility must be a part of every nursing curriculum, and in its most universal definition love is social responsibility. Loving is helping one another, being responsible for one another, caring for and about one another. Grading systems that foster separateness, competition, and exclusion of others defeat the whole concept of accountability (love) to and for the group because one is in competition with the group.[21]

Contracts for sets of criteria and the subsequent grade that accompanies the fulfilling or voiding of that contract is the surest path to teaching responsibility for one's own acts—accountability to self and consequences to self. Teachers who really care more about students than about their own sense of guilt over "failing to teach the student and enabling him to meet the contract" will be able to offer students help prior to contract commitment dates so that students who wish to fulfill contracts can do so. The extra time consumed by the instructor working with the few students who will ask for and make arrangements for help is small compared with the time spent trying to untangle a problem after it has occurred. Since any behavior can be altered by the consequences of that behavior, no teacher has the right to interfere with the consequences of unfulfilled contracts when the consequences have been specifically laid out and expressly defined.[22] Effort should go, rather, to averting the behaviors that will result in failure to meet a contract or in altering the contract.

There is no doubt reflected in the writings of modern educators that grading itself, and especially the "F" grade, serves no beneficial purpose and is probably a leading cause of a sense of failure in life.[23] In fact, Glasser's[24] eloquent indictment of grading as a method of obtaining feedback about students is so convincing that making elementary changes in institutional grading policies should be an issue in curriculum change.

Almost any method of evaluating learning can be used for establishing grades. The evaluation *methods* are not the determinant for normative or criterion referenced testing. The factor that determines whether evaluation is normative or criterion referenced is what is done with the data that are derived from the evaluation, for example, whether or not the data are used to determine if the student has attained the target behaviors or are used to determine the student's standing in the class or in comparison with other groups.

One of the most difficult decisions for a faculty to reach is the selection of a grading system compatible with the conceptual framework of the school. Many faculties compromise and use both criterion referenced evaluation for grades and norm referenced evaluation for grades within the same course as well as within the same

curriculum. The obvious difficulty in this compromise is that the two systems are devised for entirely different purposes and, when used for grading, arise from entirely different philosophical points of view. From this standpoint, then, it would seem that to combine the two systems within one course would be placing the learners of the course in a bind. The normative system communicates on one hand that the learner is being compared with his peer group, and the criteria system says that he is being compared with the objectives. The conflict between the two systems makes it clear that they are not compatible when used within the same course. Averaging normative referenced grades with criterion referenced grades mixes the messages about whether or not it is important for the learner to master the objectives or whether it is important for him to perform the behaviors specified in the objectives better than anyone else in his peer group.

Purposes 1 (to determine student attainment of the behaviors established as objectives) and 2 (to assess the success of the instructional delivery system and all of its components), as expressed on p. 192, can best be determined by criterion referenced tests.

The desirability for some norm referenced evaluation in a curriculum arises because nursing achievement tests and state board licensure examinations are normative evaluative measures. All schools are committed to acceptable achievement as rated by the National League for Nursing tests and to their graduates' eligibility to practice as attained by passing the state board examination. Some practice in objective tests that are normative graded may be desirable for this reason. The achievement test and state board examinations are used by schools of nursing for purpose 3 (to predict professional success, for example, with state boards and in the work world). Achievement tests are used by most schools to determine how well students in their program compare with other programs in the United States. State boards, using normative referenced tests in nursing, compare all students taking the examination in a state at one time.

Determining test item validity and relevance or establishing a difficulty index for test items are functions of statistical manipulations that require norming. Some tests of internal relevance and validity are necessary if the teacher asks objective examination questions partially to determine whether or not students can perform the tasks stated in the behavioral objectives. However, it is not necessary to use the findings of these statistical manipulations for grading—they can be used for the teacher's evaluation of the test itself or for comparing curricula.[25]

• • •

In summary, learning for the practice discipline of nursing encompasses not only the information of nursing subject matter but also encompasses the "living learning" process. This living learning, whether in practicum or classroom setting, is in the context of nursing. In this context each classroom is a bomb, every teacher a fuse. If the two are ever united, and by intent or accident either party strikes the spark of excitement that lies inherent in the situation, repercussions of the explosions will be heard far and wide. Torrance[26] defines creativity as the ability to formulate and test ideas and hypotheses. He also maintains that creativity can be taught.[27] The development of the ability to generate ideas, to be able to test those ideas, for example, to work through all four levels of theory building, is too often left to chance in nursing classrooms. Schrank's book, *Teaching Human Beings: 101 Subversive Activities for the Classroom,*[28] and Postman and Weingartner's book, *Teaching as a Subversive Activity,*[29] offer some alternatives to passive learning that are predicated on the feasible plan of involving learners in the excitement of learning to learn. Learning to learn is the basic process. Although risk seems high, most of the risk envisioned never materializes—learners have eager, quick minds that rapidly

surpass those of their mentors and tutors. Therein lies the hope for nursing—that today's classrooms spawn an unafraid, creative, lifetime learner who is keyed to evaluating his own behavior and performance according to his goals.

HEURISTIC

There is in every group considerable talent and strength. In many faculties, because the nature of the curriculum has directed the teaching skills of each faculty member toward certain confining pathways, members have not too clear an idea of the abilities and strengths, the interests and the inclinations of each other. Perhaps only one or two people on the faculty know that Jo Ellen's mother has suffered a stroke and a long illness, and thus Jo Ellen, usually a pediatric teacher, knows a good deal about stroke and everything there is to know about the community resources available to stroke patients in the immediate vicinity of the university. Teachers often do not know what kind of teaching strategies are used by colleagues in the classroom or in clinical conference or what kind of clinical activities are used for facilitating the learning of specific concepts. Too often faculty hesitate to come forward and say that they have a successful strategy for teaching nutrition or a magnificently interesting game for teaching interviewing. Some faculty members are excellent lecturers, some are skilled process teachers, some are good at leading seminar classes, some can program instruction well, and others are knowledgeable about commercially prepared audiovisual materials. One of the most crucial problems facing a faculty group who are beginning to plan and implement a new curriculum is to discover and tap the strengths of its membership and learn to accept each other as experts.

This heuristic is designed to help identify faculty strengths and interests and provide the information around which in-service education days can be planned using the faculty members themselves as consultants. It also will provide information about the faculty's areas of interest and indicate directions that faculty development might take. This survey will need to be done each year because faculty grow and change in skills and interest.

Heuristic: *Faculty strengths and interest survey*

Activity. A questionnaire is formulated that assesses faculty talent, strengths, and interest. The re-

Example. Faculty strengths and needs assessment form

To: Faculty
From: Task group on faculty sharing

This survey is devised to assess the strengths, talents, areas of interest, and expertise we have among us. We will approach our assessment from two angles: (1) those strengths you see in yourself; and (2) those strengths others see in you. For our report to the faculty, we will combine the two reports into one profile. Please give us the benefit of honest self-appraisals and respond to our need by letting us know what you have to share with us. The last part of the questionnaire asks what you would like in the way of acquiring new teaching behaviors or knowledges. We will attempt the following tasks with the responses you give us:

1. Provide you with a list of colleagues' strengths derived from both others' and your own perceptions.
2. Provide a list of faculty-felt needs.
3. Suggest plans for faculty sharing days.
4. Suggest plans for peer support or "colleagueship."

Questions:
1. What are your areas of nursing knowledge and expertise?

2. What special interest areas have you developed that may or may not have anything to do with your job or clinical preparation?

3. What is the teaching mode(s) in which you feel most skillful?
_____lecture   _____gamester
_____seminar   _____programmed learning
_____discussion leader   _____other (specify)
_____process facilitator

4. Can you do any of the following activities?
Write learning programs?
Make learning modules?
Think up games?
Draw or paint?
Write narrative material?
Consult learning activities?

5. In a group which role(s) do you fulfill best?
_____facilitator   _____work well on ideas that the group
_____support person, peacemaker   accepts
_____perseverer   _____detail person
_____idea person   _____organizer
                                                 _____other (specify)

Continued.

Example. Faculty strengths and needs assessment form—cont'd

---

6. Do you use any process teaching strategies in your class? If so, please describe briefly.

7. What is the thing, area, concept, specialty, and so forth that you know *most* about professionally?

8. What are the things that you want most to learn about or to do?

Peer survey:

Each faculty member's name is included in the list below, and a space has been provided for your response. Please list, under each name, those talents, areas of expert knowledge, special teaching strategies, or any abilities you know about for each faculty member. Do not feel you must write something under each person's name. We do not know each other equally well; some colleagues you know little about; others you know well. We are interested in your perceptions.

Mary Jane Smith

Tommy Jackson

Jo Ann McCall

Betty Fagan

---

sults are tabulated, published, and distributed to the faculty. Then several days of faculty sharing are set up for participatory learning of games and process-teaching tools and activities. A faculty list of people who are willing to be observed in learning situations with students is posted, and faculty are free (with consent of the teacher) to attend and see strategies modeled. Faculty who are willing make themselves available to attend class with a colleague who wishes to use a teaching strategy new to him. Peer support is requested and received as faculty attempt to implement new strategies. The faculty are reassessed every few months, since growth is rapid and new skills need to be added to the repertoire as they are developed.

Materials
1. Questionnaire
2. News sheet based on findings
3. Time for sharing
4. Mechanics for a teacher peer support system

Procedure
1. Questionnaires will be formulated by a task group of three.
2. Questionnaires will be distributed.
3. Collect questionnaires in 1 week.
4. Compile questionnaires and distribute compilation to faculty.
5. Establish task group to make plans for faculty sharing day(s).
6. Establish task group to set up mechanics for faculty peer support system.
7. Set up mechanics for reassessing strengths and needs periodically.

Puissance
1. Provides faculty knowledge of their own resources.
2. Begins process of learning to accept members of own group as experts.
3. Reinforces and recognizes creative efforts and abilities of the group.

4. Reinforces and recognizes all areas of strength and enables best utilization of faculty's special areas of knowledge and expertise.
5. Lowers anxiety as faculty begin to see how their own abilities can be used in the new curriculum.
6. Helps faculty think through abilities of colleagues.
7. Legitimizes need for peer support in venturing into new areas of knowledge or new teaching behaviors.
8. Helps decrease the feeling that faculty are expected to know all things and be all things to all people.
9. Makes all faculty learners and teachers together.

Contingencies
1. Can make weak faculty members obvious.
2. Can foment intrafaculty jealousy.
3. Can get little response and poor mileage until reinforced by seeing an actual outcome, for example, a faculty-sharing day.
4. The information can become obsolete rapidly.

NOTES

1. Carlson, Elliot: Learning through games, Washington, D.C., 1969, Public Affairs Press, p. 24.
2. Davis, Morton D.: Game theory: a nontechnical introduction, New York, 1970, Basic Books, Inc., Publishers, p. ix.
3. Tansey, P. J., and Unwin, Derick: Simulation and gaming in education, New York, 1969, Barnes & Noble, Inc., pp. 19-34.
4. Coleman, James S.: Academic games and learning, Proceedings of Invitational Conference on Testing Problems, 1967, pp. 67-75.
5. Craft, C. J., and Stewart, Lois A.: Competitive management simulation, Journal of Industrial Engineering **10:**355-363, Sept.-Oct., 1959.
6. Interaction Associates, Inc.: Strategy notebook: tools for change, ed. 2, San Francisco, 1972, Interaction Associates, Inc.
7. Carlson, pp. 24-55.
8. Sprague, H. T., and Shirts, R. Gary: Exploring classroom uses of simulation, mimeographed, La Jolla, Calif., Oct., 1966, Western Behavioral Sciences Institute.
9. Boocock, Sarane S.: An experimental study of the learning effects of two games with simulated environment, American Behavioral Scientist **10:**8-16, Oct., 1966.
10. Interaction Associates, Inc.: Strategy notebook, San Francisco, 1971, Interaction Associates, Inc.
11. Kibler, Robert J., Barker, Larry L., and Miles, Daniel T.: Behavioral objectives and instruction, Boston, 1970, Allyn & Bacon, Inc., p. 26.
12. a. Mager, Robert F., et al.: Analyzing performance problems, Belmont, Calif., 1970, Fearon Publishers, pp. 5-99.

b. McDonald, Frederick J.: Educational psychology, ed. 2, Belmont, Calif., 1967, Wadsworth Publishing Co., Inc., pp. 593-595, 606-623.
13. Anastasi, Anne: Psychological testing, ed. 3, New York, 1968, The Macmillan Co., pp. 24-27, 105-114.
14. Skinner, B. F.: The science of learning and the art of teaching, Harvard Educational Review **24:**86-90, 1954.
15. Washburne, C. W.: Educational measurements as a key to individualizing instruction and promotions, Journal of Educational Research **5:**195-206, 1922.
16. Carroll, John B.: A model of school learning, Teachers College Record **64:**727, 1963.
17. Bloom, Benjamin: Learning for mastery, Evaluation Comment, pp. 1-11, May, 1968.
18. Layton, Janice: Students select their own grades, Nursing Outlook **20:**327-329, May, 1972.
19. Hillson, Maurice, and Bongo, Joseph: Continuous-progress education, a practical approach, Palo Alto, Calif., 1971, Science Research Associates, Inc., pp. 77-80.
20. Biehler, Robert F.: Psychology applied to teaching, New York, 1971, Houghton Mifflin Co., pp. 406-410.
21. Glasser, William: Schools without failure, New York, 1969, Harper & Row, Publishers, p. 14.
22. Ibid., pp. 20-21.
23. Ibid., pp. 95-99.
24. Ibid., pp. 59-75.
25. Vanderpool, J. Allen, et al.: California Teachers Association special report on evaluation, California Teachers Association Action, pp. 7-8, May 26, 1972.
26. Torrance, E. Paul: Explorations in creative thinking, Education **81:**216-220, 1960.
27. Torrance, E. Paul: Must creative development be left to chance? The Gifted Child Quarterly **6:**41-44, Summer, 1962.
28. Schrank, Jeffrey: Teaching human beings: 101 subversive activities for the classroom, Boston, 1972, Beacon Press.
29. Postman, Neil, and Weingartner, Charles: Teaching as a subversive activity, New York, 1969, The Delacorte Press.

BIBLIOGRAPHY

Barton, Richard F.: A primer on simulation and gaming, Englewood Cliffs, N.J., 1970, Prentice-Hall, Inc.

Boocock, Sarane S., and Schild, E. O., editors: Simulation games in learning, Beverly Hills, Calif., 1968, Sage Publications, Inc.

Bruner, Jerome S., Goodman, Jacqueline J., and Austin, George A.: A study of thinking, New York, 1956, John Wiley & Sons, Inc.

Bruner, Jerome S.: The process of education, Cambridge, Mass., 1965, Harvard University Press.

Chuan, Helen: Evaluation by interview, Nursing Outlook **20:**726-727, Nov., 1972.

Connally, V.: Curriculum and instruction in nursing, Boston, 1973, Little, Brown, & Co., Inc.

Cratty, Bryant J.: Active learning, games to enhance academic abilities, Englewood Cliffs, N.J., 1971, Prentice-Hall, Inc.

De Tornyay, Rheba: Strategies for teaching nursing, New York, 1971, John Wiley & Sons, Inc.

Gagné, Robert F.: The conditions of learning, New York, 1967, Holt, Rinehart & Winston, Inc.

Gardner, John W.: Excellence: can we be equal and excellent too? New York, 1961, Harper & Row, Publishers.

Heidgerken, Loretta: Teaching and learning in schools of nursing, Philadelphia, 1965, J. B. Lippincott Co.

Langford, Teddy: Self-directed learning, Nursing Outlook **20:**648-651, Oct., 1972.

Lefrançois, Guy: Psychology for teaching: a bear always faces the front, Belmont, Calif., 1972, Wadsworth Publishing Co., Inc.

Lenburg, Carrie B.: Clinical performance examination. In Non-traditional developments in nursing education, Proceedings of the 24th and 25th meetings of the Council on Collegiate Education for Nursing, Atlanta, 1976, Southern Regional Education Board.

Mager, Robert F.: Preparing obstructional objectives, Belmont, Calif., 1962, Fearon Publishers.

Mager, Robert F.: Developing attitudes toward learning, Belmont, Calif., 1968, Fearon Publishers.

Mager, Robert F.: Goal analysis, Belmont, Calif., 1972, Fearon Publishers.

McClosky, Mildred G.: Teaching strategies and classroom realities, Englewood Cliffs, N.J., 1971, Prentice-Hall, Inc.

Miller, C. Dean, Morrill, Weston H., and Uhleman, Max R.: Micro-counseling: an experimental study of a pre-practicum training in communicating test results, Counselor Education and Supervision **9:**171-177, Spring, 1970.

Mosston, Musha: Teaching: from command to discovery, Belmont, Calif., 1972, Wadsworth Publishing Co., Inc.

Nesbitt, William, editor: Simulation games for the social studies classroom, New York, 1968, Foreign Policy Association.

Parker, J. Cecil, and Rubin, Lois J.: Process as content, curriculum design and the application of knowledge, Chicago, 1966, Rand McNally & Co.

Pfeiffer, J. W., and Jones, John E.: A handbook of structured experiences for human relations training, Iowa City, vol. 1, 1969, vol. 2, 1970, University Associates Press.

Postlethwait, S. N., Novak, J., and Murray, H. T., Jr.: The audio-tutorial approach to learning, ed. 3, Minneapolis, 1972, Burgess Publishing Co.

Rogers, Carl: Freedom to learn, Columbus, Ohio, 1969, Charles E. Merrill Publishing Co.

Schaffer, Stuart M., Indorato, Karen L., and Deneselya, Janet A.: Teaching in schools of nursing, St. Louis, 1973, The C. V. Mosby Co.

Silber, Kenneth H., and Ewing, Gerald W.: Environmental simulation, Englewood Cliffs, N.J., 1971, Educational Technology Publications, Inc.

Smith, Dorothy W.: The effect of values on clinical teaching. In Williamson, Janet A., editor: Current perspectives in nursing education: the changing scene, vol. 1, St. Louis, 1976, The C. V. Mosby Co.

Weisgerber, Robert A.: Developmental efforts in individualized learning, Itasca, Ill., 1971, F. E. Peacock Publishers, Inc.

Weisgerber, Robert A.: Perspectives in individualized learning, Itasca, Ill., 1971, F. E. Peacock Publishers, Inc.

Wilson, S. R., and Tosti, D. T.: Learning is getting easier, San Rafael, Calif., 1972, Individual Learning Systems, Inc.

8

ORGANIZING FOR AND EVALUATING CHANGE

Change is defined as altering, making different, converting, a metamorphosis, or as small coin. The key to change is "small coin." Small coin will do the job better than the "big money." The world today works on small change: vending machines, bridge tolls, children, and piggy banks. Big money is valued more than small change only because the value system places more worth on big money and therefore awards it more purchasing power. If the monetary value system were changed, perhaps money would be measured by weight instead of by denomination. If money were valued because of weight, the change for a quarter (five nickels) would be worth more than a $1,000 bill. In the hierarchical administrative system of schools of nursing, deans, department chairmen, and curriculum coordinators are considered the "big money," and faculty, students, and secretaries are considered the "small change." It is only an anachronistic value system that allows the big money to be more powerful than the small change. The small change in society feel powerless; the man on the street complains about taxes, complains about city management, and is frustrated over the lack of responsiveness of traditional democracy. For example, the ballot often offers bills that he wants only parts of, and many candidates represent no choice in political philosophy and no anticipated changes in responsiveness to voter needs. When the man on the street becomes frustrated enough, he riots, burns

a few buildings, shoots or hangs someone in a spate of citizen fury, or in some way insists that power people listen and respond. Then the big money pours on the big money (literally), and programs for change mushroom. It need not be that way, because there is small change in the air and that small change comprises organizational strategies to facilitate the participation of people planning for and implementing changes that affect their own lives.

The ways in which schools of nursing are organized lock faculties into minimally productive patterns of behavior (for example, the use of authoritative patterns of organization, the use of committee structure, and the use of parliamentary law for decision making). These practices mitigate against optimal participation, generation of the most workable alternatives, and maximum use of the talents of all participants in curriculum planning.

Schools of nursing, like their parent institutions (colleges, universities, hospitals), are organized around the military model of authoritarian structure.

In schools of nursing employees fit into a line organization that stacks in groups or units toward people with more and more power and authority. Colleges and universities compound that complex structure with a system of tenure and promotion that labels instructor, assistant professor, associate professor, and professor according to a set or established criteria. Thus

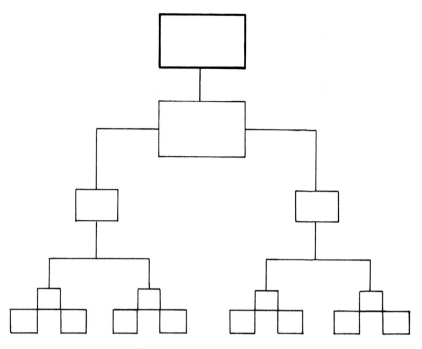

Fig. 8-1. Organizational chart.

rank and position in the organizational chart form a complex system of seniority, voting rights, committee rights, and authority. All authoritarian organizations use some modification of this military pattern. There are many variations of this format, but basically each person is responsible, at least in name, for all that occurs beneath his level in the hierarchical setup. In this way decisions become delayed while they are passed up the line for someone with more authority to make decisions to act.

Fig. 8-1 illustrates the traditional bureaucratic or hierarchical form of organization. Denial that this authoritarian pattern exists begs the problem and can place people in administrative positions of having to maintain the responsibility because of institutional organization but of having little or no authority because of the school of nursing organization. Attempting to change the system can absorb energy that would be better used in making curricu-

lum changes and can effectively delay curriculum work. Since the objective is curriculum revision or building rather than institutional reorganization, a group can (for that objective) create a faculty organization that will facilitate work; for example, the faculty can agree to try a different organizational mode for planning, creating, building, and trying out change. Formal lines of operation can be maintained for other (noncurricular change) activities.

Bureaucracies are structured to stabilize society, and both their organizational and their procedural practices reflect this stabilizing function. Traditional organizational structures almost always use parliamentary procedure for their operational tool. The very design of the organizational structure (hierarchical) and the use of parliamentary law and procedure slow the change process and mitigate against rapid responsiveness to social needs. Some of the factors that work well for stabilization and work poorly for change are discussed here.

ORGANIZATIONAL IMPEDIMENTS

Decision making that is really buck passing up the organizational chart to people away from the problem takes time and can delay change indefinitely. Power, authority, rank, salary, and tenure often depend on longevity as the primary element, and skill, knowledge, or administrative ability are often secondary elements in the selection of people promoted to power positions. Therefore these people are often opposed to changes that they perceive as threatening to the familiar pattern of existence.

Policy manuals dictate the constraints around decisions and therefore reduce the alternatives and limit the range of freedom of decision making. Procedure manuals dictate how operations of bureaucracy must be carried out lest the decision be invalidated because the procedure by which the decision was carried out was not properly followed. Procedure manuals slow the process of change and provide stabilization to the bureaucracy.

Endorsement of major or unusual decisions by bodies of people, committees, boards of regents, trustees, executive boards, etc., are major ways that changes are slowed. These groups meet seldom and are charged with stabilizing responsibilities.

Parliamentary or procedural impediments

Committee structure itself is a problem, since traditionally committees use their time in activities such as the following:
1. Housekeeping chores, for example, establishing meetings, reading, correcting, and approving minutes, selecting a secretary, etc.
2. Power struggles, for example:
    a. Building a power base for the committee and maintaining it
    b. Dividing into factions in the committee and building and maintaining a power structure useful for

delaying, fighting, and struggling with the issues that have become power issues within the committee
    c. Seducing new committee members to their point of view or their side of the power struggle
3. Doing the work assigned them

In reality, a tiny percentage of time is spent in the actual work of the committee—the largest portions by far are spent in housekeeping and power struggles.

Keeping minutes is a problem for change, since there are always one or more individuals who carry the minute books with them and say, "But we made this decision in 1908, why must we discuss it again? Can't we ever make up our minds about anything and stay with it?" They are not concerned that the conditions under which the decisions were reached or the data around which the decisions were made or even the people participating in the decisions may have changed. In a rapidly changing organization, minutes and bylaws tend to be the concrete that sets old patterns and reduces the opportunities for change. In the fast-moving society of today, decisions must alter rapidly because conditions and data—issues and context for decision making—alter daily; therefore minutes tend to freeze the action, close issues permanently, and furnish changing organizations with one more impediment. It is possible to keep, instead of minutes, a running account of the process and the discussion but not the traditional minutes with decisions.

Voting also is a problem in change. Voting does two things: It freezes decision making (often prematurely), and makes those decisions available for minutes. It carves into the history of the organization decisions that are thereby more difficult to alter, and it puts organizational members into win/lose situations with each other. Parliamentary law precludes discussion without a motion; motions immediately mean that one must vote yea or nay or make an amendment. The free flow of al-

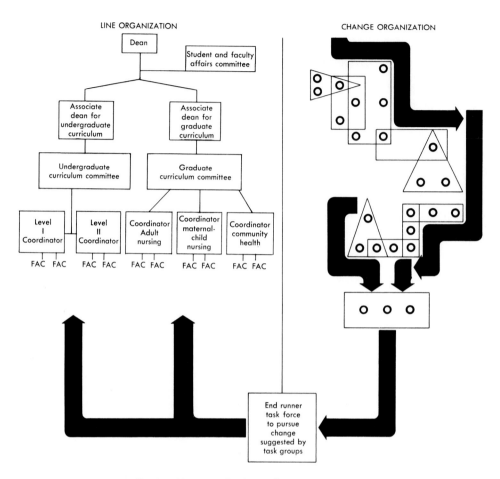

LINE ORGANIZATION

CHANGE ORGANIZATION

Fig. 8-2. Line organization—change organization.

ternative ideas that are seeking win-win solutions is immediately suspended, and battle lines for arguments, for and against, are set. Once set, they are difficult to break and become power struggle situations.

These and other procedures that work so well for the smooth operation of bureaucracies and are effective in stabilizing organizations are the very ones that mitigate against rapid change and social responsiveness. One obvious answer to this problem is the establishment of a parallel organizational structure. Faculties in the process of changing can maintain the usual bureaucratic structure for the ongoing work of the school and create a parallel organization for change that would plan and develop the new curriculum and then

send the selected changes back through the legitimate organization for acceptance and validation. The same people work in both organizations, but they change modes in the curriculum work. Ordinary routines, procedures, policies, committees, minutes, voting, and parliamentary law are suspended during curriculum change work but are utilized for ongoing operations. (See Fig. 8-2.)

The organizational problem is twofold: how to get maximum participation by the total group involved with curriculum change, and how to make the curriculum flexible and responsive to society's (students' and clients') needs. There are three categories of change factors that facilitate the two goals just listed: (1) basic organizational patterns, (2) basic planning strategies, and (3) basic ground rules. "Basic" is used because the suggestions here are beginning ones: For each phase of curriculum building activities, the group may wish to add, change, delete, or suspend some of the organizational modes, ground rules, or planning strategies, depending on the needs of the moment.

BASIC ORGANIZATIONAL PATTERNS

Organizations can take a variety of organizational patterns or structures. The focus described here will be traditional nursing school, modified traditional, or "linking pin," Collegia, and functional team organization. (See Fig. 8-3.)

Traditional or bureaucratic systems (Fig. 8-3, A) are typical of nursing school organization. Hospitals, colleges, and most business and governmental agencies in the United States function under hierarchical structure, and nursing schools are characterized by all six characteristics listed by Bennis[1] as typical of authoritarian organization:

1. They have a division of work that is based on functional specialization (not only teaching/administration but clinical specialization).
2. They have clear-cut channels of communication and hierarchy of authority and responsibility.
3. They are characterized by rules, laws, and job descriptions that cover the rights, duties, responsibilities, and relationships of members.
4. They have predetermined procedural specifications and directions for handling work situations.
5. There is a certain amount of impersonality in the relationships between levels of the hierarchy.
6. Tenure and promotion are based on longevity, ability, or technical competence.

The modified traditional, or linking pin, organizational system (Fig. 8-3, B) has many of the characteristics just listed. It varies somewhat in that the groups within the organization have some autonomy, leaders may be appointed or elected and are not necessarily chosen because they are professors or associate professors, leadership can rotate periodically, and one or more members of each group belong either to another group or to a central executive or advisory board or group, thus linking each group and providing continuity, liaison, and communications. Procedure manuals, job descriptions, and other marks of bureaucratic organization are still in evidence.

On the opposite side of the continuum is a very loosely knit organizational pattern called a collegia (Fig. 8-3, C).[2] In a collegial organization, individual accountability is an earmark, and roles are almost completely blurred and can shift and change with the task to be accomplished. Small groups assemble and shift in membership based on the needs of the group to accomplish an objective. Group membership is temporal as is group leadership. Leadership is almost always by ability to facilitate, knowledge of the part of the task being worked on, sudden inspiration or insights, and other transient phenomena. Investment of energy is toward the task, and no energy is committed to stabilizing the group. The "job" or "task" to be accomplished can be envisioned as being like a basketball that is passed back and forth among the players according to their place on the court, the pattern of play, or their particular talents. The group moves the ball down the court, throwing it from one person, or small group, to another until at last someone puts it in the basket and the job is finished. If the ball hits the backboard, bounces back into play (feedback), reworking occurs until the ball is finally put through the basket and the goal is made.

The type of organization that offers most for curriculum change in schools of nursing is a modification and synthesis of the collegia and linking pin approaches—the functional team or task group organization.[3]

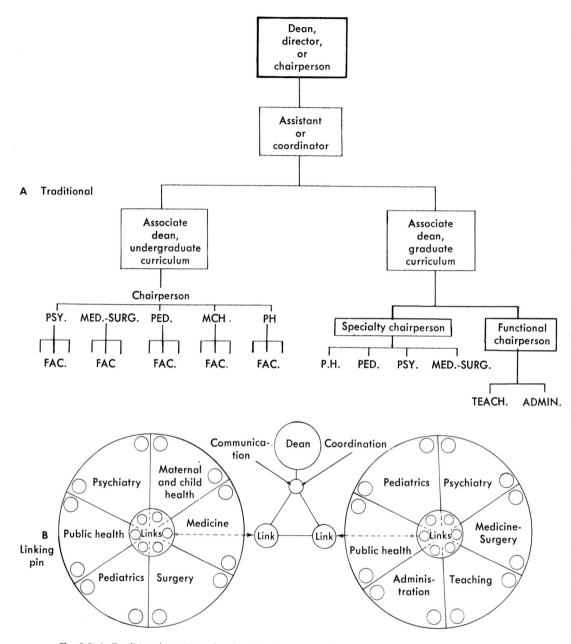

Fig. 8-3. A, Traditional nursing school organization: direct up-and-down flow of authority; membership and job by rank, position, or tenure. **B,** Modified traditional, using "linking pin": one person from each group "links" with other units to provide channels of communication; membership is fairly long term; many rotate positions periodically; rank, position, and tenure are important but can be circumvented within limits. **C,** Collegia: objectives are clear cut; participants collaborate with whom they need to at the time in order to achieve the goal; lines are temporal. **D,** Functional team: groups or task forces are established and dissolved around tasks that need doing; membership is by ability to contribute to the task; role blurring occurs; rank, position, and tenure are unimportant; all participate equally.

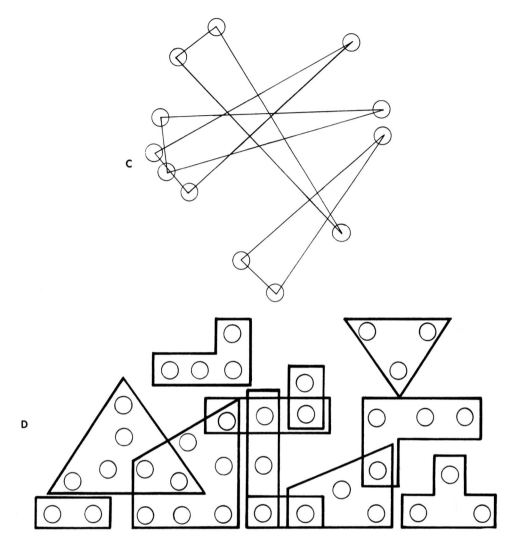

Fig. 8-3, cont'd. For legend see opposite page.

In functional teams (Fig. 8-3, *D*), groups or task forces of from two to five participants are organized around specific tasks. Membership on the task force lasts for the duration of the job to be done. Once the job is accomplished, the task force dissolves. Role blurring occurs, and task force members participate on equal footing according to their ability to contribute. Leadership in the group evolves from group needs and is not imposed on the group from without. Ground rules may change from task to task or from day to day within the same task force, since they, too, are generated in response to the needs of the task and not on a permanent basis. Completed work can either be sent to another task group (called an alter group, as in alter ego, or a feedback group) for critiquing or be submitted to the whole group. Reworking or revising, based on the feedback, may be done by the same task force or may be altered by the critiquing group, depending on the agreement between the groups.

Working in task groups using a task analysis as a basis for organizing for cur-

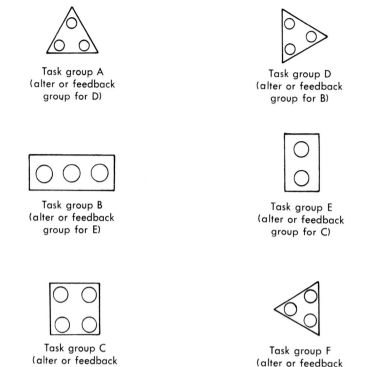

Task group A
(alter or feedback
group for D)

Task group D
(alter or feedback
group for B)

Task group B
(alter or feedback
group for E)

Task group E
(alter or feedback
group for C)

Task group C
(alter or feedback
group for F)

Task group F
(alter or feedback
group for A)

Fig. 8-4. Typical task group organization pattern with feedback or alter group assignments.

riculum change accomplishes some of the following:

1. Explicit and definitive task analysis provides client systems with an overall view of goals and steps that must be taken to reach the goals.
2. Established target dates enable change participants to pace their work realistically.
3. Temporal organization keeps the faculty and students job or task oriented and decreases focus on power.
4. Participating in task groups outside the area of immediate skill widens the horizon of individual members' views of nursing, decreases tunnel vision, provides scope, and brings fresh ideas from people not necessarily locked into a single system or way of accomplishing a goal or viewing a concept.
5. Working with people outside of the usual committee structure broadens the base of working relationships and

decreases fantasies about what colleagues are like; it establishes new communication habits and patterns.

The task force organizational pattern allows implementation of a format for change that facilitates optimal participation by all people involved in change. How to organize task groups is found in Heuristic 1, examples 1 to 5. It is congruent with a task analysis framework for organizing curriculum change and enables tasks that are small enough to be handled in a short time span to be assigned to a specific group for a specific purpose. Power struggles have little time to develop, and compromise is often delayed until adequate numbers of alternatives have been generated. Groups are small enough so that each member can generate possibilities and alternatives and bring them to the group for critiquing. The group can then put together the task from individual contributions. Fig. 8-4 is a model of a typical task group organization pattern with feedback or alter group assignments.

Task groups are transitory, membership expectations are for a temporal existence, work is task oriented with no energy given to maintaining the group, and dissolution is natural when the task is completed.

Many nursing faculties have lost faith in committees. Committee work tends to move slowly, power struggles develop and are perpetuated over each new issue, little creative work is generated, and compromises are made that pull the teeth from changes that looked promising and exciting. Traditional committee structure connotes "power," and committees tend to structure themselves so as to continue to work and perpetuate their own existence. Committee membership becomes a prestige item, and changes that threaten the power, existence, or membership of the committee are resisted.

When curriculum changes are planned using the functional team or the task force approach, lines of authority become somewhat obscure. Every school of nursing has an administrator, a dean, a chairman, or a director. This person is, in the eyes of the institution, accountable to superiors for the activities of the faculty, for the curriculum, and for the success or failure of the curriculum change enterprise. Thus no curriculum changes of major dimensions can occur without the consent and participation of the ranking person(s). Since ranking persons have and can exercise veto power or can influence administrators up the line to exercise veto power, the veto ability needs to be made explicit to the planning group. Inclusion of administrative persons in work (task groups, heuristics, findings, and so forth) decreases surprise, keeps them involved with the changes being planned, and decreases the chance that vetoes will occur.

SOME PLANNING STRATEGIES FOR CURRICULUM CHANGE

The work of building or revising curriculum, when viewed as a whole, looks so impossible both in magnitude and complexity that just the thought of it inspires delaying tactics. Since curriculum building is a process and since processes can be systematized and systems have tasks that can be analyzed, one strategy to cope with the problem of magnitude is by "task analysis"—taking a big job and breaking it down into small bits that are of a size and nature to be handled. Focusing on the job to be handled offers some reassurance that at least some part of the job can be successfully achieved. Success breeds success, and the reinforcement of completing one small bit of the total task motivates and energizes the group for the next job.

Early in the book (pp. 24 and 25) an overall task sequence was suggested for curriculum change. In each of the sequence components an analysis of tasks for that component must occur before that phase of curriculum building can be successfully organized and accomplished. Each group will need to analyze the tasks as they are necessary to the curriculum change patterns of individual nursing schools. One heuristic at the end of this chapter is an example and/or format model of a task analysis for a tiny bit of change and the task group assignments for that series of tasks.

The second planning strategy that is most useful is to provide for feedback prior to total faculty consideration. Feedback is provided by task groups called alter groups. These critiquing groups provide checks and balances so that the creators of an idea, or task, can have the benefit of objective feedback. For example, it adds validity for noninvolved persons to examine the work, ask questions, suggest clarification or elucidation of specific parts, look at congruencies between parts, suggest revisions, and provide other feedback. The use of an alter group not only improves the product of the task group and helps to prepare it for total curriculum group discussion but it widens the base of support through investment. When a second task group becomes involved, they have already participated in the accomplishing of the task and therefore are prepared to speak to it and support, at least in some measure, the group who were originally assigned that task. The more people there are who participate in the creation of an idea or the completion of a task, the more balanced the discussion of that suggested alternative is likely to be.

The third basic planning strategy suggested here is the generation of more than one alternative for every phase of, or task in, curriculum building. Choice is perhaps the most important aspect of facilitating change, and one of the reasons preplanned change can be so effective is that groups need not be faced with having to take an alternative because it is the only one available. Group planning for change includes at every phase the assigning of more than one task group to a task, with directions to work independently of each other, and the consequent offering of more than one alternative plan to the total curriculum building group. The consequences of having a choice are: (1) groups tend to be more stimulated as they look at alternatives and discuss the potentialities and liabilities of each plan; (2) congruence and/or incongruence of parts of the plans with the conceptual base of the curriculum are brought to light; and (3) the best parts of the alternatives can be pooled for developing a plan that meets the needs of the curriculum as viewed by the group.

Rewards and reinforcers

Another important strategy for change involves an obvious and explicit reward system. There is reward inherent in creating curriculum changes that are workable and are tangible manifestations of yesterday's visions. *The more emphasis that can be placed on the continuity of the road from the past (what individuals wished to accomplish in the curriculum) to the present (what the total group has accomplished) the greater will be the feeling of successful accomplishment.* Beyond the reinforcement of accomplishing the total group goals is the individual group member's contribution to that goal. Often work on curriculum becomes a synthesis of so many people's ideas that individual contributions are lost, and an anonymity develops which makes the curriculum itself impersonal and easy to disown as not being a part of each contributing faculty member.

There are some things that curriculum planners can do to keep the personal element in the curriculum without destroying the holism by reverting to clinical specialty area recognition. For instance, when a task group of three or four people collaborate on a special project and generate a piece of the curriculum puzzle that is particularly fitting for distribution to other faculty, students, other schools of nursing, or for publication, it is highly rewarding to give recognition to the people preparing the product. By-lines such as "Prepared by Tamara Beecroft, Kenny George, and Sue Dianne Nichols, in collaboration with other members of the College of St. Simion School of Nursing under the auspices of the School Curriculum Development Endeavor" are expressive of the individual work, the contribution of the "whole," and the motivating factor, and thus give special credit to the authors without detracting from the general credit due the group. Other reinforcing activities include the following:

1. Encourage and facilitate publication of materials generated.
2. Provide letters, encouragement, and active support for tenure and promotion of faculty.
3. Speak to "power" people, such as deans, presidents, and other administrators, of specific contributions that individuals have made.
4. Promote publicity for innovative curriculum endeavors through local newspaper, college newspaper, faculty newsletters, and so on.
5. Celebrate milestones of accomplishment with small parties (this activity interrupts flow and marks progress and thus provides a point of reference).

6. Save early work as a starting point marker to make comparisons and provide perspectives on where the group has progressed in curriculum building.
7. Send general congratulatory letters periodically when particularly effective results have been achieved.

These activities are useful for role modeling the process of valuing the contributions of individuals. Too often faculties tend to devalue their own work and value that of outsiders. Any activity that provides patterns of behavior that establish the value of "home town prophets" builds self-confidence and helps the group make it legitimate to use each other as consultants.

Basic ground rules

Group work is facilitated if there are some basic operational ground rules for the accomplishment of objectives. Faculties working together for curriculum change need to develop ground rules that facilitate change and promote healthy group relationships. It is possible to achieve both ends. Most often faculty working relationships have established patterns of interaction—some patterns that are facilitative and some that are inhibitive of functional communications. There are, on any faculty, committees or groups who are powerful. Immediately on the opening of an issue, pro and con groups draw their battle lines and win-lose conflicts are generated. With people who have worked together for long periods of time, the "red flags" or "buttons" that will elicit known predictable reactions are familiar and assessable. Button pushing and red flag waving can be a favorite pastime or a smooth way to sidetrack an issue.

There are no easy answers to the problem of establishing communication patterns that are more supportive, more productive, and more useful for facilitating change. An outside communication facilitator is invaluable to any group considering curriculum change. Neutral facilitators can help group members look at transac-

tions and interactions, analyze the communication factors, and establish more effective ways of communicating. The following list suggests ground rules that groups might like to consider for curriculum change communications: Each group should evolve its own list and add to it as it is used.

1. Try to have no surprises. Let everyone know in advance plans that are under way. Peep previews, preliminary reports, and agreements to check out rumors will keep surprises at a minimum.
2. Provide as much informational input as possible. Part of the backbone of any planned change is the collection of data phase. Handouts, consultation with experts, training sessions, television, movies and other audiovisual materials, circulation of helpful articles, and data discussion sessions prior to the time the information must be used help to provide the data necessary to planned changes.
3. Make conflicts explicit and legitimate. Bring out hidden agenda items so that real issues can be handled. Legitimacy of conflict makes it possible to look for alternatives that meet every group's goals rather than locking into win-lose power struggles.
4. Identify high investment areas (areas of high feelings), and elicit the help of a neutral facilitator either from within the group or from a source unrelated to the problem or issue itself. This enables all factions to struggle or fight "fair," since a facilitator will ensure each participant's rights.
5. Make risks legitimate, and failure salvageable and acceptable. Operating in small task areas, or bits and pieces, allows greater risks to be taken because if one small part fails, the whole system of changes is not likely to fall apart. Backup systems are alternative ways of handling the problem if an original plan fails.
6. Make change in the middle of a trial

run acceptable. Then if a plan being instituted is not working, alterations in the plan can be made without violating the group's preconceived notion that a trial run *has* to be run all the way through.

7. Try to make it necessary to analyze failure or the reasons a part of a program is not working so that alterations and changes are not precipitous or without fair trial or so that the parts of a plan which may be the cause of the problems can be changed.

8. Agree to respond to each other's contributions to the group: comments, needs, and behaviors. Acknowledgment of entering into the group process reinforces and encourages continuing contributions and provides feedback. To go unacknowledged or be consistently erased leaves one having few behavioral cues, with a feeling of impotence and powerlessness and of being very alone in the group. Other participants are aware of nonresponsiveness and are reluctant to risk contributing and not receiving a response. A simple agreement to say "amen" or use some body language that is an obvious acknowledgment is necessary to a developing sense of group power.

9. When complete win-lose deadlocks occur, agree to some form of action that will allow unlocking and saving of pride. Delay the issue or shuttle it to another time if necessary so that the group can be explicitly charged to look for alternatives which will meet criteria for a solution which pleases all. One way is to say, "What do we want in the solution that will fulfill the needs of both groups?" Then brainstorm for criteria. Try never to make a voting decision while in win-lose situations.

10. Delay decision making of final decisions. Make tentative decisions, take a consensus, decide on a trial basis, or accept something as a "provisional" or "working copy." Voting and recording in the minutes creates a feeling of finality that makes it more difficult for some members of the change group to accept alterations. Minutes become laws and members refer to them to win battles. If records are needed, call them "notes on the conference on _____" or "record of discussion."

PROCESS OF CHANGE APPLIED TO CURRICULUM BUILDING

In Chapter 1, changing is listed as one of the processes chosen to illustrate the throughput aspect of nursing.

The process was broken down into the three components of all processes: purpose, organization (or system), and creativity. The organizing propositions[4] presented in the synopsis of the process of changing will be adapted to the process of curriculum change and elaborated on here to provide an example of the direct application of the change process to the process of curriculum building. Utilization of the two processes together will illustrate the characteristic that all processes are interrelated and naturally inclusive and provide a conceptual base for curriculum change.

Purpose. To anticipate and solve the problems of curriculum with maximum efficiency and effectiveness and with minimum disruptions.

System

1. Curriculum change occurs when needs arise with which standard procedures and courses cannot cope. When new factors arise and when many variables become part of a formerly stable organization, new coping mechanisms are necessary to ensure the continuity, quality, and efficiency of educational responses. Organizations, institutions, and individuals who find a modus operandi that works for them tend to "fix" or "solidify" that modus operandi because the very fact that it works is reinforcing. Consequently, when things in the environment or the needs of the system of education change, the curriculum fails to respond by modifying its standard mode of operation, and thus efficiency

decreases, needs go unmet, purposes are not achieved, and the decay of the curriculum begins.

For instance, when the structural components of the conceptual framework change, the school of nursing may or may not respond to those changes. If the curriculum does not alter with each new need or new variable, the changes begin to accrue and affect the relevancy of the curriculum. Eventually, the variables, such as changes in the ethnic composition of the student group, shifting emphasis in the numbers of clients cared for at home rather than in the hospital, number of clients seeking nursing care, changing laws affecting nursing education, and greater participation of clients in their own health care, pile up. The school of nursing must either respond to those changes or stay rigidly unresponsive and therefore become increasingly irrelevant. When this happens, the faculty spends most of its time coping with a series of crises that are generated by poor curriculum adaptation. Nursing historically has had few variables, since many factors were stable and dependable and standard procedures and stylized curricula were the ways used to cope with those conditions. Now health care as a national concern is the focus of the energy of consumers, legislators, and health professionals. The variables are so many and the stable factors so few that standard, previously learned modes of operation will no longer serve. The cues in the nursing world that used to be stable points of reference no longer exist. Nursing will either decay as a discipline, or it will devise more flexible and versatile programs of service and therefore of education.

2. The breakdown of effectiveness of standard procedures and traditional organization causes an increase in anxiety of the individual, faculty members, and students. Anxiety is the signal of readiness to change. Even though mild anxiety is the natural state of an organism, a rise in the normal level of anxiety makes for discomfort, and faculty seek to return to a more comfortable state of being. If curriculum change procedures are not instituted that will enable better coping with the new factors, anxiety will continue to increase until total efficiency is affected. Some faculty do not institute plans for changing until there are a limited number of alternatives, and change is then a matter of crisis. In this instance, change that is planned for long-term goals must be delayed while crisis intervention occurs, panic is controlled, or extreme anxiety states are lowered.

Crisis is a time when intense learning can occur and rapid changes can be made. However, a change agent must be available during crisis to participate with the faculty in crisis intervention activities. Curriculum changes are easier when faculties preplan and work out changes in advance. But when curriculum crisis occurs because of legislation, administrative edict, student demands, or changes in the faculty group composition (for example, the death or resignation of a faculty member), that crisis can become the useful vehicle for curriculum changes.

3. Anxiety provides a need to change or adapt that is accompanied by an increase in individual and collective energy. People in the anxiety need-to-change sequence exhibit greater work output. However, if there is no articulation of goals, the work output takes on the form of "busy work," of trying to make the obsolete system work successfully, or of vicious circles. If the next phase of planned change is instituted, energy is available for work toward planning change. Faculties in the anxiety state are open to alternatives and can learn new behaviors for planning and implementing changes. Change agents who can provide options, models, cues, and stimulants and otherwise facilitate solution-directed activities during anxiety help the group use their energy in positive ways. This phase of anxiety (when the energy output level is increased) is "prime time" for changing.

4. Need to change or adapt stimulates fantasies of solutions or the anticipation of the achievement of objectives. Everyone who is troubled dreams a dream of "trouble free." Fantasies occur such as "If only this and that were so, all would be right with heaven and earth," and "If we had this or that in our curriculum, the millennium would be here." Everyone anticipates longingly the achievement of his private vision of how things could be better. One of the difficulties is that visions of how things could be improved and visions of objectives are *private*. As private objectives, they have the connotation of illegitimacy or being unacceptable. People fear offending other people, power people, vested interest groups, and some friends. If the goals are shared at all, they are shared with a few chosen friends.

5. Free exchange of ideas about goals and subgoals helps establish specific and legitimate goals and collaboration for their achievement. Visions of the future can be translated into group objectives only if the group provides a time or a mechanism for articulation of ideas and fantasies about the future so that goals for work and criteria for changes can be established.

The ability to talk freely together as a faculty-student group involved in changing promotes the realization of group goals through the mechanism of *making goals and the means for reaching them legitimate, explicit topics for discussion*. Participation of those affected by changes at every level—administration, faculty, and students—generates a commitment to the change process itself and makes collaboration for specific tasks possible and desirable.

Group commitment to the change process itself instead of specific changes enables continuing investigation, growth, and improvement. Groups who organize for change and proceed to plan and implement change can devise together a desired change that gets frozen into decisions of total commitment. Commitment to the specific change, rather than to changing,

is a trap. Using words like provisional, tentative, trial, and interim communicates the concept of change as a process—continuing and progressing forever. Faculty-student commitment to flexibility, innovation, and creativity becomes real only with use. The process-of-change concept is actualized by building a framework for change that provides for and necessitates constant use of feedback for making continuous alterations to the whole curriculum. For instance, no public health nurse would make a plan for a visit and act on it regardless of the conditions encountered on the visit. The conditions encountered on arriving at the client's home would become rapidly gathered feedback that would probably quickly be utilized to alter the preconceived plan. The same habit of gathering and utilizing feedback and alteration of plans becomes an activity habit, whether or not one is dealing with matters of curriculum or patient care.

Conditions of change

For change to occur, certain conditions must be provided. The change agent seeks, in collaboration with others, to establish these conditions so that planned change can proceed. These conditions are as follows:

1. *Key organizational people must support and participate in the change.* In school curriculum change, directors, department chairmen, deans, curriculum coordinators, and key power people must support the idea of planned change as a total group effort. Since this means relinquishing some power to the group and exposing oneself in the group on a peer basis, it may be, at first, only a beginning acquiescence and become a growing commitment. However, trust, collaboration, peer relationships, and free exchange of ideas are *learned* phenomena, and with a skilled change agent any group can learn these behaviors.

2. *The processes employed in change must be congruent with the philosophy, processes, and goals of change.* The ends

do not justify the means, and the means employed for change must be of the same kind and caliber as the change that is desired. People learn as much from models as they learn from any other learning mode, and the means for obtaining curricular changes furnish a behavior model for groups in the process of change. If an authority figure resists changes and if subterfuge, underground tactics, deviousness, and dishonesty are used to obviate the authority structure, the planned changes will contain the same group tactics; thus the seeds of failure for the new curriculum are sown.

3. *Participation in change is a voluntary commitment, as is opposition to change, and the battle must be freely joined.* The implications of this condition are (a) that the only pressures existing on individual participants are peer group pressures, and (b) only in discussions where differences are aired openly without authority pressure for a particular previously determined outcome can there be true resolution through the examination of available alternatives. In addition, (c) mutual agreement must be reached within the change group and not be imposed by an authority figure.

4. *All relevant or interdependent units are involved or oriented to the fact that the process of change is occurring in one of the groups so that changes will not damage, shock, or interrupt other contingent units.* For instance, if students wish to change the learning strategies in a section of a course in an attempt to make their learning more relevant, teachers of other sections and all authority people involved should be notified so that shock, threat, and articulation problems are anticipated and minimized. Organizational patterns undergoing change in a curriculum situation need to be communicated to other departments which are interconnected with nursing so that others can aid and abet the changes instead of blocking them and so that the changes do not interrupt or decrease the effectiveness of others. If a school of nursing decides to require a bac-

teriology course different from the one that has previously been required and changes the prerequisite without involving the biology department, students may be unable to get the required course because of lack of sufficient number of sections, space, or other problems. The faculty and/ or administration may question the feasibility or workability of the new plan, and the plan may fail, not because the changes are ineffective but because the proper "other" people were not consulted, alerted, oriented, or included in the planning phase.

5. *Change participants who learn to consider each other's ideas and opinions using interpersonal communication principles develop a growing trust in participating individuals and in the group process. Concomitantly, the group learns to solve problems with increasing effectiveness.* Free exchange of ideas is not possible without an atmosphere of trust. Trust is basic to the mechanisms of planned change and is developed through consistently respecting the rights and limits of others and in meeting the needs of the group and the individuals in the group. Continuing communication requires a set of changing, evolving, colleague-oriented, equally participative ground rules. In autocratic systems, loyalty is given to the institution or group, the employer or "boss," the dean, supervisor, department chairman, or head nurse. Peer group relations are marked by competition and a win/lose attitude in the suggesting of goals or solutions. One mark of successful changing is that loyalties shift to nursing, the university, and the school. The win/lose problem may not disappear, but the lines of battle are drawn around issues, not personal loyalty to an authority person.

In a group in which the safeguards of ground rules have been established, in which each group member assumes the responsibilities for the group's work and is accountable for the quality of the group's communications, several things occur:

1. Individual faith in the ability of the

group to produce successfully increases.

2. Individual respect for members' ability to participate increases.
3. Trust in the group process increases.
4. Group skill in problem solving increases.
5. Win/lose discussions decrease as the group becomes increasingly skillful at designing a multiplicity of win/win alternatives.
6. Essential support for individuals becomes possible without sacrificing the goals of the group.
7. Loyalty to colleagues and to nursing begins to replace loyalty to local schools or authority persons.

Some change leaders try to induce groups to commit themselves to change prior to involvement in change activities. This is scary to groups and is seldom successful. Commitment is an after-the-fact feeling—it comes after investment of time, energy, brains, and emotions. Investment of these things is purchasing power, purchasing ownership of and commitment to the change.

Evaluating curriculum changes

Evaluation so frequently comes at the end of books and at the end of events that it would seem that it is a way of looking back to see where and how one came to be where one is. However, evaluation is not a looking back; it is a prophecy. Evaluation (feedback) dictates the road ahead because past events cannot be changed.[5] Evaluation should not come at the end of things but rather at the beginning and continue throughout any process. The essence of process itself, the secret ingredient that makes an entity a process, is feedback—sought or unsought, intentional or accidental, preprogrammed or random. The use of feedback (evaluation) is process.[6]

Curriculum evaluation is similar in its relationship to other aspects of the curriculum in the same way as the old song about the bones: "The head bone connected to the neck bone, the neck bone connected to the shoulder bone, the shoulder bone connected to the back bone. . . ." In curriculum it is, "The philosophy connected to the conceptual framework, the conceptual framework connected to the objectives, the objectives connected to the content, the content connected to the outcomes, the outcomes connected to the evaluation." Any evaluation not so connected will have little relevance to the curriculum and therefore will be of limited use to the faculty and students. Most sources tie evaluation directly to objectives, which is the most common and useful way to proceed with curriculum evaluation. However, this is so only if the objectives are directly related to the *setting, student, and knowledge* aspects of the conceptual framework.

Curriculum evaluation precedes change, planning for change, and setting goals and establishing programs. To have evaluation that is programmed for optimal service to the curriculum, baseline assessments must be made.

There are several aspects of curriculum change that must be evaluated to furnish maximum feedback for the ongoing curriculum building process. Therefore planned evaluation must do the following:

1. Reveal whether the behaviors of graduates are similar to the behaviors desired of graduates as specified in the objectives. If so, how? If not, how not?
2. Tell how graduates of the program compare with previous graduates.
3. Indicate how graduates of the program compare with graduates of other comparable programs.
4. Disclose whether the behaviors of graduates are those expected by the professional organization for the type of program, and if they are different, in what ways they are different and whether the difference is an intentional one.

The key to all four aspects of curriculum evaluation is the determination of the exact behaviors desired of graduates and finding ways to ascertain if and to what extent those objectives have been met. All other comparisons are subsequent to that fundamental comparison. Determining how graduates under a new program compare with an old program only matters in the areas where the two programs have similar expectations. The comparison of graduates of one program to other comparable programs is important only in those areas where the programs have similar expected behaviors for graduate nurses. The extent to which graduates meet the behaviors specified by the professional organization for the type of program only matters insofar as the program objectives are specifically intended to be similar. In other words, the value judgment of "better or worse" than before, than others, than specified by the professional organizations is important only if the faculty makes it important. Following are the key questions: Are the graduates different? In what ways? Are those differences desired differences? Are they specifically reflected in the program objectives?

There are basically two kinds of evaluation—formative and summative. Formative evaluation is taken during the operation of the process or the curriculum. It is used to determine how to reach the goals better and helps to focus on things that must be done to achieve goals. Formative evaluation is usually frequent and is done periodically throughout the time the students are in the curriculum. Formative evaluation can be done on students and their learning and behavioral changes and on all of the other factors that must be evaluated that contribute to student learning. The primary reason for the existence of formative evaluation is to furnish feedback to the system while the system is in operation and ongoing so that changes can be made which correct the system to achieve the goals.

Summative evaluation is taken at the end of a period of operation or learning to determine if the goals were achieved. It is a general assessment of the extent and degree to which the desired outcomes or goals have been attained. Summative evaluation comes periodically at the completion of activities, courses, or a curriculum time span such as quarter or semester. Both of these types of evaluation are used for student and curriculum evaluation.

Evaluation of student learning is used for curricular evaluation in that student learning is the purpose of the curriculum. Whether or not students learn what they are supposed to learn is the key to all evaluation. For curriculum evaluation purposes all the factors facilitating or impeding student learning are examined, as follows:

I. Setting factors
   A. Materials
      1. Textbooks, learning resources, practice paraphernalia, and other learning materials such as media, models, equipment, dolls, beds, etc.
      2. Reality practice resources, agencies, patients, nurses, ancillary workers, etc.
      3. Teachers, available and appropriately skilled
II. Knowledge base
   A. Goals
   B. Content
   C. Learning activities
III. Student
   A. Entrance characteristics and behaviors
   B. Interim achievement
   C. Exit behaviors
   D. Achievement tests
   E. State board
   F. One-year postgraduation behaviors

Evaluation of all these factors, formatively and summatively, provides a thorough curriculum evaluation program. Each of these factors must be evaluated using the program objectives and the student behavioral objectives. Since most curriculum evaluation endeavors center around the program and student behavioral objectives, the objectives of the curriculum are the first factors to be evaluated. In other words, are the objectives indeed the desired objectives of the program? Are they in keeping with the trends in the profession? Do they reflect the conceptual framework? Are they measurable? These are the questions that must be answered prior to proceeding to other phases of evaluation.

When a group establishes program objectives, it establishes criteria of evaluation, not only for student success but also for evaluating the success of the revised curriculum. For instance, program objectives usually contain objectives about the following topics:

1. Learning how to learn (independence in the learning process)
2. Being instrumental in the process of changing:
   a. In the health care systems
   b. In the social and political systems
3. Continuing education
4. Being socially responsive or responsive to needs of society (nursing care advocate)
5. Being creative in giving nursing care
6. Being expert decision makers
7. Leading others
8. Planning, giving, and evaluating nursing care
9. Collaborating with others in delivering health care.

There are basically four curriculum evaluation questions to be answered about the program objectives:

1. How well do students meet these objectives on entry to the program?
2. How do they progress toward meeting the objectives during the program?
3. How well do students meet the objectives on graduation?
4. In what ways that are consistent with program expectations as expressed in the objectives do graduates function on the job after graduation?

When planning an evaluation program for curriculum change, one needs to hypothesize what objectives for the program will be established so that baseline measurement of students, and faculty if desired, can be taken before contamination occurs. Once program objectives are discussed and tentatively established, people tend to put some of them into nursing courses that are being taught regardless of whether the new curriculum is implemented at that time or not, thus contaminating the sample. One can easily formulate a hypothesis about the topical content simply by constructing a topical list of concepts that have a high probability of being covered by the faculty when objectives are established. Once this is done, an evaluation blueprint can be drawn up.

Measurement. Evaluation is a much broader and more inclusive term than is measurement, but it is often used to include measurement. Measurement refers to the quantitative analysis of something. For evaluation purposes measurement means to reduce data to a number. Evaluation, on the other hand, includes both quantitative (numbers) and qualitative (values) factors. Since evaluation is the process of providing feedback, it goes on constantly, either explicitly or implicitly. Whether or not the receivers of feedback (the evaluators) accept and use the data is another question, but feedback is available. Measurement, on the other hand, must be deliberate; it is never implicit. To measure, the evaluator must quantify qualitative data. For instance, all personal characteristics inventories are measurements of qualities, for example, dominance. The strength of these characteristics is measured by determining the strength of the characteristics in a "normal" or standardized population. Normal is used as a reference point, and each individual's strength (of dominance, for example) is measured according to how much he exhibits this characteristic in comparison with the normal group. The human need to reduce data to numbers is very great. A surgical operation is judged by a patient's neighbor not by how much it hurt, how awful the cause, or how disrupting the illness to the family but by how many stitches it required. A fish is evaluated not by how hard he fought, how much fun he provided when he struck, how he glistened in the sun when he jumped, or how brightly colored he was but by how many inches long he was or how much he weighed. "I love you two pounds and three ounces' worth" is only slightly more ridiculous than "a bushel and a peck, and a hug around the neck." Even Elizabeth Barrett Browning wanted to "count the ways" of love. Qualitative data can be quantified, and human beings are extremely clever at finding means and methods for reducing descriptive data to numbers.

Design. The design for evaluation needs to follow the principles of good research design in that checks and balances, controls, controlled testing conditions, validity, reliability, and relevance must be of vital concern. The difficulty with basic curriculum evaluation, especially for nursing, is that there is a dearth of tested reliable tools which one can use to show achievement of goals definitively. Most tools available to the evaluator are, at best, only indicators of direction or clues to attainment—not proof positive of results. This handicaps the evaluator but cannot be used to relieve him of the responsibility of searching for indicators of changes.

Designs for evaluating curriculum changes can be either experimental or non-experimental and still provide valid, reliable data to the faculty. The basic disadvantages of the experimental design (for curriculum evaluation) are the necessity for tight control of the variables and the need to establish a rigid design for the study. This prevents ongoing utilization of feedback. Nonexperimental designs (for curriculum evaluation) are easier to conduct, are cheaper, can be done by people less sophisticated in the ways of research, and promise findings that are equally if not more broadly representative of the needs of the student groups.[7] These designs allow continuing utilization of feedback and ongoing curriculum changes. The difficulty with the nonexperimental design is that it lacks the ability to establish cause-and-effect relationships with any degree of confidence.[7] However, in curriculum evaluation, direct cause-and-effect relationships are hard to establish defini-

tively because of factors other than design. For instance, objectives are often interrelated, and content usually contributes to the attainment of more than one objective. Therefore conclusive evidence about what curriculum omissions, errors, or misconceptions contribute to the failure to meet which program objectives is hard to obtain. In curriculum evaluations, conditions are taken as they exist, or as they have been created by the curriculum developers, and evaluative studies are oriented toward defining and describing the conditions and determining the consequences or results of those conditions. This approach is not the most useful one for the generation of a well-founded conceptual construct or for the developing of new theories.[8] This is not to say that new theories of nursing or new conceptual constructs do not arise from nonexperimentally designed curriculum studies; they do, but they remain in the realm of "hunch" or untested hypotheses and are unlikely to gain as much general acceptance and respect as "true" or "pure" research. However, curriculum builders have long faced that difficulty because experimental research designs for curriculum development and evaluation are rare and often as inconclusive as nonexperimental and/or nonresearch designs.

An experimental research design often will necessitate having two parallel curricula using a separate group of students and separate faculties within the same educational setting. This design makes good research but is detrimental to the faculty progress as a unit of growing teachers evolving a common framework and a common teaching skill pool. The group of teachers involved in new or innovative curricula will, through a program of faculty development that is a deliberately structured part of a new curriculum, begin to grow in educational expertise and develop innovative teaching strategies and different evaluation methods. The group of teachers involved in the status quo curriculum are not exposed to problems and experiences that promote professional development in the areas necessary to the new curriculum. In this way the seeds of discontent are sown, and different levels of faculty development, power groupings, and thus ultimate failure or impediments to progress may result.

Each group dealing with curriculum development must make some decisions about evaluation design. Some of the data that will contribute to evaluation decision can be obtained using these questions:

1. Who is available to formulate and actualize evaluation. What are their strengths and abilities?
2. How much time is available to the person or group designated as responsible for evaluation?
3. How much money is available for evaluation purposes? Consultation time? Computer time? To contract out all of the formal evaluation tasks? For faculty release time?
4. How much student time is the faculty willing to make available for evaluation activities? For standardized test? For questionnaires? For "raps" or discussion groups?
5. How great is the faculty's desire to have the program replicable and exportable to others? If program components are exported, contamination of the sample is inevitable.
6. How strictly controlled can the group be? Is it possible or desirable to run two different and uncontaminated groups?

Tools. There are several tools available for curriculum evaluation, and an evaluation blueprint that is thorough and effective will contain a mixture of several types of tools. What one tool may evaluate well, another may not assess at all. Since curriculum building is conceived as a process that is ongoing and constantly dynamic, constant feedback, while learning is in progress, is an absolute requisite for curriculum evolution. Both formative and summative evaluation are essential and can be mutually reinforcing. The wider the variety of evaluation methods and tools

used the more reliable will be the data that can be extracted from the results and the more usable will be the conclusions drawn. Some tools are designed to reveal the kinds of objectives that have been achieved, and some are designed to determine how graduates function in relation to other programs. These measures may be constructed on a pretest and posttest basis and are of little value for giving immediately usable feedback to the curriculum builders.

Some of the methods for curriculum evaluation are listed here with a short discussion of the data that might be provided by the device and the use to which the data might be put.

Student raps or discussions. Organized, scheduled student rap groups containing fifteen to twenty-five students and two or more teachers provide opportunities for students to give direct feedback about program strengths and weaknesses in relation to meeting their needs as individual learners and as a group of learners. At first, trust is a problem in student raps, but trust is developed by teacher responsiveness to student needs. When needs are exposed by the students and teachers respond with rapid changes, trust is reinforced. Students can tolerate teachers saying "no" to a request made in rap sessions as long as the "no" is accompanied by adequate, clear, and rational explanation. Responsiveness to student comments in raps does not have to be a "yes" or "no" but must be some kind of respectful treatment of the feedback. Instant solutions during raps are dangerous. Notes of student feedback can be taken, and faculty can ask for suggestions for altering the program in ways that would more fully meet student needs or take care of the identified problem. However, no solutions should be offered until an appropriate task force (student and faculty) can look at the problem and offer alternatives for solution. This needs to be done as rapidly as possible. Often the tendency in rap sessions is to make it a "griping ground." Griping has evaluative as well as other benefits if it leads to constructive discussion. Raps have the capacity to provide students with the opportunity for free-flowing ideas for change or with reinforcement of things to retain. Student raps (and individual student conversations) provide one of the best sources for instant "fingertip" feedback from the educational consumer's point of view. For optimal use, student evaluation must be treated as consumer evaluation and not as the total (only) source of evaluation. Student feedback must be weighed with goals, total program, other evaluation methods, and administrative problems and constraints about which students may not have information.

Teacher rap sessions. Organized, scheduled times for faculty to discuss problems, practices, strengths, and weaknesses of the developing curriculum are necessary to provide a constant source of feedback useful for guiding the direction of curriculum change. The same kinds of programs for faculty rap can be devised as just described for student raps.

Performance test checklist. A set of definitive program objectives can be further reduced to course and task objectives so that the steps necessary to attain desired graduate behaviors reflect the requisite progressive levels of attainment. From such a sequential list one can easily evolve behavioral checklists for determining mastery of specific learning levels. Such a list enables the teacher and student to define, develop, and evaluate true growth of the individual student.[9] This growth record can reveal how rapidly the learner moves toward the achievement of the goals and thus is an indication about the success of the curriculum in facilitating student mastery of the program objectives. The outcome of such an evaluation tool is a record of achievement rather than of grades. Because of their specificity for the objectives, records of achievement are more useful in curriculum evaluation than grades, which represent a wide variety of variables and as a standard of achievement are known to be unreliable.[9] Specific behavioral objectives can be utilized as performance criteria.

Homemade data collection instruments. Homemade questionnaires are a valuable source of data for the curriculum evaluator. Much of the data provided by evaluation will be quantitative (numerical), and much will be qualitative (descriptive). Qualitative data appear to be more subjective than quantitative data, but both are somewhat subjective. Some sources that are descriptive include (1) opinions of teachers, (2) opinions of students, (3) evidence in changes in attitudes and level of commitment, (4) changes in values, (5) the kind, quality, and quantity of recommendation for changes from teachers, students, and employers, (6) compliance with group decisions, (7) group morale and perseverance, (8) faculty attrition and the reason for it, and (9) students' success rate and attrition and the reasons for that attrition. These clues or evidence about the curriculum will enable faculty to evaluate and describe what is perceived or happening. Perhaps these data will be just as useful in providing a basis for continued change as any of the objective or quantitative data obtained. There are several types of questionnaires that can be adopted to obtain curriculum evaluation data. Most frequently, questions on evaluation tools are geared to student and faculty ideas, feelings, and experiences about the educational program.

The easiest type of instrument to develop and score is one that can be machine tabulated. One type of instrument provides several responses from which the respondent can choose the one most like what he feels or thinks. Another type provides statements accompanied by a Likert-type scale. The respondent selects a place on a numerical continuum that most nearly reflects his feeling. When beginning to learn to devise and test data instruments, the evaluator may wish to try several types and select those which provide him with the most data for a given purpose.

Forced responses of an open-ended nature are helpful in providing data unanticipated by the evaluator. The responses must be sorted into categories suggested by the data themselves. For example, the student can be asked to list the five most helpful aspects about a given learning strategy or the five most annoying things about a course. He can then be asked to rank those five items in order of priority from most to least in a two-stage response.

Data generated in this way are nonexperimental, survey-type data useful only as clues to curriculum impact. They should be treated with the full knowledge of the dangers inherent in accepting the findings as conclusive evidence of curriculum success or failure, but they can, however, be most helpful as supplementary data about directions for continuing curriculum development and valuable to those planning for change. These data can be used in conjunction with other types of feedback, both formal and informal.

An evaluation of the total learning milieu is most useful for restructuring curriculum and the learning environment. One popular device is the Nursing School Environment Inventory.[10]

Normative measures. Normative measures are those tests which are computed to show similarities and/or differences of one individual, or group of individuals, when compared with others. They can be content measures such as the National League for Nursing Achievement Test Series, personal characteristics measures such as the California Psychological Inventory, Shostrom's Personal Orientation Inventory, and the Edwards Personal Preference Inventory, or interpersonal relationships measures such as like the FIRO, FIRO B, and FIRO F series. One must search to find tools for testing some areas covered by objectives. The Torrance Test of Creative Thinking has usefulness in determining success in the student's ability to generate innovative alternative solutions to problems; the Chapin Social Insight Test shows some promise for helping to assess problem-solving ability. The Bass Orientation Inventory may hold some promise for

assessing the personal orientation (self, other, task) of students. Any good test and measurements' source can aid in finding measuring tools for analyzing student changes.

It is possible to generate some testing devices that can be reliable indicators of change. Homemade tools can prove to be indicators of student growth or change, but they lack the standardization and rigid norming that occurs with commercial instruments. However, they can serve a purpose and be exciting to generate. Normative tests indicate how students in one setting differ from an established norm. They can be used to measure one student's similarities and differences or to measure similarities and differences among all testing samples. Given as pretests and posttests, they provide indications of changes.

Blueprints for evaluation. When trying to design an evaluation plan for curriculum change, it is helpful to devise some means of looking at data-yielding tools to obtain a sense of those areas of objectives which can be easily evaluated and those which will need further measuring.

Fig. 8-5 shows one method for looking at the whole. Possible test and measuring devices or techniques are listed as well as topics for objectives. An "X" is placed in the appropriate box if there is a possibility that that device or technique holds promise of generating data which may be useful in indicating curriculum impact. There need be no conclusive evidence—only a belief that clues may be extracted from the data. For instance, there is little evidence that the Edwards Personal Preference Inventory provides conclusive evidence of leadership ability, but it is hard to believe that a person who tests high in dominance, perseverance, achievement, and change would not exhibit nursing leadership behaviors. Such conclusions on no more evidence than has been accrued to date would not be justified, but coupled with other data (performance checklist and so forth), grounds are provided for making deductions that may be placed in the "strong possibility" list if not the "conclu-

	Questionnaires	Performance check list	Chapin Social Insight	California Psychological Inventory	Edwards Personal Preference Inventory	Torrance Test of Creative Thinking	Myers-Briggs	National League Achievement Tests	Raps	Mass orientation	FIRO Series
Learning	X	X							X		
Changing	X	X		X	X	X			X		
Continuing education	X	X									
Socially responsive	X	X					X			X	X
Creative	X	X				X					
Problem solving/ decision making	X	X	X			X	X		X		
Leading others	X	X		X	X	X			X	X	X
Giving nursing care	X	X				X	X	X	X	X	X
Collaborating	X	X		X	X		X		X	X	X

Fig. 8-5. Data yielding inventory—an example of evaluation blueprint.

sive evidence" list. Once the table is completed, tools can be selected from those on the list which promise the most conclusive and corroborating evidence and those which provide the most data for the expenditure of time, energy, and money.

Another evaluation blueprint approaches the design directly from the conceptual framework and lists aspects from the three areas of the conceptual framework (setting, student, and knowledge) as headings for what must be evaluated. Across the top of the grid are placed content topics derived from the conceptual framework, objectives, and course content. In the grid, boxes can be placed how the topics will be evaluated and what test, checklist, person, or tool will be used to pursue the evaluation. (See Fig. 8-6.) Only a few examples of content topics will be used, since this is individual to each school.

Choosing evaluation tactics and devising

an evaluation blueprint that is appropriate to the objectives, provides comparisons with other programs, shows differences between present graduates and former graduates, and discloses whether or not graduates have behaviors similar to those deemed important by the professional organization are extremely difficult and occupy the curriculum evaluator's time prior to changing the curriculum. How many measures to use, what kinds, and how often to evaluate are the key questions that evaluators ask. There are no pat answers. It is hoped that plans are well made and time is not wasted collecting data which are unnecessary for the final analysis. However, the evaluator is not obligated to use all that he has collected. If there is real doubt in the evaluator's mind about the need or value of a tactic, the general rule of thumb is to collect the data, and if it is not needed for final evaluation, omit

	AFFECTIVE CHARACTERISTICS	Assertiveness	Leadership	Creativity	Philosophy	Self-awareness	Responsiveness	COGNITIVE SKILLS	Problem solving	Assessment	Problem identification	Planning	Implementation	Evaluation	Maturation	STAGES OF DEVELOPMENT	Assessment	Problem identification	Planning	Implementation	Evaluation	STRESS RESPONSE	Assessment	Problem identification	Planning	Implementation	Evaluation	COMMUNICATION	Written	Verbal	Sending messages	Clarifying skills	Validating skills	Expression	Body language	PSYCHOMOTOR SKILLS	Physical assistance	Crutch walking	Transfer to wheelchair	Walking weak people	HYGENIC CARE	Bed bath	Evening care	Skin care	Mouth care	Simple, daily	Unconscious patient
SETTING																																															
Materials																																															
Textbooks																																															
Media																																															
Software																																															
Hardware																																															
Paraphenalia																																															
Models																																															
Equipment																																															
Practice resources																																															
Agencies																																															
Patients																																															
Nurses																																															
Ancillary workers																																															
Teachers																																															
Available																																															
Appropriate skills																																															
KNOWLEDGE																																															
Goals																																															
School																																															
Level																																															
Course																																															
Learning activity																																															
Content																																															
Input																																															
Learning activity																																															
Reality practice																																															
STUDENT																																															
Baseline																																															
Characteristics																																															
Demography																																															
Achievement																																															
Values																																															
Motivation																																															
Formative																																															
Classroom																																															
Clinical																																															
Summative																																															
Exit achievement test																																															
Final examination																																															
Classroom																																															
Clinical																																															
State Board																																															
One year after graduation																																															

Fig. 8-6. Data-yielding lists.

it. One need not use all the data that are collected. However, if additional data are needed, it is impossible to go back in time to re-collect it. This general rule must be applied with constraint because student, teacher, and staff time is costly, and time should not be spent gathering data that will be useless in the end.

Process is the utilization of feedback to make changes that are adaptive. Curriculum building is not a process if continuing and varied evaluation feedback loops are not built in so that the curriculum process has the same opportunity for growth which all living things must have. Obtaining feedback, which becomes input, which alters the whole, is vital to all processes.

HEURISTIC 1

Finding an organization pattern that permits every faculty member to participate in change to his capacity or desire to participate and that allows for free flow of ideas and rapid alteration of plans requires a strategy that breaks with the traditional hierarchical organizational pattern without destroying the formal organization or rendering it useless. Faculties have habit patterns of operating within the system of authoritarian structure, and utilization of the established organization can not only limit participation to certain "elected" members of committees or councils but can also stifle creativity and the ability to change quickly. Some groups have suffered autocratic leadership in administrators whose despotism created reactions in the faculty so that when democratic leaders did arise, the faculty placed such tight controls on their process for change as to almost guarantee no movement. Committee structure, voting on every idea for change, generation of detailed documents in the total group, and leadership that dictates rather than facilitates are automatic progress stoppers. Commitment to change comes after the fact, not before it, and total involvement in the process through definitive tasks is one way to achieve commitment to change.

Simple changes in organizational structure and participatory decision-making tactics can turn a group of bogged-down faculty into a group of quick change artists. The need to change and grow is in every group. The knowledge about how to organize for change, how to allow the need to change to be realized, and how to facilitate the changes that the faculty wishes to make can be learned. This heuristic is a simple organizational strategy that does not ensure success but certainly makes it a more realistic expectation.

Heuristic: *Task group formations and operation as a change strategy*

Activity. In this activity the job to be done is analyzed for its components. The components are divided into manageable tasks and grouped as a unit. Task forces are organized by placing emphasis on the following criteria for assignment:

1. One person who knows the content area under discussion very well (two if necessary to deal with several content areas)
2. One person who is good at facilitating the group
3. One person who is a good "idea" person or has a good grasp of the conceptual framework

These task force members need not be different persons. Often the person who knows content is also good at making the material generated by the group consistent with the conceptual framework, and so forth.

Other considerations when forming task forces include the following:

1. Compatibility of members. People with known power struggles, personality clashes, or personal vendettas for each other should not be placed on a working group together. Time to resolve long-standing feuds must not be taken out of the assignment.
2. Keeping a balance of those who produce and those who tend to drag or be unproductive. All the freeloaders in one group may indeed deserve each other's company, but it hardly gets the task accomplished or facilitates their growth by isolating them.
3. The size of the group. Three or four members are sufficient. If members with expertise not available in the group are needed, they can be

called in as expert consultants and asked to participate on a short-term basis.

4. Putting people who are fairly committed to the task completion on the task force. At least one or two persons who consider that they are intimately involved because of teaching assignment or personal interest need to be a part of the group. However, commitment because of personal bias or vested interest is not necessarily a reason for inclusion or omission from a group. Since two task forces can be assigned to a single task to generate alternatives, it is possible to put vested interest people on a task force or on a feedback group so that their ideas can be aired and valued.

Once task force work is complete, critiquing by the alter group takes place. When the alter group has given feedback, the originators of the work need to be given time to utilize the feedback in reworking the plan if they so desire. Presentation of alternatives to the faculty and tentative agreement on one plan or a composite plan conclude that phase of activity.

To keep the work in smooth operation and to increase the potential of finishing tasks in time for implementation deadlines, a fairly clear target date schedule must be established. There is never enough time for tasks to be accomplished. Work always takes the time allotted and more. Once target dates are known, the groups need to know all of the contingencies so that constraints on the group about deadlines and needs can be discussed realistically from the first day of the assignments.

One of the most crucial components in the organization of task forces for specific tasks is a definitive set of directions about the task, describing what needs to be done, what the outcome of work needs to contain (not in content but in factors), and what is to be done with the product.

Materials
1. Target date schedule
2. A task analysis
3. Task group and alter task group assignments
4. Definitive and clear task directions
5. Any ground rules that differ from the usual

Procedure
1. Identify the next group(s) of task(s) to be done.
2. Analyze each task for its components.
3. List the components in a loose task analysis sequence.
4. Assign task forces using criteria listed under "Activity."
5. Assign alter groups.
6. Establish realistic target date schedules.
7. Write task group directions.
8. Distribute task packets to faculty.
9. Arrange for first meeting (or mechanics for meeting to be called).

Puissance
1. Allows participation of everyone in some phase or aspect of curriculum planning.

Example 1. Tentative tasks and target dates

	Date for presentation to feedback (alter) group	Date for discussion by faculty	Date for finalization
Group 1 Tasks			
Acceptance of curriculum format	Done	Done	10/2
Teacher use and number of sections for 12-unit load within college formula	Unnecessary	10/9	3/20
Prerequisite and nonnursing courses	10/9	10/23	
Nursing electives	10/9	10/23	11/13
Group 2 Tasks			
Content sequence of pivotal course Nursing I	10/16	10/30	11/13 A.M.
Learning experience sequence of individual courses (fairly detailed course outline by semester)	12/11	12/18	1/8
a. Nursing I, II, and III courses and practicum	9:30-10:30 A.M.	9:30-10:15 1:00-3:00 Meet to combine as directed	
b. Skills courses	12/11 10:30-11:30 A.M.	12/18 10:15-11:00 1:00-3:00 Meet to prepare for finalization	1/8
c. Problem-solving stimulation courses	12/11 1:00-2:00 P.M.	12/18 11:00-11:45 1:00-3:00 Meet to combine as directed	1/8
d. Communication course	1/22 A.M.	1/22 P.M.	1/8
Open curriculum (RNs and LVNs)	12/4 P.M.	12/11 P.M.	1/8
Course outlines	4/23	5/7	5/21

Example 2. Task group assignments

Task Group A	**Task Group B**	*Task:* Prerequisite and nonnursing courses
R. Jenkins	C. Wadsworth	Task Group K (alter group)
H. Stubbins	M. Rogers	P. Spencer
J. Walker	K. Gardner	M. Deal
S. Funk		
Task Group C		*Task:* Teacher load, course section, size, and number
C. Thomas		
M. Joseph		
M. Williams		
Task Group D	**Task Group E**	
F. Wheeler	G. Christopher	
M. Jones	E. Harper	
H. Wilson	L. White	
Task Group I (alter group)		
A. Bevis		
M. Walker		

Example 2. Task group assignments—cont'd

Task Group F	**Task Group G**	*Task:* Nursing electives
T. Delacorte	D. Blume	
D. Bumgartner	J. Lawrence	
B. Jackson	M. Bowman	
Task Group J (alter group)		
L. Martinez	J. Lombardo	

Example 3. Sample tasks analysis for task groups A, B; alter group H*

Task: Prerequisite and nonnursing courses

General overview and purpose of tasks. Now that we have devised our general curriculum format for nursing major courses and have at least a beginning course description and beginning content outline, we need to establish the following:

1. What courses are necessary as prerequisite to the nursing courses as we have developed them
2. What courses are necessary to fulfill college requirements for general education, and what kinds of courses we think are necessary to enable our graduates to better meet the program objectives

Background data. We established some basic guidelines as desired characteristics of the kind of things we wanted in our prerequisite and nonnursing courses in our meetings in the past. These are summarized as follows:

1. Provide the student with as much flexibility as possible so that every unit is not specified.
2. Within an area of desired content try to allow choice, for example, rather than a course in growth and development, a choice among several courses perhaps offered by the Department of Home Economics, Psychology and Health Education.
3. Leave as many completely free electives as possible, and provide a list of courses that would have content helpful to nurses so that students who wish (and/or have no concept of nursing) can have some idea about helpful areas of knowledge, for example, "The black family," "Social issues," "Native American history," or "Health in the Mexican-American community."

Task components and suggested operational sequence

1. Specify any behaviors or cognitive input necessary to the learning of nursing.
2. List the *areas* of knowledge basic to the behaviors specified as program objectives.
3. List all courses required by the college regardless of the major of the student.
4. Determine what courses not already required by the college contain those knowledges basic to the behaviors listed as program objectives. List all of them from every department by area of knowledge as determined in item 2.
5. From catalogue descriptions, contacts with the teachers teaching the courses, and/or contacts with students who have taken the courses determine the content in the listed courses as accurately as possible.
6. Determine if the courses listed have prerequisites or concurrent courses that are required.
7. In each area of knowledge delete those courses that (a) require too many prerequisites, and (b) are terminal (will not transfer to other institutions).
8. Establish priorities among the courses of one subject area and designate preferences by ranking numerically. Give rationale for priority setting.
9. Make a plan to present to the feedback group. The plan should contain (a) those which should be positively required with no options; (b) those which should be required by subject area (e.g., a course in social problems, social issues, or cultural conflict); (c) those which are recommended as prerequisite to graduate study (e.g., statistics) and are therefore optional; (d) recommended electives; and (e) those which are required by the college.
10. Summarize the units in each category and make a summary sheet including the 45 units designated for nursing major courses.
11. Give work to alter group to examine.
12. Meet with alter group and receive feedback.
13. Make alterations in plan using feedback based on group decisions.
14. Present plans to faculty on designated date.

*This will be the only tasks analysis example offered for the tasks represented in this heuristic.

Example 4. Curriculum planning

Task group A and B

Strategy for preparing tentative plans for prerequisite and nonnursing required courses

Organization. Two task groups of three teachers each

Resources. Take data collected from teachers and other relevant resources (bulletin and curriculum guides available to you) and prepare the nonnursing course tentative plans.

Directions

1. Organize the plan so that it shows General Education courses, required electives, prerequisite to the majors, and so forth. If courses must be taken in a specific order, state the order of preference. Prepare the tentative plan using a format that might be used in academic counseling.
2. Real course numbers should be used. If nonexistent courses are desired, describe them in detail, including which department would need to offer them.
3. State the total number of units required for graduation under the tentative plan. Example: 124, 128, or 132 units (124 units minimum, 132 units maximum allowed by college).

Sequential order of work plan

Use tasks order suggested.

Both task groups will formulate plans independently (obtaining information and opinions from anyone they wish). Tentative plans will be submitted to a third group who will examine them for feasibility. The third task group is expected to critique and return the plans to the original task groups with suggestions of the areas needing further work or polishing.

Task group three will pronounce the tentative plans ready for submission to the faculty.

The faculty will then react and return the plans to task group three, who will act on the faculty's suggestion and formulate one tentative plan pleasing to the faculty.

After the plan has been tentatively accepted by the faculty, it will be submitted to the usual administrative channels as part of the curriculum package.

Task groups D and E

Strategy for preparing tentative plans for content sequence of Nursing I, II, and III

Organization. Two task groups of three teachers each

Resources. Collect data from any source. Suggest review of project materials and curriculum material from previous years; WICHEN material, that is, "Defining Clinical Content Series," and "Essential Content in Baccalaureate Programs in Nursing," and so forth.

Rationale. The nursing courses constitute the epicenter of the nursing curriculum, and the other courses will "cue" their content sequence to this course.

Sequential order of work plan. Same as for task groups A and B.

Task groups F and G

Strategy for preparing tentative plans for nursing electives

Organization. Two task groups of three teachers each

Resources. Collect data from any source and consult with any faculty member(s) not assigned to this task. Suggest a review of project and curriculum materials from previous years.

Rationale. Faculty desires nursing electives so that the student may have a choice within prescribed limits in pursuing an area of interest. Choices will be limited by reality factors such as faculty availability and community resources. The following two faculty comments are worth considering:

1. Specific electives do not have to be offered every semester but only one semester per year or on demand.
2. Some electives should be clinically oriented and some classroom only.

Sequential order of work plan. Same as for task groups A and B.

Feedback (alter) groups

Composition and purpose. Feedback groups are formed in pairs. Each pair is assigned to peruse the work of both of the task forces in each of the three tasks under study.

The purpose of these feedback groups is to listen to the task forces and ask whatever questions are necessary to promote ease, clarity, and efficiency of presentation.

Rationale. We wish to decrease the amount of time the total faculty is involved with the consideration of one aspect of curriculum development. Task group presentation of work to a feedback group who will ask questions and make suggestions will facilitate clearer and more comprehensive presentation to the entire faculty.

Example 4. Curriculum planning—cont'd

Methodology. Feedback groups are to meet with task groups of their assigned topic separately. Two task groups and one feedback group make a rather large number of people, and meeting with groups together may make for task contamination. Allotted time should be limited.

Task groups should have all materials prepared and the presentation planned to expedite work. Any handouts, illustrative materials, or photocopies may be made by the secretary, so let me know and I'll arrange the details with her.

Feedback group composition

Group K: Penny, Mary   *Task:* Prerequisites and nonnursing courses
Group I: Margaret, Ann   *Task:* Content sequence of Nursing I, II, and III
Group J: Laura, June   *Task:* Nursing electives

2. Decreases individual's feeling of powerlessness over direction of curriculum change.
3. Strengthens product because it uses each person's strengths.
4. Allows each person to participate eventually in every course and therefore gives each faculty member a knowledge of the whole curriculum instead of some small part.
5. Increases commitment to the whole.
6. Decreases proprietary feelings about one course and increases proprietary feelings about many courses.
7. Dilutes the impact of blockers and nonproductive members.
8. Allows some flexibility in task components and goals and makes possible alterations based on task group discussion.

Contingencies
1. Groups can flounder in the following ways:
   a. No leader arises.
   b. A power struggle develops.
   c. Misunderstandings about task surface.
   d. Task group membership does not "jell."
2. A piece of the curriculum puzzle can go skewing off on tangential things, or arbitrary changes in content or direction can be made without informing or consulting with the other groups.
3. Overall coordination of all groups is hard. Someone must attempt to keep everyone informed.
4. It is time consuming for reports, hashes and rehashes, checking out, and clarifying.
5. As the work gets heavy and time grows short, task group anger can be directed at the person or group making assignments, doing task analysis, and communicating deadlines.

HEURISTIC 2

The problem of surveying graduates to determine their current status, occupation, educational activities, and so forth is one that confronts all curriculum evaluators. Every nursing program that seeks accreditation by state and national groups or seeks to determine how relevant the nursing behaviors being taught in the curriculum are to the nursing behaviors being practiced needs to take a survey of graduates. There are several problems that confront the surveyor. This heuristic addresses itself to two of them:

1. What are the current addresses of the graduates?
2. Out of all the information we would like to know, what questions are most relevant to ask?

The first question is a matter of time and detective work. Secretaries and student volunteers can trace down untold "lost" students by writing and calling classmates and relatives of students whose addresses are unknown. This task needs to be started several months before the survey is scheduled to occur. The second question is more difficult. There are always more questions the surveyor would like to ask than is feasible. The reason for curtailing the questionnaire is a general principle of surveying: The more succinct the questionnaire and the easier it is to respond to the more likely one is to get a response. Try to keep the questions to fewer than forty, and try to keep the answers short or numerical.

There are several ways one can go about mailing questionnaires and increase the probability of getting responses:

1. Avoid mailing the questionnaire near a major holiday such as Christmas. It is too likely to be mixed in with holiday mail or laid aside until there is more time to answer.
2. Include a postage-paid, self-addressed envelope with the questionnaire.

Example 5. Alumni survey form[11]

Directions
- Circle the number of the answer that applies to you.
- You may omit any question(s) that you prefer not to answer.
- If your address is incorrect, please correct it when you return this questionnaire. You will be sent an up-to-date list of all your classmates whom we have been able to locate and their addresses.

Name_____

Personal data

_____ 1. Year of graduation: (1) 1958. (2) 1959. (3) 1960. (4) 1961. (5) 1962. (6) 1963. (7) 1964. (8) 1965. (9) 1966. (10) 1967. (11) 1968. (12) 1969. (13) 1970. (14) 1971. (15) 1972. (16) 1973. (17) 1974. (18) 1975. (19) 1976.

_____ 2. Sex: (1) Male. (2) Female.

_____ 3. Age: (1) 20-25. (2) 25-30. (3) 30-35. (4) 35-40. (5) 40-45. (6) 45-50. (7) 50-55. (8) Over 55.

_____ 4. Ethnic origin: (1) Afro-American. (2) Caucasian. (3) Mexican-American. (4) Oriental. (5) Philippino. (6) Other, specify _____.

_____ 5. Marital status: (1) Single. (2) Married. (3) Divorced. (4) Separated. (5) Widowed.

_____ 6. Children: (1) Yes. (2) No.

_____ 7. Number of children: (0 +)_____.

Professional data

_____ 8. License state: (1) California. (2) Western. (3) Midwestern. (4) Northeastern. (5) Southeastern. (6) Not licensed.

_____ 9. Currently working in nursing: (1) Full-time. (2) Half-time or more. (3) Less than half-time. (4) Not working in nursing.

_____10. Working (for remuneration) in position other than nursing: (1) Yes. (2) No. (If yes, please write us a note stating how you are employed and why you left nursing.)

_____11. Employer: (1) General hospital. (2) State psychiatric hospital. (3) Private psychiatric hospital. (4) U.S.P.H. Service. (5) City or county health department. (6) Public school system. (7) Physician's office. (8) Private industry. (9) Army. (10) Navy. (11) Peace Corps. (12) Nonnursing employer. (13) Housewife. (14) Self. (15) VNA. (16) Home care agencies. (17) Extended care facility. (18) Other, specify _____.

_____12. Employment location: (1) California. (2) Western states. (3) Midwestern states. (4) Northeastern states. (5) Southeastern states. (6) Outside United States.

_____13. Those who are employed in California—location of employment: (1) Santa Clara County. (2) Greater Bay Area. (3) Santa Cruz County. (4) Northern California (other than specified). (5) Los Angeles area. (6) Southern California (other than specified).

_____14. Position: (1) Staff nurse. (2) Head nurse. (3) Supervising nurse. (4) Coordinator. (5) Administrative (director or asst.-assoc.). (6) In-service instructor. (7) Public health nurse. (8) Liaison nurse. (9) School nurse. (10) Teacher in baccalaureate program. (11) Teacher in A.A. Program. (12) Teacher in hospital program. (13) Independent practitioner.

_____15. Specialty area: (1) School nursing. (2) Medical-surgical nursing. (3) Psychiatric nursing. (4) Public health nursing. (5) Maternal-child nursing. (6) Pediatric nursing. (7) Private duty. (8) Operating room. (9) Outpatient. (10) Industrial nursing. (11) Office nursing. (12) Other, specify _____.

_____16. Are you nursing in: (1) Acute hospital. (2) Community. (3) Day care center. (4) Convalescent hospital. (5) Clinics. (6) Other, specify _____.

_____17. Have you been employed in an acute hospital as a staff nurse (R.N.) at any time since graduation? (1) Yes. (2) No.

_____18. If yes and hospital nursing was your first job after graduation, circle appropriate time interval spent there: (1) 1-6 months. (2) 7 months-1 year. (3) 1-1½ years. (4) 1½-2 years. (5) 2-3 years. (6) 3-5 years. (7) More than 5 years.

_____19. If yes and hospital nursing was not your first job but another intervened, circle the amount of time you spent employed in nonhospital nursing: (1) 1-6 months. (2) 7 months-1 year. (3) 1-1½ years. (4) 1½-2 years. (5) 2-3 years. (6) 3-5 years. (7) More than 5 years.

_____20. If you left your job (either item 18 or 19 above), did you do so to: (1) Take another job in nursing. (2) Go back to school. (3) Become unemployed for a time. (5) Take a job out of nursing.

Example 5. Alumni survey form—cont'd

Educational data

_____21. Are you currently enrolled in a program leading to an advanced degree or certification: (1) Second baccalaureate. (2) Certification in some area of psychiatric therapy. (3) Secondary school credentials. (4) Growth and development credential. (5) Master's degree in nursing. (6) Master's degree in field other than nursing. (7) Ph.D. degree program. (8) Doctorate in nursing. (9) Nurse specialist. (10) Ed.D. degree. (11) M.D. degree.

_____22. Since graduation have you attended any professionally oriented educational programs? (1) None. (2) Continuing education. (3) Workshops. (4) In-service programs at place of employment.

_____23. If you are enrolled in a formal educational program, indicate where: (1) U.C.S.F. (2) U.C.L.A. (3) California State University, San Jose. (4) Other California State University. (5) Other in-state institution. (6) Out-of-state institution.

_____24. If you have graduated with another baccalaureate or higher degree since you completed your program at San Jose, indicate which one you have finished: (1) A.B. (2) B.S. (3) M.S. (4) M.N. (5) Ph.D. (6) Ed.D. (7) D.N. (8) D.N. Science. (9) M.D.

_____25. If you have graduated with an advanced degree, indicate where: (1) U.C.S.F. (2) U.C.L.A. (3) California State University, San Jose. (4) Other California State University. (5) Other state institution. (6) Out-of-state institution.

_____26. If you have graduated with advanced degrees, indicate when: (1) 1968. (2) 1969. (3) 1970. (4) 1971. (5) 1972. (6) 1973. (7) 1974. (8) 1975. (9) 1976. (10) 1977. (11) 1978. (12) 1979. (13) 1980.

_____27. Plans: (1) Return to nursing when children are older. (2) Return to school for master's degree. (3) Return to school for doctorate. (4) Change jobs. (5) Continue as is. (6) Not to return to nursing.

_____28. Publications: (1) None. (2) Nursing journal. (3) Public health journal. (4) Other periodicals. (5) Pamphlets and booklets. (6) Books.

_____29. Research: (1) None. (2) As a part of degree requirement. (3) Other than degree requirement. (4) Independent. (5) As part of team. (6) Participated in another person's research.

_____30. Professional membership: (1) None. (2) ANA. (3) NLN. (4) STT. (5) CSEA. (6) ABH. (7) CTA. (8) Other.

Civic activities

_____31. Civic activities: (1) One. (2) Two. (3) More than two.

_____32. Type of civic action: (1) Nursing oriented. (2) Health oriented. (3) Political. (4) Other.

---

3. Accompany the questionnaire with a newsletter explaining something about why you are conducting the survey and why you need the student's participation.

4. In the newsletter give some news about the institution of general interest to all alumni, for example, personal items about faculty, students who have achieved remarkable distinction, new curriculum, grant information, new buildings, or other interesting items.

5. Promise something in return to those who respond: a short report of the survey or an up-to-date list of classmates' addresses.

The survey is an easy way to gather data about the kinds of things alumni are doing. The questions must be directed toward determining if the behaviors of graduates are congruent with the expectancies spelled out in the program objectives.

Heuristic: _Alumni survey_

Activity. This survey involves the task of constructing questions that will elicit the information necessary to the total evaluation of curriculum. Formulating the questionnaire is a process of the following factors:

1. Setting down the topic to be covered
2. Formulating questions and answers that can be computerized
3. Getting feedback from a small sample group about the ease of answering
4. Obtaining feedback from faculty group about the content of the survey form
5. Getting an accurate mailing list

6. Involving alumni and/or student volunteers to address and stuff envelopes
7. Keeping the responses in an organized way
8. Getting the computer cards punched
9. Interpreting and summarizing the printout
Materials
1. Addresses of the graduates
2. Self-addressed, postage-paid return envelopes
3. Mailing envelopes
4. Letter to alumni
5. Questionnaire
6. People to address and stuff envelopes
7. Task group to compute responses and write up data
Procedure
1. List the topics covered using the objectives as guides.
2. List additional information needed and obtainable with this survey.
3. Devise questions in each category.
4. Have questionnaire critiqued by a group of peers.
5. Test out questionnaire on small sample to see if it is clear and answerable.
6. Have enough questionnaires printed to accommodate the number of graduates.
7. Use up-to-date, recently validated alumni mailing list.
8. Address and stuff envelopes with (a) letter, (b) self-addressed, postage-paid return envelope, (c) questionnaire with directions.
9. Collect responses in a central file by class and in alphabetical order.
10. Keypunch responses for a computer that is available to the school of nursing.
11. Obtain printout of responses.
12. Interpret and write description of findings.
Puissance
1. Obtains large amount of data in one operation.
2. Can be computed on a machine and thereby decreases time spent in hand tabulation.
3. Leaves small room for multiple interpretations about the meanings of responses.
4. Can be slanted directly toward the objectives of the program.
5. Can obtain personal, professional, educational, and civic activities data simultaneously.
6. Involves student volunteers and/or alumni in evaluation activities. This increases investment and heightens interest in the program development and changes.
7. Yields excellent data that are easily interpreted statistically.
Contingencies
1. May get less than 30% response and may be statistically less reliable than desired.
2. Is time consuming, especially for finding out the current addresses (and names) of alumni.
3. Is a time-consuming job to address and stuff envelopes.

4. Requires someone with some computer skill and an available computer.
5. Needs statistical computations.

NOTES

1. Bennis, Warren G.: Changing organizations, New York, 1966, McGraw-Hill Book Co., p. 5.
2. Ibid., pp. 200-202.
3. Taba, Hilda: Curriculum development: theory and practice, New York, 1962, Harcourt, Brace & World, Inc., pp. 462-474.
4. Bennis, pp. 81-94, 99-108.
5. Honor B. Dufour, verbal comments, 1972.
6. Shepard Insel, verbal comments, 1971.
7. For descriptions of experimental designs see Abdellah, Faye G., and Levine, Eugene: Better patient care through nursing research, New York, 1965, The Macmillan Co., pp. 160-167.
8. Ibid., p. 168.
9. Hillson, Maurie, and Bongo, Joseph: Continuous-progress education, Palo Alto, Calif., 1971, Science Research Associates, Inc., pp. 78-79.
10. Lysaught, Jerome P.: An abstract for action, New York, 1971, McGraw-Hill Book Co., p. 465.
11. This is an adaptation of a survey format developed at the University of California, San Francisco, School of Nursing, under a United States Public Health Service Division of Nursing Curriculum Research Grant (No. MU0072). It is used with permission of Dr. June Bailey.

BIBLIOGRAPHY

Abdellah, Faye G., and Levine, Eugene: Better patient care through nursing research, New York, 1965, The Macmillan Co.
Beauchamp, George A.: Curriculum theory, ed. 2, Wilmette, Ill., 1968, The Kagg Press.
Bennis, Warren G.: Changing organizations, New York, 1966, McGraw-Hill Book Co.
Biehler, Robert F.: Psychology applied to teaching, Boston, 1971, Houghton Mifflin Co.
Bloom, Benjamin S., Hostings, J. Thomas, and Madaus, George F.: Handbook on formative and summative evaluation of student learning, New York, 1971, McGraw-Hill Book Co.
Conley, Virginia C.: Curriculum and instruction in nursing, Boston, 1973, Little, Brown & Co., Inc.
Drucker, Peter F.: The effective executive, New York, 1967, Harper & Row, Publishers.
Ebel, Robert L.: Encyclopedia of educational research, ed. 4, New York, 1969, The Macmillan Co.
Gronland, Norman E.: Measurement and evaluation in teaching, New York, 1976, The Macmillan Co.
Havelock, Ronald F.: A guide to innovation in education, Ann Arbor, Mich., 1970, Institute for Social Research, University of Michigan.
Hillson, Maurie, and Bongo, Joseph: Continuous-progress education, Palo Alto, Calif., 1971, Science Research Associates, Inc.

Scriver, M.: The methodology of evaluation, AERA Monograph Series on Curriculum Education, No. 1, 1967.

Seiler, John A.: Systems analysis in organizational behavior, Homewood, Ill., 1967, Richard D. Irwin, Inc.

Taba, Hilda: Curriculum development: theory and practice, New York, 1962, Harcourt, Brace & World, Inc.

Tyler, Ralph, Gagné, Robert, and Schriven, Michael: Perspectives of curriculum evaluation, Chicago, 1967, Rand McNally & Co.

INDEX